The Firstborn

EXPERIENCES OF
EIGHT AMERICAN FAMILIES

The Firstborn

Experiences of Eight American Families

Editors

Milton J. E. Senn, M.D.

and Claire Hartford

A Commonwealth Fund Book

Harvard University Press

Cambridge, Massachusetts / 1968

Distributed in Great Britain by Oxford University Press, London
Library of Congress Catalog Card Number 68–25619
Printed in the United States of America

To the memory of
Ernst Kris and Katherine M. Wolf

colleagues whose creative talents
were matched by their compassionate regard
for children and parents

Foreword

Human behavior is still a largely uncharted area that offers an inexhaustible challenge to behavioral scientists in their quest to know man and his ways of living. The search for such truths takes forms as varied as the complex modes of behavior characteristic of each human being.

To the investigators responsible for the studies that appear in this book it seemed that important aspects of individual and family psychodynamics, especially in relation to the specific events of childbirth and child-rearing, would be revealed through close examination of families *in situ* over a span of several years. Their objective was to collect, assess, and report data on family life, beginning with the first pregnancy, with special interest in the development and rearing of children in the family.

The in-depth methods of the study precluded a large sample, and the research team did not make a quantitative analysis of the data, such as factor analysis. It is hoped, however, that in providing these detailed family studies, the investigators have made available a source book of materials that may be of use and interest to research workers and practitioners in the fields of medicine, education, and the social sciences—indeed, to all those concerned with child behavior and development.

This book is the first long report to utilize the large amount of data collected in a study begun in 1951 at the Yale University Child Study Center. Some of the material has already been used in papers published in scientific and professional journals. A psychoanalytic study of two families (not included in this book) is now being prepared by other members of the research team.

In telling the stories of individual families, the authors do not propose to present *all* available material, however intriguing it may have been. They are primarily concerned with illustrating certain premises which they consider vital to a child's development and integration within his family. These factors are pointed up in a comparative way, by presenting the biographies in juxtaposition with one another, and later, in summarizing the material.

This book is testimony to the perseverance and dedication of the many people who worked on the study over the years. We acknowledge and honor their profound contributions and call attention especially to Dr. Ernst Kris, noted psychoanalyst, who headed the research team and who was joined by Dr. Katherine Wolf, specialist in child development. The untimely deaths of both these important contributors interrupted their own major works based on this study. A good portion of the psychological observation material on infants came directly from Katherine Wolf's descriptions, in which she had the devoted help of Anna Marie Leutzendorff.

We are indebted to Jennie Mohr, Albert Wessen, and John Mabry whose manuscript provided substantial material for the frame of reference, theory, family narration, and the comparative summary. Their considerable contributions form much of the foundation upon which this book is based.

We also call attention to the many people whose particular professional capacities were engaged in working directly with the families, especially Rose Coleman Lipton, Sally A. Provence, Samuel Ritvo, Albert J. Solnit, Marianne Kris, John McDevitt, Grace Abbate, Charlotte Gill, Gladys Lack, Audrey McCollum, Janet Brown, Laura V. Codling, and John Doris.

We gratefully acknowledge the assistance of the Child Study Center's technical staff, particularly Paul H. Hartmann, Ruth Parker, Jennie J. and Demetra Parthenios, and Elizabeth M. Towner.

Integral to the study was the sustained financial support by the Commonwealth Fund, which enabled the work to continue uninterrupted for several years, even in the face of slow returns in the form of publications. It provided a base of confidence which is indispensable to the morale of any significant endeavor.

Above all, we recognize our gratitude to the families themselves, whose identities and rights to privacy are carefully protected but who nevertheless allowed us the privilege of coming into their lives in the interests of scientific understanding.

M.J.E.S.
C.H.

New Haven, Connecticut
December 1967

Contents

Introduction

The psychiatric clinics of our nation are crowded with people whose histories refer their symptoms back to the first years of childhood, to something that "went wrong" in family living at that time. There is an increasingly strong feeling among physicians that a major task of preventive medicine is the improvement of family living. Many books on sociology and psycho-social development have been written to explain the components of family living, to minutely examine the multitude of phenomena incorporated in family living.

Popular literature on child care reflects abundant concern with the problems of individuals and especially with the problems attendant upon socialization of the first child. We presume to know a great deal about the conditions under which individuals form families, the significance of family living for individuals, and factors relating to the achievement of "marital happiness" and the "success or failure" of marriage.

In this vast array of literature the family per se is regarded as the context within which significant events of child-rearing take place, or as the environment which determines whether the child will develop normally or pathologically. Yet because the family has served mostly as a "background," scientific attention has not been focused upon the earliest reciprocal values established in the new family. We have few formal scientific descriptions of the mechanics and dynamics of day-to-day family functioning. The latter deserve more examination than they have hitherto received.

The objective of this book is to present material illustrating the family climate preceding the firstborn, the "personality" of the neonate as he enters the family orbit, the action of the environment upon the infant and the infant's impact on his milieu — the beginnings of the child-parent-family integration. We want to look at what happens when the "twosome" becomes a "threesome" and to describe some of the everyday qualities of "average" American families. It is hoped that this study will contribute to the general knowledge of how early family experiences can, and indeed do, affect the development and early personality of the child.

Also, it seems appropriate to mention that the years intervening between the time these families were studied and the current report have produced no conclusive answers for human behavior and development. Yet the findings have supported the concept of cause and effect in human relationships and have provided greater insight into, and acceptance of, certain basic premises. It is as important to provide reaffirmation and substantiation of existing concepts as it is to disclose entirely new premises. We believe this book will serve such a purpose.

Eight American family histories are presented to show the dynamics of life and parental climate from early pregnancy through the first two years of the child's life. The parental history and background, as learned mainly from the mothers (and occasionally fathers or other family members), are included because of their relevance to the entire study.

In order to protect the identity of the actual families, pseudonyms have been used and a variety of minor alterations have been made in the sociological setting. Such alterations were made most carefully to avoid any distortion of the families' histories.

It would be virtually impossible in a book of manageable length to give an hour-by-hour account of the individuals or of family proceedings. But even if people lent themselves to constant observation via specially contrived living arrangements, it was not felt that this would reliably reflect the nuances of child growth and family development. In fact, the study group believed that behavioral research could not readily be fashioned by laboratory techniques without some loss to its integrity.

Because we were seeking explanations for certain specific elements which we regard as crucial to a child's individual development and to the formation of his family's integration pattern, we have included in the family stories only that material which sheds relevant light on these elements. We know that this material can at most present only clues, which may either support or invalidate the significance of these elements. And certainly we are under no illusion that an eight-family sampling may justify all-encompassing generalizations; we believe only that it may suggest worthwhile areas of specific study

SIGNIFICANT ELEMENTS IN CHILD DEVELOPMENT AND FAMILY INTEGRATION

We believe that there are six distinct areas, each with integral components, which may give significant clues to the catalytic forces that operate on the child and his family in their patterns of integration and development.

These concepts and factors were selected from the works of American sociologists and psychologists. They do not represent any one perspective or school of thought *in toto* but were considered by us to be salient aspects of the study.

A. EXPECTATIONS

1. Maternal expectations;
2. Specificity of expectations;
3. Motivational orientation;
4. Role of child in fulfilling mother's expectations;
5. Paternal expectations.

B. BEHAVIOR

1. Communication;
2. Regularity and flexibility of scheduling;
3. Techniques of management;
4. Relation of expectations to behavior;
5. Paternal behavior.

C. SOCIO-CULTURAL INFLUENCES

1. Socio-economic status and values;
2. Extended family;
3. Spatial arrangements and values.

D. FAMILY RELATIONSHIPS

1. Marital;
2. Mother-child;
3. Father-child.

E. PERSONALITY CHARACTERISTICS

1. Handling of anxiety and hostility;
2. Dependency and the sense of security;
3. Feelings of adequacy or inadequacy;
4. Planning and impulsiveness;
5. Self-assertion;
6. Recapitulation of past experiences.

F. EMERGENCE OF FAMILY INTEGRATION PATTERNS

1. Family structure;
2. Division of labor and balance of power;
3. Development, achievement, and social behavior of child;
4. Prospect of siblings;
5. Status of family in community;
6. Types of parent-child adaptation.

A. EXPECTATIONS

By the time of marriage each of the partners already has a pretty well-established structure of expectations concerning many areas of life. This structure was built year by year from recognized and unrecognized wishes, needs, hopes and fears; from cultural and personal values; from feeling and acting; from hearsay and past experiences. These expectations may be borne out in most events of daily life, or for various reasons they may be altered by the behavior of other family members. Moreover, situations may arise for which there are no adequate expectations, or anticipated circumstances may not even occur. Thus the dynamics of life exert a modifying influence on expectations and are a basis for changes in the family situation.

Although the characteristics of the new family which is created by the birth of the first child are largely predetermined before its advent, the experience of creating a family begins with the development of anticipations of the child and of parenthood during the pregnancy period. Such anticipations will be molded by the family cultural blueprints and by the experiences of the parents in their own families of orientation.

Furthermore, probably from the time of their marriage and certainly through the months of pregnancy, both husband and wife will have developed many expectations of how they will raise the child and of what they will do as a new family. The daily course of pregnancy, the process of labor and delivery, and the beginning of life with the newborn are the realities of experience against which these expectations are measured, by which they are sustained or modified, and from which further expectations arise.

Certain aspects of these expectations merit special attention. The family, as the unit of living and of social status in our society, is basically affected by the level of aspiration held by its members. Therefore, we may expect to find the structure of the new family to be strongly colored by the level of socio-economic aspiration held by the parents both for the long and the short range.

Equally significant are the role adjustments which accompany the transition from "couple" to "new family" and the relation between the couple's expectations of what "life with baby" will be like and their actual experience of it. This means that as the child grows, parents must constantly adjust their expectations and behavior to his changing capabilities. The extent to which they are able to adjust — to learn to accept changes in the child's capabilities as they come — is variable.

All families have certain experiences in common: care for the child's physical needs; relationships created through physical and emotional interaction; management of routines of family living; modification of husband-wife relationships and behavior; socialization of the child, and so on. The process of integrating the individual child into the family is accomplished through such events and experiences. But the character of such experiences is unique for each family.

It is obvious that many of the experiences of this period are not anticipated; in many areas there are no expectations to guide the parents in directing their course. The experiences, in turn, give rise to new expectations; behavior and expectation will continually modify one another. It is probable that the realistic or unrealistic character of expectations of parenthood, the anticipations of success or failure, and the ideas about modes of behavior that will be needed to fulfill such expectations will largely be influenced by comparable features of past experiences. The mother will manifest this in the feelings and ideas she has toward and about the child, in her expectations of sources of satisfaction or dissatisfaction, and in her response to the particular individual characteristics of the child.

Shifts in expectations and knowledge occur. New learning takes place; old learning is modified through experience. This leads to new activities, new orientations, new structural characteristics. The study of the changing expectations of parents with regard to family living will be an important key to changes in family structure. We learn to have the expectation that two plus two equals four. Hence, we act on this assumption, confident that if we do, we will be "right," and that if we do not, we will suffer adverse consequences. This crude example points up several important points. First of all, expectations are learned — either by trial and error, by experience, or more normally through participation in the culture. Secondly, expectations have a motivational component; one must have "confidence" in them if they are to be effective guides to behavior, and they are related to some goal the individual wishes to achieve. Thirdly, expectations tend to become normative; not only do they frequently come to have the sanctity of the "ought" but because they influence behavior they often partake of the character of a "self-fulfilling prophecy."

Presumably every conscious rational act is based upon some expectation where that behavior is not random. It is thus theoretically possible to describe an individual's role in terms of a series of discrete expectations, just as it would be possible to describe his body of knowledge in these terms. It is through the discrete learned expectations that the cultural determination of behavior takes place.

But expectations are not learned once and forever. Like all

learned items they are subject to reinforcement or extinction, to modification or obsolescence. Only if an expectation "pays off" in reality will it ordinarily continue to guide behavior. Expectations thus are subject to modification in terms of the consequences of behavior just as they determine it originally. It is this interaction between expectations and behavior which is the stuff of much of an individual's "reality testing."

Moreover, expectations are psychologically meaningful in that they provide a person with a feeling of security, of manageability of his situation. Insofar as a person can expect or anticipate what will happen, he can exert some control over it and function effectively. But the strength of human desires and motives is such that expectations can be distorted as well. Because a parent wants her child to be a "little adult," she may really expect that he be so as an infant. And the strength of distorting motivations may be such as either to cause the persistence of unrealistic expectations or to preclude learning from taking place. Expectations, like any other human tool, may be maladaptive as well as adaptive.

In practice people do not always communicate their expectations, even under questioning in an interview situation. And they vary greatly in the amount and number of expectations that they divulge, either spontaneously or otherwise. We cannot, therefore, take verbally reported expectations as an indicator of the baseline in knowledge of an individual's behavior.

We can only use reported expectations as a means of gaining some fragmentary knowledge on this point. But any communication has an expressive function, and the expectations an individual is willing to express will yield some insight into his psychological situation. The mother who expects the worst of the experience of childbirth may thus be communicating something of her anxieties about the maternal role rather than just her understanding of her future reality situation. Seen in this light, expectations can be useful in understanding individuals as well as their actual behavior.

B. BEHAVIOR

The daily course of family living presents an ever-increasing variety of parental experiences as the anticipations of pregnancy give way to the reality of dealing with the newborn. Expectations previously held come up against the reality of constant contact with the child. The parents are occupied with many tasks necessary for satisfying the baby's physical needs. They comfort him when he is in distress, protect him from real or suspected dangers, play with him, discipline him, control his behavior. In turn, he provides them with pleasure, anxiety, frustration, satisfaction. The pattern of family living changes, and in varying degrees the child becomes a determining factor in the creation of the new way of life.

It is not enough merely to describe what the parents set up as desirable or undesirable behavior or how they go about trying to achieve these ends. The variation from one family to the next in how they accomplish daily tasks is indicative of differences in outlook, personalities, effective experiences, sources of satisfaction or frustration, and concepts of self in the parental role. All of these are factors in their actual behavior.

Behavior may be viewed as having two major functions. One is instrumental behavior, which is directed toward the management of a situation, the carrying out of activities which provide the child with food, physical conditions for growth, play, and learning. The second is expressive behavior, or spelling out to the child the emotional dimensions of love, pleasure, anxiety, displeasure, satisfaction or dissatisfaction, which are significant features of the behavior of a mother toward her child. The child's behavior, too, may be seen as either instrumental or expressive.

Instrumental and expressive behavior may or may not occur together, and the same act may or may not serve either or both functions. But the distinction between them is important for an understanding of the ways in which the child is nurtured, and the quality of his relationships with his parents. The extent and character of a mother's affective expression toward the child and the emphasis she places on performance and activity determine to an important degree the character of the human and physical environment in which the child lives.

Whether instrumental or expressive, the varieties of behavior which constitute the daily interaction between mother and child may be evaluated in certain broad categories: permissiveness, diversion or substitution, accommodation, restriction, avoidance.

They are not mutually exclusive, as any mother may use a variety of methods in relation to any one or more areas of activity.

Some of them apply to the mother's own activity, others have to do with how she engages the child in behavior she considers appropriate or desirable. In not all instances are these two points clearly separable; both involve interaction between mother and child. In varying degrees the patterns of family life may result from the parents' own kind of activity, or from their placing responsibility on the child from the earliest period in his life. Also it is significant to observe shifts in techniques which are the response to the growing abilities and initiative of the child, and to assess the suitability of the methods used for the development of harmonious family organization and the satisfaction of individual and group needs.

In summary, however, we feel that one general type of behavior is based on the recognition of the child's desires as he expresses them, or as the mother anticipates that he will express them. It is child-focused behavior in the response to the child's wishes; or willingness, or attempts to create willingness, in him to do as the mother requires. The other type of behavior is parent-focused, involving restrictive or avoidant action characterized by the mother's attempt to ignore or override the child's desires or performance, whether they are expressed or not. These two groups, for our purposes, may be designated as permissive or tolerant; and non-permissive or non-tolerant.

The amount of detailed reporting by the mother or the staff observers varies widely, both from family to family and from time to time. Therefore, the actual number of observations available may not correctly represent the frequency with which specific kinds of behavior actually occur, or the emphasis actually placed by the family on one or another area of daily experience. Another limitation has to do with the non-specificity of reporting which sometimes produces uncertainty about the particular area of activity or the exact type of behavior described. We assume, however, that the evidence available from the mother's reporting and from the two-year observation period generally does represent the relative importance of different areas of activity for the family.

The mother's ways of behaving with her child in the every-day course of events will also provide us with some indication of the extent to which her expectations are realized. When expectations are concerned with specific behavior patterns of mother and/or child, we may look for some consonance between expectations and behavior. Even when expectations are general in character, the behavior may demonstrate specific ways of fulfilling them in specific areas of family activity.

C. SOCIO-CULTURAL INFLUENCES

The integration of the firstborn child into a family takes place within the potentials and limitations posed by the interpersonal and socio-cultural environment of the infant's parents. Not only does each infant have emotional and physiological needs; his parents also have their individual needs and life goals. By considering the personality and familial needs of the infant's parents, we are calling attention to the fact that the incorporation of the child into the family takes place within a variety of family structures and social-psychological climates.

These social-psychological climates include both environmental circumstances and personal relationships. The circumstances that influence them include the presence of extended family members, socio-economic status, and physical environment and housing arrangements. If grandparents share the living arrangements, there are present additional potentials, as well as limitations, for the growth and development of the new family. The presence of other adults in the family may complicate matters.

Another circumstance that we wish to consider is the socio-economic status of the family, an important determinant of the social values of the parents. It particularly manifests itself in the extent to which they appear to prize material possessions and economic achievement or use their children as objects upon which to drape their status symbols of prestige and accomplishment. The extent to which families are upward-striving and the extent to which they manage their income in order to meet the goals associated with upward mobility are both extremely important aspects of the environment into which the child is born.

Somewhat contingent upon socio-economic status and the presence of extended family members is the quality of the physical environment itself. This involves not only the arrangement of rooms and the provision of space for necessary life activities, but more important, how effectively the parents are able to arrange the space that is available to them in order to accommodate their child. The most significant thing is how the parents themselves view the use of space; the limitations and rights they impose upon the available space in the home.

D. FAMILY RELATIONSHIPS

It is apparent that the relationship between husband and wife assumes a crucial importance in the life of the new infant. Marital relationships may be viewed as having both ego-supporting and ego-threatening aspects; such relationships cannot be considered as either exclusively supporting or threatening. Rather, most marital situations involve a relative balance between these two kinds of psychological conditions.

When we speak of families characterized by marital compatibility, we mean that such relationships are more frequently emotionally satisfying than threatening. By marital incompatibility we mean that there is more frequent dissatisfaction than emotional comfort and feeling of well-being. We should add parenthetically that there are wide individual personal differences in how husband and wife may view themselves and each other as well as in defining what a "happy marriage" means to them. In other words, a marital relationship that is satisfying to a parent with one kind of personality may not be satisfying to one with a different personality.

We speak of the triadic integration of the child into a family to define the behavioral "togetherness" of the family. We say that a three-person family group shows behavioral "togetherness" when there is a great deal of sharing among all three family members in play, trips, household organization, routines, rituals, and ordinary day-to-day living. Behaviorally, the child is said to be a part of a triadic family when he is included in activities involving both parents at the same time.

It is apparent that such a relationship, if it is to emerge at all, will involve dyadic relationships between the child and each of the two parents, although the mother-child relationship may be considered of fundamental importance. The emergence of a triadic family organization most decidedly does not imply the absence of, or unimportance of, dyadic relationships. Rather it implies that the separate mother-child and father-child relationships have provided a basis for togetherness involving all three family members. On the other hand, while the mother-child and father-child relationships may be well developed, a triadic relationship may still be excluded because of jealousies and feelings of exclusion on the part of one of the parents.

Since the behavior of parents with their child involves their personalities, it is apparent that we must also consider emotional togetherness along with behavioral sharing. Consequently, the triadic integration of the child into the family involves the emergence of a family sense of "we-ness" and appreciation for the needs and feelings of one another. If parents are inclined to perceive "we" as meaning mother-father-child then we say there is a psychological integration of the child into a triadic family relationship which involves the perceptions, attitudes, and behavior of the parents as well as of the child. It is the prerequisite for unitary family development.

If one or the other of the dyadic relationships (marital, mother-child, or father-child) is so impaired that it operates against the possibility of family togetherness and excludes mutual balancing of attitudes and behavior, the family integration can only be segmental.

E. PERSONALITY CHARACTERISTICS

We have previously indicated that certain personality characteristics are intimately associated with the parents' attitude toward their baby as well as with the mechanisms of behavior involved in child care. While the postscript information on the families was prepared from follow-up records which used psychoanalytical insights and application, our emphasis in this study is rather upon the more surface aspects of personality as revealed by attitudes, beliefs, and on-going human behavior.

First, we are interested in the extent to which parents may show feelings of inadequacy or adequacy in terms of self concepts or interactions in the broader world of human relations around them. Secondly, we are interested in behavioral evidence of the effect of past personal or social history of the parents upon their present functioning. It is part of our basic theoretical orientation that past socialization experiences have a direct influence upon the adult personalities of the parents. Such influences may often be shown by the extent to which parents incorporate their past experiences as children into their present child-care practices. We have seen that parents may violently react against their own childhood experiences or, on the other hand, may strive to continue past events into their present handling of the child.

Thirdly, the various ways in which parents customarily handle dependency, anxiety, anger, and hostility feelings which are inevitable parts of human life, strongly influence the course of the family itself. It is necessary to make a clinical judgment about the effectiveness of their modes of handling these feelings even though we are well aware of the difficulty that this kind of judgment entails. Ideally such a judgment should rest on two considerations: first, the amount of such feeling with which a parent must cope; and second, the nature of the coping mechanism itself. Because we are not attempting to analyze the psychodynamics of the parents' behavior, our judgment is limited to the observation of the presence of anxiety and the ways in which it is handled in terms of the family functioning as a unit.

Fourthly, the parents' handling of their own dependency needs is a crucial element in the child's incorporation into the family. Again, our chief interest is in how dependency needs are handled and whether or not they appear to intrude upon child care and family functioning. Fifthly, we are interested in the extent to which planning and pre-arrangement mechanisms represent a basic way of expressing a personality characteristic. It may range from compulsivity at one end of a continuum to impulsiveness at the other. Although we do not discuss the psychological significance of compulsively planned behavior, it is quite clear, for example, that such behavior becomes an important aspect of child care and the process of family integration. Finally, we shall review again the extent to which parents may focus upon the child as either a chief source of satisfaction or dissatisfaction.

We have said that family organization represents an area of interacting personalities, each with a psychological-social history, and we recognize that the parents have come to be the way they are as a result of past experiences. This combines with the social and psychological demands of the present to create the themes which influence both child care and emergent nuclear family structure.

In the emergent family structure which assumes a unitary or segmental pattern, we shall be interested to see which, if any, of the above personality characteristics are decisive factors.

F. EMERGENCE OF FAMILY INTEGRATION PATTERNS

In the foregoing our assumption has been that the family structure pattern is a logical outcome of several distinct factors: the expectations held by parents, their own ways of behavior, the socio-cultural influences upon them, their intra-family relationships, and their own unique personality characteristics. Commentary on why a specific cluster of these factors may result in a unitary family integration while another combination of factors tends to produce segmental family integration is the subject of our final chapter.

We continue to use the concepts of unitary and segmental as ideal types, that is, we do not assume that any one family would be characterized by either complete unity or complete segmentation. We will see as the family histories unfold that they range along a continuum from unitary to segmental with the differences between any two families being largely ones of degree. A closer examination of the qualities characterizing these two polarities of structure may have significance in explaining the dynamics of family orientation.

If the expectations towards having a child and building a family are pleasurable, does it then follow that the behavior pattern and web of relationships automatically make for a unitary organization? What role do the personality characteristics of the parents and their socio-cultural influences have upon the family integration? How does the child himself, his development, achievement, and social behavior influence the family integration? What is the manner in which the different family types handle day-to-day living problems? Are the families uniquely different from each other?

These and other questions will be measured against our yardstick: that the unitary organization involves the experience of shared values and a structure of relationships involving all members, both behaviorally and psychologically, in a single web of mutual interaction; that segmental organization contains the existence of some disparity in life values between family members, that it denotes the primacy of dyadic relationships over a more comprehensive unity and the existence of a loose pattern of interaction where members are minimally involved in the family group.

The situation is not in fact that one family may have a "lucky" combination which leads to unitary integration, unalloyed happiness, and favorable child development, or that another family may be saddled with an unfortunate combination which precludes happiness or favorable child development. We hope to show that neither is the unitary family totally free from problem areas nor is the segmental family totally devoid of satisfactions and functional adaptability.

Our basic goal, then, is to evaluate the groundwork which may have portent for the family future and the development of the child. We shall see that in these widely different kinds of family organization all the children did finally manage to adapt, in varying degrees, to the familial environment to which they were exposed. Only time will tell whether the diverse kinds of family patterns have a markedly different influence on the child's personality as seen in later childhood, adolescence, and the adult years.

Design of the Study

The challenge of the study was to "see and hear" the families adequately and accurately, with verification from several points of view. Therefore, the technique was kept flexible and unstructured, ready to fit naturally and realistically into the on-going home and family environment. Further, many of the interviews and examinations were reported separately by members of different disciplines. Information was acceptable only after discussion and agreement by all the represented disciplines.

Since there was no desire for a quantitative study, involving large numbers of people, from which one could glean broad generalizations, a small but representative sampling of families was considered adequate for the purpose in mind. The advantage of a small group was seen in the opportunity for intensive and personalized concentration on each family, hopefully resulting in better understanding and communication. The value to the Child Study Center was in terms other than quantity, averages, or predictive values.

DATA COLLECTION

Data were collected through a combination of clinic and home visits, discussions, observations, tests, and services. The number and type of these contacts for the first two years are outlined in the following table. They began during the mother's pregnancy and continued over the course of the study. The postscripts are derived from subsequent data.

An important element of the study was providing services to the families in the course of gathering research data. This was a decision based on several factors. First, because the staff wished to engage the families in discussions and observations involving circumstances where services would be needed, they felt obliged to respond to these needs as they arose. In the interest of the study it was better for the same pediatrician to see the baby when he was well and when he was ill. This proved its worth many times over through the insights it provided into the families' lives.

Secondly, the study depended on a close relationship between the staff and the families, which was best brought about through extending the services. Also, the study itself benefited from such a relationship, since services to the families were repaid by their willingness to give information about themselves and to provide access to their daily lives.

Number of Interviews and Observations

Family	Hospital visit[a]	Home visit[b]	Well-baby clinic[c]	Office visit[d]	Total
Harris	8	24	21	15	68
Cyrenski	3	27	16	7	53
Silver	3	22	15	8	48
Bjornson	5	19	18	—	42
Fallon	1	26	14	15	56
Neville	3	22	18	13	56
Grasso	3	20	17	11	51
Callini	3	18	19	8	48
Total	29	178	138	77	422

[a] Visit of interviewer or pediatrician to mother at time of delivery.

[b] Visit of interviewer or pediatrician to the family's home.

[c] Observations made by interviewer of the mother-child-pediatrician interaction at time of well-baby clinic, or pediatrician's developmental tests and physical examinations of the child and interviews with the mother during well-baby clinic.

[d] Visit of mother (and occasionally father) to office of interviewer or pediatrician.

SELECTION OF THE STUDY GROUP

Women in early pregnancy coming for their first visit to the obstetrical clinic of the Grace-New Haven Hospital* were screened by

* Now Yale-New Haven Medical Center.

the head nurse to select white married women in their first pregnancies, between the ages of 18 and 35, who expected to remain in New Haven for a number of years. The research project was explained to them, and if they were interested in participating, one or more interviews were held to discuss the program at length. The mother was encouraged to talk it over with her husband to decide on the family's participation.

One cannot examine the factors that led to selection of these cases without considering the importance of motivation on the part of those consenting to participate. The reasons why individuals want to join such an undertaking are important and varied. Some of these reasons became more apparent in time.

The pediatric and educational services to be provided were incentives to some, if not all, of the research subjects. The prestige attached to a university study project was another. Some anticipated the opportunity to share in the latest scientific information about child care and family life.

One further motivating element, which appeared with increasing clearness as contacts during pregnancy continued, was the sense of need on the part of some mothers for help and support in the assumption of the maternal role. In some instances, this was related to anxieties and difficulties in the mother's total life situation. The possibility that individuals will turn to such a proposal for the satisfaction of a variety of needs, some of which may not be directly related to participation in the study, may have an important effect on the character of the sample chosen for the study and consequently of the results.

CHARACTERISTICS OF THE STUDY GROUP

Ages of the mothers ranged from 20 to 29 years, and of the fathers, from 26 to 36 years. The social, economic, and religious characteristics are varied. Two mothers and one father were foreign-born. The majority were second-generation white Americans. Backgrounds included Northern, Western, and Eastern European nationalities, with a predominance of Italian and Eastern European families.

Five of the eight families were Roman Catholic, one Protestant, and two of mixed religious faiths, one Roman Catholic and Protestant, and the other Protestant and Jewish. Both the ethnic and the religious distribution of this small group of families generally followed the characteristics of the community. The educational background of the parents ranged from grammar school to postgraduate university training. Employment included skilled and unskilled industrial work, and white-collar and professional occupations. It can be said that the eight families provide a wide range of contrast among the major sociological variables which might affect patterns of family integration.

GENERAL PROCEDURES OF THE STUDY

The procedures of the study and the types of contact made with the family members were the result of the combined service and observation orientation of the project. They included prenatal obstetrical and laboratory procedures, psychological testing and psychiatric social work interviews, delivery and hospitalization, full pediatric care and periodic examinations, developmental testing by pediatricians and psychologists, observation of the child at well-baby clinics, pediatric consultations for the mother, and casework help, as the occasion required, by the social worker who was the mother's interviewer.

The reports are based on the observations and clinical judgments of the research team. A considerable degree of objectivity was achieved, since all evaluations and judgments were based on detailed records written from notes made at the time of data collection and transcribed as soon as possible. Reliability and validity were sought by the continual convening of research conferences, in which the family events, individual descriptions, evaluations, and interpretations were discussed not only by the observer, social workers, and the pediatricians but also by psychoanalysts, psychiatrists, and psychologists in the research group.

Sustained contact with the families was maintained through two pediatricians, three social workers, and an educational psychologist. Other staff-family contacts included those of the psychologist who administered psychological tests to the mother (and, in a few instances, to the fathers) and a staff member who sometimes provided transportation for mother and child to the well-baby clinics. The records of all staff members were combined in a single record for each family.

SOURCES AND METHODS OF OBTAINING DATA

Initial interviews with the prospective mothers were conducted by the psychologist and social workers at the obstetrical clinic. During the early stages of pregnancy these were held at monthly intervals, but they became more frequent as pregnancy progressed. The number of ante-partum interviews ranged between a minimum of five and a maximum of fourteen for each mother. They involved discussion between the mother and the interviewer on aspects of the mother's past history and current activity related to her experience of pregnancy and the anticipation of motherhood. During this period a feeling of rapport was established with the mothers. In the eighth or ninth month of pregnancy the pediatrician was introduced to the mother. Visits by both the interviewer and the pediatrician were made to the mother and child during the lying-in hospital period.

After the baby was born, the task of the interviewer in home visits was to combine the gathering of data through conversation with the mother and observation of the home, the infant, and the child-mother interaction. At times, family situations were observed as other family members were present. Home visits were made by the psychologist or social workers throughout the study and were timed to take place monthly during the first year and at six-week intervals during the second year. Although the pediatrician's home visits were made for the purpose of caring for the child, they also provided information through conversation with the mother and with other family members and observations of the home situation and the care of the child.

In the first year of the child's life there was monthly attendance at the well-baby clinic; during the second year this took place every six weeks. These were timed halfway between the home visits. The well-baby clinic provided developmental testing, physical examinations, and pediatric interviews, during which matters of importance to the mother concerning the care and development of the child were discussed. On occasion, the interviewer who conducted the home visits also observed at the well-baby clinic in order to evaluate the mother-child interaction in a highly structured situation as compared to that of the home.

In some instances, fathers accompanied mothers and children to this clinic. On the whole, however, the fathers' participation was limited because of their work, their reluctance to become involved, and their expectations that the study primarily involved mother and child. The study was able to accumulate only limited data on the fathers.

The developmental tests at the well-baby clinic provided data on the child's development and indicated the child's capabilities and progress in relation to the expectations and activities of other family members in his environment. At times of testing, mothers were always informed of the presence of observers behind the one-way mirror. Besides interviews and observations at the well-baby clinic, the pediatrician's contact with the family included home visits during occasions of illness and extensive telephone conversations.

The alternate spacing of well-baby clinic and home visits sometimes departed from schedule because of illness or unavoidable interruptions, which caused some gaps and overlapping in the data-gathering. However, this did not seriously affect the study.

Casework services varied from family to family, and from one period of time to another. Although the families had not originally come to the clinic because they specifically sought such help, they nevertheless began to look to the social worker as a person who could be appealed to because she was interested and understanding of them. Since her discussions centered around feelings, expectations, and events which had strong emotional significance for them, they sometimes called upon the social worker for specific help.

When urgent problems arose, there were more intensive periods of casework, but such help was not offered unless a family member requested it. Casework was limited mainly to dealing with immediate and short-term problems which became intensified during specific situations or home crises. The same event, for instance, might be discussed by the mother with the pediatrician or the social worker, or both. In this way the data-gathering techniques were varied, and it was possible to compare assessment of the same item by different disciplines.

In conferences of the whole study staff these items were viewed from several positions, which provided an enrichment of the material and a more thorough understanding of it. On the other hand, when more time was spent on a special family crisis, there was less time to observe and secure factual information on day-to-day interactions of parent and child. These losses, however, were more than balanced by acquisition of other relevant material and by greater understanding of the meaning of particular facts and events to the family.

Staff members were also aware of the social and cultural environment as it pertained to child-care practices, patterns of family living, and the development of the individual. The data-gathering tried to encompass sociological as well as psychological material and a fullness of observation in terms of both physical and human environment

THE ROLES OF INTERVIEWER AND PEDIATRICIAN

For purposes of reference the term "interviewer" refers to the social workers and psychologists, as distinguished from the pediatricians. The interviewers were mainly concerned with the broader social and psychological aspects of the family and the integration of the child within it, while the pediatrician was primarily concerned with the elements of child care and maintenance in a sound doctor-family relationship. The quality of the relationships which were gradually built by each of these staff members with the families would materially affect the kind of data obtained.

The roles of pediatrician and interviewer were not always clearly differentiated in the mother's mind because both disciplines stressed that they were concerned with the total family situation. And, in fact, their areas of concern were often overlapping. However, the pediatrician's role was more understandable to the mothers than was that of the interviewer.

The interviewer's role was complicated by the fact that the mothers had no preconceptions of the role in the first place. Unlike the clear-cut services they could expect from the pediatrician, the parents did not immediately understand the interest of the others. As the interviewer explained her role in talking about aims, experiences and problems of parenthood, in time it became more understandable, although it lacked the authoritative nature of the pediatric service.

In the study the pediatrician was the major source of information about the development of the child; practices, problems, and pleasures of child care; and management of daily life with the child in times of health and illness. As the child's doctor, the pediatrician established a relationship with the family that was primarily child-centered, although her concerns were also with all aspects of the wider family circle.

The social worker was primarily mother-centered as related to understanding of the family environment, the relationships among the various family members, the impact of the child on the established family organization, and helping the mother deal with some of her own problems. This involved attitudes, feelings, expectations, and behavior of the mother.

The primary distinction made by the staff members, therefore, was between the child-orientation of the pediatrician and the mother-orientation of the social worker. This was not a sharp or rigidly defined distinction. However, when one staff member was working on a particular problem, the separation of roles needed to be clear in order that there would be no intervention or disturbance in the handling of the specific situation. Each had to be fully aware of what was going on in order to contribute to, and not inhibit, the work of the other. Staff and research conferences aided in this demarcation.

The mothers varied considerably in the ways they related to the two individual roles, and in how they provided information or requested help. Some of the mothers maintained a minimum of involvement in their relationship with the staff. They welcomed the pediatric services and advice, were willing to provide a certain amount of information if solicited, but maintained distance in home and clinic visits. Other mothers turned eagerly to the pediatrician, at times becoming dependent on her for support, while merely tolerating the social worker as a condition of the study. Still others looked to the social worker for specific help, and in such cases there developed an active casework relationship between interviewer and mother.

How the mothers looked at the two roles was demonstrated in

the ways of reporting the same material to the pediatrician and to the interviewer. When records were compared, it was occasionally found that the same event or circumstances assumed quite different emphasis and proportion when told to the different staff members. The interviewer learned about difficulties with the baby's sleeping or feeding, but to the pediatrician there was a denial of any such problem. Perhaps the mother was trying to convince the pediatrician that she had no problem in functioning adequately. Or the pediatrician might learn of a meaningful event in the mother's past history which was not given the same significance in her talks with the interviewer. Perhaps the mother could not tolerate too close an examination of a painful experience in her discussion with the interviewer. Consideration must be given to the strong defensive barriers in some mothers against the recognition of anxiety, and in others an appeal for an ego-supporting relationship. Still others turned primarily to their families and their own resources for help in meeting the difficulties they encountered in the new experience of motherhood.

NATURE OF HOME INTERVIEWS

The home interviews were highly unstructured and of widely varying character in order to explore areas that appeared to be of significance and to allow the mother to open or close subjects as she felt the need to communicate or withhold. The pediatrician's interviews were more structured because of the mother's customary emphasis on discussion of specific child-care problems and procedures. The social worker was alert to the need for the acquisition of research data and for exploration of specific areas in order to get comparable data on all the cases. But this was balanced by the mother's freedom to talk about whatever seemed important to her at that particular time.

The mothers varied considerably in their articulateness and response. Some talked freely about the pregnancy period itself but revealed little of their past history until later. Others talked much about their own life history but avoided discussion of their pregnancy until shortly before the child was born. Some showed a readiness to communicate, while others were inhibited. Skill or discomfort in verbalizing, and ease or lack of ease with the interviewer, were other contributing factors. Despite these differing degrees of communication, the combination of verbal interchange plus observation of the mother in the home and interaction with the child provided the data required for the study.

The character of each interview was modified by factors such as housekeeping activities, the presence of other family members, and the activity of the child. Sustained discussion of problems or events of importance was usually possible. Some mothers treated the social worker more as a social visitor, others resorted to household activities as a deterrent to an involved discussion. The social worker adapted her interviewing to the situation. Length of interviews ran from three-quarters of an hour to one and a half hours.

Another important factor to be considered was the extent to which the social worker became instrumental in changing some aspect of the family situation by initiating subjects and focusing on problems. This involved a degree of participation and was recognized as one of the possible elements in such an on-going research project. Similarly, when the pediatrician gave medical care or advice in respect to the child, this, too, was a degree of participation. However, since service to the family was understood as a feature of this study, it could not be avoided. In each instance of such involvement, the interviewer reported on her own participation and was as objective as possible in her observations.

In summary, the home interviews covered three aspects: (1) active interchange with the mother in obtaining specific types of information; (2) observations of the mother in the home, attitudes and behavior toward the child, the physical surroundings, physical management of the child, and the responses of the child to such management; (3) observation of, and interaction with, the child, especially as the infant grew and was more frequently present and participating in the interview. In this respect, choices sometimes had to be made by the interviewer concerning her concentration on interaction with the mother, observation of the child, or of the mother and child together.

Participation of the fathers in the home interviews and the entire study was unfortunately sparse. Historically, fathers tend to regard such things as "the wife's domain." Further, hours of work made it difficult to see the father often in the home setting. Occasionally fathers visited the social worker in her office or were present in evening home interviews. Also, fathers occasionally came to the well-baby clinics and were at home sometimes during the pediatrician's visits. Contacts with other family members were meager except where the families resided with the extended family group. Considering the importance of the relatives in the life of the child, the absence of such material is a marked limitation of the study.

ANALYSIS OF DATA

There were several levels of information in the interview records: (1) the observed behavior of the mothers and other family members; (2) the reports by the mother of attitudes, feelings, and events; (3) the interaction between interviewers and mother; and (4) the evaluations or judgments of the staff on what was seen and heard.

A set of categories was established in the records to cover past history, characterization of family members, parental expectations, behavior of the three family members in relation to one another and in specific areas of family life, and behavior in relation to the extended family and the community. Subcategories provided for more specific identification of information within these broad areas. The system of itemizing the data was planned to help locate each category for each family. The itemizing and categorizing were done by two members of the staff and were tested by independent analyses of the same interviews.

No attempt was made to quantify the categorized data or to employ the methods of content analysis. Because this study is mainly concerned with a process, it was important to know that certain types of ideas or behavior were prominent at one period and minimal at another, or that certain problems engrossed the family at one time and became relatively insignificant at another time. The use of such terms as "more" and "less" gave indication of which aspects were stressed or minimized; discussed frequently or ignored. Only descriptive use was made of these relative terms and they were not translated into numbers because it might tend to confuse the reporting with the experience.

A mother might have referred a number of times to an experience because of the impression it made on her, but this did not mean that the experience recurred. If there were difficulties in child sleeping patterns, this mother might dwell in many detailed descriptions of the battle over sleep, while another mother might dwell little on equally significant material. It should also be recognized that the real significance for a family of an event or situation may not be revealed by the frequency with which it is mentioned. The intensity of feeling attached to a single comment may overbalance in importance the frequent discussions which consume time and attention but have relatively little significance for the family. A question which was barely touched upon may in fact be of the utmost importance, yet may be masked for various reasons. Hence, quantitative content analysis methods seemed inappropriate for this study

LIMITATIONS OF THE STUDY

As noted above, plans for obtaining material did not specifically include the sociological aspects of the problem, and the staff were more responsive to the psychological data. It turned out, however, that the material had both psychological and sociological importance and was amenable to study as a totality and not exclusively from one or the other point of view. Because of the staff's interest in psychoanalytical theory, the data were principally obtained on the mother-child relationship, since this interaction is the child's most important experience in the early years.

Yet the lack of information about other family members, especially the father, was certainly an important limitation of the data. Expectations of the father and his behavior with the child were known to quite different degrees in the eight cases studied, and it has therefore been impossible to draw extensive comparisons or to delineate patterns of father-child activity with completeness. What we have learned about the fathers came primarily from the mothers. This fact must be considered in evaluating the meaning and importance of such data.

In a number of cases family members other than the parents were significant and constant figures in the life of the child, and limitations in this respect should certainly be considered. The ways in which the influence of the older generation persisted in the course of the family's development and the effects of the social patterns on the parents in these families was not very well known, certainly constituting a cultural gap in the study.

The problem of the frequency, timing, and completeness of reports is a difficult one and the determinants of data-gathering are multiple. Some lie within the meaning or importance of specific data for the particular family members. Others lie within the observer. Her role as participant as well as observer influences what she sees and hears, and what she selects for recording. It also influences, at times, the actual course of events in the family, though this influence may not be adequately understood or sufficiently taken into account. It should be pointed out, however, that this influence probably acts in the direction of making available fuller and more meaningful data rather than in the direction of distortion. We have indicated that the clinical knowledge and experience of the observers in this study made for depth and clarity of observations, even while their influence was recognized and reckoned with.

The Fallon Family

A MOTHER'S AMBIVALENCE

"My harelip affected everything that happened to me. Before I began to wear makeup people reacted to the sight of my face with shock." This was stated in an offhand manner with a nervous laugh, but its validity was unquestionable. Mrs. Fallon had a disfiguring congenital fissure of the upper lip which had been repaired but had left a contorting scar extending from the mouth well above the nostril. Although it was carefully covered with makeup, it still remained conspicuous and omnipresent, marring the appearance of this otherwise attractive, sturdily built woman of 28 years.

It was the reason Hilda Fallon had thought she could never have a husband, home, and children. And she used to brood that "people who want things too much are unlucky and never get them." She had always felt insecure and inadequate, certain that others didn't really like her and were "shocked" by her disfigurement.

Hilda's childhood had been difficult. She was "right in the middle" of seven children coming in close succession. Two had died in infancy, but there were two older and two younger siblings. Times were hard for her immigrant Austrian parents, and as a child she had known poverty and emotional turmoil. During the Depression they were never on charity but mighty close to it.

Under the burden of supporting the family her mother often flared into a temper, and Hilda feared her mother's anger. The father, nine years older than his wife, left home when Hilda was fourteen. He went out of state to a town where his brothers managed to secure a job for him. Although he sent money home, he never visited or wrote the many years he was away. He became ill and was hospitalized but then disappeared with no word of his whereabouts. He was at last located, and finally the family succeeded in bringing him home.

At home he sat in his room having nothing to do with the family except for occasional outbursts of temper. He refused to wash or keep himself clean. Hilda's memories of her childhood were of loneliness, of constant yelling, and of awakening terrified in the dark and quiet night.

She reported that she was good at school subjects and took part in the mathematics club but did not participate in social activities. She felt that she was "good at things where you have to use your head." Going to church always meant a great deal to her, even though her parents were irregular in their attendance and her siblings tried to avoid it.

As she grew away from the dolls with which she played until twelve or thirteen ("older than most girls") she began to think of boys. She never had any real boyfriend of her own but would go out on blind dates arranged by her girl friends. Apparently her girl friends didn't think the harelip was so terrible and they included her in their dates. Although she felt badly about getting dates this way, she realized that she wouldn't go out otherwise. So she came to terms with it.

While dates gave her some pleasure, none of them ever materialized into anything that looked like a prospect of marriage. Often her friends assured her that the boy "wasn't good enough" for her anyway. She didn't mind dates at night with a new boy, because with careful makeup and dim lights he might not notice that something was wrong with her face. But she always refused daytime dates such as picnics, especially if they involved swimming, which would affect her makeup.

The story of her courtship and resultant marriage was an important one for Hilda Fallon. One of her girl friends had a cousin with whom she arranged a date for Hilda. At first, all the dates with Charlie Fallon were at night, and it was not until some time later that he learned about her harelip from his cousin. After that he saw her in the daytime. Until recently he had never admitted that it bothered him considerably at that time. But as he came to know Hilda better, he began not to think about it or notice it.

In the beginning their relationship was on the basis that he liked to go places, have a good time, and spend money freely, while on her part she enjoyed the casual fun. But after she had been out with him several times she realized that she liked him "too well" and wondered whether to stop going with him. "I had a feeling that it wouldn't last and sure enough it didn't."

Around this time she was offered a temporary job in Oregon by the insurance company for which she worked. Part of her reason for deciding to take the offer was that she was so upset at having broken off with Charlie. He wrote her and she debated for some time whether to answer. When she finally replied, she received no answer in return.

Trying to find a way out of this humiliation, she went on a weekend trip and sent numerous cards to friends, including Charlie. This evidently inspired him to write, as she had hoped it would. But then she was careful not to repeat the experience and did not write again.

Upon her return they started to date once more and in a few months became formally engaged. During the engagement her fiancé pressed to have premarital sexual relations, but she refused. She had been "brought up strict" and it was impossible for her to have sexual relations outside of marriage no matter how much she liked him. They had argued about this and when he said he'd have to find other girls, she told him to go ahead. Again she had the feeling that her relationship with Charlie wouldn't last, but finally they were married when she was twenty-three years old.

Mrs. Fallon emphasized that the marriage meant a great deal to her. "I didn't simply marry the first man who was interested, but married a man I really wanted." Her friends said that he wasn't good enough for her, but the girl who was most critical of Charlie's reputation married a man who "everybody knows runs around with other women."

Mrs. Fallon commented, "We get along very well as far as sexual relations are concerned because I give him what he wants." She guessed that sex was more important to men than to women, but unlike her friends, she did not feel that sexual relations were a duty rather than a pleasure. "I sometimes wonder if I'm normal because I don't find this part of marriage any burden."

In any event, she certainly wouldn't let her husband know if she felt like that about sex. "Maybe that's why the husbands of my friends seek other women." However, just before she became pregnant she did have a diminished interest in marital relations, "but I didn't tell my husband." She said, "I cater to Charlie, which my friends say is foolish." She even planned her meals to take into account his likes and dislikes. "His preferences always come first."

And Mr. Fallon wanted special consideration from her. Before their marriage he resented any attention she paid to girl friends. When they quarrelled she was always the one to make peace. As far as she was concerned, "getting along is more important than pride," and in any event, she felt that she got what she wanted this way.

Mrs. Fallon felt that her husband had "inferiority feelings" dating back to his early childhood. He was a "problem child," she said. Laughingly she pointed out, "Sometimes I try to be an amateur psychologist. I've read about such things and I give thought to why people act as they do."

She said that when Charlie was about three or four years old he went to live with an aunt and uncle in California for some reason. When he returned home he seemed to feel very strange with his family and couldn't straighten out the relationship to his own parents or siblings. He would ask if his father were also father to all the other children as well as himself. Mrs. Fallon thought that being so far away at so young an age had made him feel that he didn't belong to his own family any more, which started his inferiority feelings.

She wondered why it was that he always had to be the center of attention. She characterized some of his ways as "a misplaced sense of humor" and mentioned that "sometimes people misunderstand him." "When Charlie is out with a crowd he's always the center of the fun, but he gets upset and jealous if someone else is the center of attraction." Even his own family admitted that "he always has to be on the top, the favored one."

Another important factor was that Mr. Fallon was "something of a worrier, and his nerves are not so good." He was in service during World War II but was soon released on medical discharge. His feeling was that if things didn't happen the way they did, he would certainly have been killed in the war. As it happened, before he was to be shipped out he had an automobile accident which put him in the hospital. There was an injury to his head and afterward he was quite nervous. Now he constantly complained of a variety of aches and pains. Both his father and grandfather died of heart attacks, and "he is always sure there is something wrong with his heart" despite repeated medical assurance to the contrary.

Mrs. Fallon felt that it was difficult to cope with her husband's attitude towards money. He had always made pretty good money and spent it freely. As a warehouseman for a board and carton company, he was subject to job fluctuations. Often he was on part time or temporarily laid off. But he had a habit of boasting about big pay checks which came from overtime work and never mentioned the many weeks he earned nothing at all.

She felt that this put her in an embarrassing position with friends and family because they think "I'm stingy if I buy only a small present when my husband earns so much money." In her opinion, the boasting about money was tied up with the inferiority complex.

Mr. Fallon couldn't resist the temptation to spend money impetuously, according to his wife, so they had agreed that he would turn the money over to her. She had little budget envelopes for rent and various bills. "I never borrow from them for anything extra that I want, but if Charlie runs out of his allowance money I give him some of mine." She didn't like the thought of her husband going without money in his pocket, and "this way of working things out together is much better."

When the Fallons first married they lived with her mother and decided against having children until they had a place of their own. When they moved out of her mother's apartment about a year ago they considered starting a family, but she hadn't expected to become pregnant so soon. "When you avoid pregnancy for a while it makes it harder later to become pregnant." Although she was Roman Catholic, Mrs. Fallon was not unduly concerned about contraception and religion. "It doesn't bother me at all, because every one has to work out what they want to do themselves." She said that even the Church wasn't consistent. "We're told that sex is for the purpose of having children and not for pleasure so we shouldn't prevent conception. But then they give us rhythm charts so you can avoid sexual relations when you can get pregnant. So then you would have sexual relations for pleasure only." Therefore she did not see the difference between the Church's approach and any other kind of contraception.

This was not something she and her husband had talked over,

but in any event the religious angle would not be any problem to him. Although he was brought up in the Church, he didn't go now, and his family hoped she would be a good influence to get him started again. But Mrs. Fallon felt that "people have to make up their own minds about such things." She wouldn't permit him to stop her from going to church, and she wouldn't try to make him go when he felt otherwise. However, both of them agreed that children should have religious training. "I go to confession regularly, and it means a great deal to me." Mrs. Fallon recalled that when she was growing up, some of the other children tried to avoid church, but she always wanted to go.

Prior to becoming pregnant, "we didn't use anything in particular, but I just douched and things like that." She also added that they had been practicing coitus interruptus. When Mrs. Fallon became pregnant so quickly she wondered "whether it might be a tumor or something." "You know how such thoughts go through your head." When she missed her second period she was sure she must be pregnant. When she began having pains at the time her third period was due she became afraid that something was going to happen.

She hadn't noticed any changes in her body since an initial breast enlargement and wondered whether she was "built differently inside than other girls." She could really begin to think about the pregnancy only after being reassured by the doctors. Shortly after this, she fell in the bathtub and hit her chest. This worried her very much and she went for a chest X-ray. Since then she had read that the worst thing for a baby was for the mother to have an X-ray. "I would not want to do anything to hurt my baby." She wondered why she had so many doubts and whether other girls had them.

When she was frightened by a mouse early in her pregnancy her husband said she shouldn't get upset, because it might hurt the child. "I know that's just superstition but maybe people who want a baby so much are not so lucky." Then she broke off to say, "I know it's silly to talk like this."

Physically she had not felt very well and was quite nauseated. She vomited usually when she first got up before she had eaten anything. The main thing was, "I'm so very tired at night. Maybe it's because I'm still working." She had tried staying home for a few days to see if that would make a difference, but she had felt even worse. She thought it better to be with people and talk to them "even though they give all kinds of advice but never answer the questions I really want to know." She worried whether the way she felt "is the way it ought to be or not."

Her husband was not very sympathetic towards her. He said that "other women have babies and don't talk of every little pain they have." She answered, "You're not married to other women and they don't tell you about their pains." One thing she noticed in herself was that she was much more emotional and got upset over "the least little thing." When her husband said something, she blew up. Then the next day she couldn't see why she should have gotten so upset. Her family always told her, "You're dramatic and like to play-act and exaggerate things."

But doubts about herself still cropped up. Sometimes she was unsure that she could handle a tiny baby or keep it from being injured. "I know that there are classes where they teach you how to do these things, but I'm afraid it wouldn't do any good with my own baby."

Mrs. Fallon told of a girl friend who had never wanted a child and had said so from the beginning. When she became pregnant she was actually angry and said she would hate the child. But when the baby was born it was a beautiful boy who was absolutely perfect from birth and she never had a moment's worry with him. Now her friend said that she loved her baby too much. Mrs. Fallon hoped she would be that lucky.

In addition to experiencing nausea and vomiting, she felt miserable otherwise. It did not surprise her because she "always anticipated trouble." Her appetite was very poor and she actually had a weight loss at the beginning of pregnancy. "I used to get so much enjoyment from eating and liking everything but now I go to the store after work and can hardly think of anything I'd like."

One of the things that became a constant problem for Mrs. Fallon throughout pregnancy was a vaginal discharge which the doctors were not able to overcome. She was treated with douches, jellies, gentian violet, etc., with variable but at best temporary success. Mrs. Fallon complained that the clinic doctors gave her "the brush-off," saying there was nothing to worry about. At one time she expressed the hope that if she came to the clinic more often, the discharge would be controlled. But at another time she expressed irritation at having to come so often for fear she'd lose her job.

The discharge made her feel unclean and she bathed frequently. She carried extra panties to change if necessary and worried that there might be an offensive odor. She was unable to wear sanitary pads all the time because they were too irritating, and she was unable to use tampons because she couldn't insert them properly and they were too uncomfortable.

She wondered what it was, why she had it, and why it did not clear up. She knew a number of girls "who had a discharge and they were very nervous people." She said her discharge began after marriage, but she didn't think it was related to sexual intercourse. At first she had been afraid that it was a venereal disease but had been reassured about this by doctors. When it began, her husband developed a rash on his penis and he angrily "accused" her of giving it to him. But the doctor told her, "It's more probable that he gave it to you." The doctor had explained how a certain organism can lie dormant under the foreskin of a man for a long time without affecting him but that it reacts on the woman. He had explained that part of the trouble was because her husband was not circumcised.

Mrs. Fallon thought that she would be a very poor patient because she "makes such a fuss" when she is sick. Her husband kidded her, saying, "What are you going to do when it comes time for your delivery?" In a joking way she had replied, "I made up my mind to give the baby one hour to be born because I think I can stand it for that long. But if the baby doesn't cooperate, it can just stay where it is."

Mrs. Fallon liked her job and regretted that she would be unable to return to it because they had no maternity leaves. But she was not concerned because she didn't think she wanted to work after she had a baby. Money was no problem either, because Mr. Fallon had a decent job even though there were frequent layoffs. However, she said she would work in an emergency because "at times like that women can get jobs easier than men since they're lower paid and don't have to think about permanency or the future of the job."

The kind of planning that now concerned Mrs. Fallon was in

relation to the household, and how much of her time would be taken up by the baby. A dinette which they did not use could be a future bedroom for the baby. But for the present there was a little room closer to their bedroom which would be suitable. She thought it best to keep the baby in a separate room.

Somewhat apologetically Mrs. Fallon explained that she was getting a small crib from her sister, whose child was now six years old. The crib was in very good condition and the baby would need it only for a short time. Later they would use their own money for a large-size crib. Her sister also had a lot of baby clothes which Mrs. Fallon would utilize. She laughed as she said that someone was even giving her a small washer mainly for baby clothes. Eventually she wanted an automatic machine, "but if I had one I'd be expected to do all the washing and I don't want that."

Rather angrily Mrs. Fallon contrasted herself with her husband's sister, who was also pregnant and insisted on getting everything new for her child. She felt that though she had economized to the point of taking "hand-me-downs" for the baby, it had served no purpose. All the money she had saved by this was forced to go for repair of their automobile, which Mr. Fallon's brother had accidentally smashed. It seemed to Mrs. Fallon that she always "got the short end of everything" and that things never turn out right for her.

Early in her pregnancy Mrs. Fallon indicated that she didn't want rooming-in at the hospital by which the baby would remain side by side with her. Her friends had told her that she would need all the rest she could get and she could learn how to care for the baby when she got home. After much discussion and when she was near term, she decided in favor of the rooming-in arrangements.

During her fifth month Mrs. Fallon seemed to feel somewhat better. She had gained a little weight and her appetite had improved. She was even glad that she hadn't gained more because she didn't like the increased size of her waist and abdomen. Although she felt fine during the day, she was still tired and listless at home at night. Her husband wanted her to leave her job because she was too tired to get things done around the house. But she dreaded staying at home and wanted to postpone it. "I'm so clumsy at home that I'm always dropping things." It was different at the office, where she could get the most difficult job done well and efficiently. "At home I spend too much time on the phone instead of doing the necessary things, which just pile up."

Even though she sewed very well and had made her own clothes since she was young, Mrs. Fallon hated darning. Her husband complained that his socks weren't darned and buttons were off his shirts. He told her not to be fussy and just "darn them up any old way." But she said, "I have to do it right or not at all."

Mrs. Fallon's doubts and fears concerning the baby remained in evidence. One of her thoughts was, "I want a baby so much that maybe it won't be perfect." She discussed a nearby couple who had had a child with a large birthmark although they were "perfectly normal." She said the doctors had told her a harelip was not hereditary, so she was not going to worry about it.

During this period Mrs. Fallon's father was hospitalized for a severe cerebral vascular episode with extensive paralysis. At her family's insistence she did not visit him, because she might become upset. Consequently, each member of the family told her different stories about him and she didn't know whom to believe. After a short period when his condition was critical, he made a good recovery with some residual paralysis and was sent to a convalescent home.

Mrs. Fallon guessed that "the doctors were glad to get rid of him" and that they evidently thought "he was insane because they called in a psychiatrist to see him." She also commented on how very aged her father seemed at seventy-one compared to men older than he.

In her sixth month Mrs. Fallon quit her job. While she still dreaded staying at home, she planned to keep herself busy. Her vaginal discharge was worse and she hoped more frequent medical visits would help. She asked about circumcision if the baby were a boy and thought that it was automatic for all male babies because "it avoids trouble." Her husband, she said, has had a lot of trouble, and his brother had to be circumcised in the army because of difficulties.

Since her last visit, Mrs. Fallon reported, she had gained eight pounds and "have just let myself go." Her husband thought she was awfully large, but she told him he ought to see some of the other women at the clinic. A few days later she reported a total weight gain of twelve pounds along with the doctor's admonition that she was gaining too much. "People think I'm lucky that I can eat and not gain too much but they don't give me credit for how hard I work not to gain." Her husband had complained that he got no desserts other than jello or fruit, and she told him, "If I can diet, so can you." She guessed that he was just beginning to realize that this was his baby too and that he had to do something about it.

The visiting nurse had asked whether Mr. Fallon would be willing and able to wash the diapers for a few weeks after delivery. Mrs. Fallon thought this was hilarious. "He's the most helpless thing you can imagine around the house." The nurse then suggested diaper service, but Mrs. Fallon thought it might be too expensive. However, when she told her husband that he would have to wash the diapers, he readily agreed to diaper service. Then Mrs. Fallon was plagued by indecision as to which service to use and about their relative merits.

She was similarly plagued by indecision concerning help when the baby came. Initially she thought that neither her own nor her husband's family would be able to help her. Then her mother offered to take two weeks off from work to help, but her sister advised against it, saying that she had been of little actual help with her baby. Finally a girl friend who had had a baby offered to help. Hilda thought that it would be a comfort to have someone around who knew what to do, even if she didn't help much.

The Fallons had already selected both a boy's and a girl's name. Mr. Fallon wanted a boy, but Mrs. Fallon preferred a girl. "If I'm going to have more than one child, I wouldn't care about the sex but if there's only one, I want a girl." Almost superstitiously she predicted, "It will probably turn out to be a boy, just because I'm so set on a girl."

The question of Mr. Fallon changing his job arose in the seventh month of pregnancy. While he was making very good money, his work was subject to fluctuations and layoffs. His six years of service gave him seniority and a certain security, but it had limitations. Mrs. Fallon thought her husband was "a fool to work so hard and put in extra time whenever his boss asks," especially since he was constantly worried about his health. However at a recent examination the doctor had told him that his aches and pains were just "nerves."

In the meantime Mrs. Fallon had heard of examinations being

given by the city for prospective employees in her husband's field. She persuaded him to take the tests even though he was reluctant to do so because he was sure that he wouldn't pass. To his surprise and pleasure they said that he had demonstrated ability for certain kinds of work and would be put on the list. As time went along he became cynical and thought they just wanted to make him feel good.

But then Mr. Fallon received a phone call from the city to set up an interview for a possible opening. The new job would mean starting at considerably lower pay than Mr. Fallon earned, but it would be steady. With periodic raises and extra benefits he would soon make a very good wage. Mr. Fallon showed some interest and his wife began "working on him," since she was convinced that it was important for their future.

The need to make a decision weighed heavily on Mrs. Fallon, and she was unable to eat or sleep normally. She laughed as she said, "I'm usually constipated, but with this problem I have lots of bowel movements and urination." In great detail she presented the difficulties involved in making such a change, but she felt able to manage on the decreased income and said she would not mind too much. After all, she said, "I was brought up knowing hard times."

To her the imponderable was how her husband would take the financial limitations, as "he can't stand being without money in his pocket." Mrs. Fallon said that she wanted him to feel that it was really his decision, and if hardship were involved, she could always go back to work somewhere on a part-time basis.

Charles Fallon discussed the job matter with many people, all of whom said "he'd be a fool not to take this opportunity" because security was worth a whole lot more than the temporary high wages he was making. Nevertheless, both of them had been plagued by indecision the entire week. At night her husband was sure he wanted the city job, but in the morning he again had doubts. Finally he decided to accept but added, "If they don't offer the job I won't be too disappointed because then the decision will be out of my hands." To which Mrs. Fallon fervently commented, "Then it would be fate."

She was expressly troubled by the fact that making a decision was so hard for her. Repeatedly she asked, "Am I normal? Is it normal to be so uncertain about what you want to do or what would be the best plan to make?" This was tied to her up-and-down mood swings. One week she was way down, and the next she was "on top of the world." It seemed as though she was never at a happy medium but always on one extreme or the other. This was true before pregnancy but was even worse now. "There was a whole month when I simply hated my husband. I felt that I couldn't stand to have him around." But this was not really the way she felt about him, she added. When she looked back at one of these "down" moods, she wondered how she could ever have felt that way, but at the time it was very real.

At a later date she reported on her husband's job interview. Nothing had come of it and now that the whole thing was over, she was just as glad because the financial situation would have been too difficult. Mrs. Fallon seemed to dismiss the whole thing as a closed episode and didn't refer to it again.

Mrs. Fallon thought that one of her troubles was, "I'm too sensible in the way I handle things." Then when something upset her plans she felt frustrated. She said that she was often uncertain about her own feelings and "sometimes looked at things in a mixed-up kind of way." "Is it normal for me to talk so much?" she asked. "I can't keep things to myself. When something upsets me I must get it off my chest." Her sister told her that she never listened to advice even when she asked for it. But the reason she did this, Mrs. Fallon said, was because "I'm different from my sister and when I talk things out I can understand them better, about myself and about other people."

In this connection, she discussed with the interviewer her reaction to various doctors at the clinic and wondered if her reaction to a particular doctor was because he was Chinese. She didn't feel that she had racial prejudice nor did she question his competency. But she hoped he would not be the one to deliver her baby because "he's not interested in me." A Negro girl had expressed similar sentiments, and Mrs. Fallon said that "surely the Negro girl couldn't have been prejudiced racially."

Mrs. Fallon was eager to discuss the contradictions she felt within herself, and to seek answers for them. "If I have less than others I complain, and then afterwards I feel guilty about complaining so much. But if I have more than someone else, then I feel guilty about their bad fortune." She felt that she kept wanting "more and more" because formerly she used to think that she couldn't expect to get out of life what other people did. "I thought that way because of my harelip and it certainly did affect everything that happened to me." But now "it doesn't matter at all and other people are more concerned about my appearance than I am."

Mrs. Fallon had seen many doctors in an effort to correct her harelip, and always her friends or relatives would urge her to try somebody else and something new. Even after she had grown up she had come to the hospital at the insistence of a friend who had learned of some new skin-grafting technique. But, of course, the answer was always the same.

She said that both her mother and her husband objected to her going without makeup around the house, and she supposed she ought to wear it regularly "just to protect other people from shock." To show how little she cared about her appearance now, she said that she didn't even plan to bring makeup to the hospital when she had the baby "because no one will care how I look anyway." But her husband and her mother were insistent that she bring makeup.

One of the things that Mrs. Fallon still hoped to achieve, which had been on her mind for years, was to own her own home. Since she had indeed secured a husband and was about to have a child, that too now seemed within her reach. "Maybe it sounds silly since my husband only earns a weekly wage, but it's part of the feeling that the more I have, the more I can look forward to."

Sympathetically she mentioned that maybe her pregnancy was hard on her husband sexually. He had heard from other fellows at the shop that "women become real passionate when pregnant," but so far he had been waiting in vain. During the first few weeks she had felt so sick that she had had no interest at all; then when she got over being sick, it still wasn't important. "And now I'm at a point when I'm not supposed to have intercourse at all." So she guessed that "he's just out of luck." She said that in the evening he didn't want her to sit near him or get too affectionate because "it's much too hard on him." But she didn't think he needed to seek out other women, and he could wait for her.

The balancing of her relationship with Charlie Fallon was not easy for her. He talked about taking two weeks of vacation to help her after the baby was born. But then he worked out a plan to take on an extra job for those two weeks in order to earn more money for his family. "I know he's doing it for me, but I'd just as soon he wouldn't."

She pondered at length about how much she usually did for her husband and said she had warned him that when the baby arrived there wouldn't be much time for him. She had heard that some husbands resent a new baby and are even jealous of it. She didn't know if that would happen with Charlie, but "he always expects special consideration from me." While Mr. Fallon said that he understood, Hilda pointed out that "deep down there's a world of difference between understanding and actually feeling a thing." She feared that she would have to neglect one or the other when the baby came, but that the baby must come first.

One morning in her ninth month Mrs. Fallon had a very slight "show," and thought that she was ready for the hospital. She described how upset and excited she became. First she cut and set her hair. Then she "went through the whole house and vacuumed everything in the place." By the time she had finished, there were no further signs so she decided to relax. She started to get breakfast and became annoyed with her husband because he hadn't left the bed or made any effort to help her. But he only laughed and asked for his coffee in bed.

On the other hand, Mrs. Fallon made reference to the fact that she thought her husband would like a large family, now that he had gotten used to the idea of having a baby. She too would like to have more than one child, but she would want "a little time in between." She said, "Charlie does an awful lot of kidding and sometimes I don't know whether he's serious." Once he had said that he was going to "teach the kid 'a real vocabulary.'" Hilda remonstrated that he mustn't teach their baby bad words, that he had to set a good example and "act differently."

For instance, he "shouldn't sit around the house in his shorts and shock people that way." Sometimes when her girl friends were over he would come into the room with only his shorts on. Or he would call a warning, "Girls, don't look. I haven't got anything on," even though he was completely dressed. Then he laughed at their embarrassment.

As time went on, and delivery came close, Mrs. Fallon resolved her feelings about the doctor she had disliked. Now she felt that he was nice, knew his business, and she had lots of confidence in him.

The reason for her change of heart was that he had talked with her at length about the vaginal discharge. He had had laboratory tests done and was able to assure her that it was not a fungus but a yeast (monilia). Also, he had allayed her fears about the possibility of its affecting the baby, saying that this was most unlikely. She liked his frankness, "because if a doctor cannot be certain of something, it's better to say so."

The doctor painted her with gentian violet because it was too late in pregnancy to douche. While he was doing this, she had "the very funny thought that if the baby were born right then, it might come out all purple." She added that "this was silly" because she knew the baby was well-protected in the way it grew and was born.

Finally the doctor had also talked to her about breast feeding and said it would be better for her physiologically even if she did it for just a short time. This made her uncertain again of what to do. She was sure that she didn't want to breast feed, that she wouldn't like it at all, and had been relieved when the pediatrician told her it was all right not to breast feed. But now the obstetrician brought back her indecision.

It was also difficult for Mrs. Fallon to refuse to comply with suggestions from those she liked. Since she now liked the obstetrician, she was loathe to refuse his suggestion, but she also liked the pediatrician and wanted to follow her recommendations. "I'll decide after the baby is born and see how I feel then" was her compromise.

Hilda Fallon seriously questioned her own adequacy to do the right thing either for the baby or for her husband. She felt that she would be willing to make sacrifices for the baby but that her husband would be unwilling to do so. "He's not even sympathetic with my aches and pains. When I complain he says 'you wanted the baby, so shut up.' "

Two days later the delivery took place. When Mrs. Fallon noticed that the membranes were ruptured, she prepared for her trip to the hospital. She was poised, courageous, and efficient and made all the preparations herself, since her husband was too excited to help.

During labor the obstetrical and nursing staff were impressed with Mrs. Fallon's "excellent emotional attitude." She was apprehensive only at times, rested comfortably, and cooperated well, relaxing adequately between contractions. The labor lasted six hours and fifteen minutes. But immediately after her son was born, a most dramatic change took place.

After checking that the baby had all the proper fingers and toes, Mrs. Fallon became quite detached and apathetic. She didn't ask any other questions or even look at him. At the nurse's invitation to put the baby to the breast, her answer was simply "No." When the nurse placed the baby in her arms, she said, "Take that thing away."

This so upset the nurse that she couldn't help remarking, "After all, it's your baby." To the nurse's satisfaction, however, Mr. Fallon seemed delighted with the birth of his son, Ross. His wife's reaction to his enthusiasm was, "The way he carries on, you'd think he produced the baby all by himself and that I had no part in it."

The study staff, however, found little cause for rejoicing and were rather non-plussed by the baby. They felt that here was a "poor specimen," a baby who distinctly gave the impression of wanting to be left alone in a world which was too difficult for him, even without their intrusion. This feeling was supported by the sluggishness of his reflexes, the bad turgidness of his skin. While he was not considered premature, some of his features reminded one of a premature baby. While no birth injury was assumed, there was yet a vague clinical impression that something was awry.

Ross's activity remained consistently under the median, and his response to outward stimulation was comparatively unreliable, even for a newborn. His reactions reflected discomfort, but the discomfort was not well-defined in terms of movement or crying and could not be soothed by the usual handling. The movements of his extremities and the movement impulse itself appeared interrupted, less swift and smooth than was usual at birth. The impression remained of greater passivity than one ordinarily saw, and a speculation was voiced about his preparation for the experience of actively making his wants known.

Crying was not continuous nor overly loud or agonized. It was rather a repeated whimpering, moaning, or grunting which reflected a discomfort rather than a despair, a deeper-than-surface disturbance, which could not be easily comforted by human ministration. His moans and whimpers indicated that he was always uncomfortable, but that he could not "cry it out." And just as his physical movements were not vigorous enough to discharge his tension, neither was his crying forceful enough to serve the purpose of adequate communication.

Even in the typical hand-mouth contacts of the newborn, Ross's patterns seemed more accidental than purposeful. His hands circled more or less around his face, and when they came into contact with his mouth there was no appreciable change to show that the tension was relieved or that a focusing had been achieved. All the usual channels seemed deficient to provide Ross with comfort. His movements and his crying did not serve to discharge his tensions, his environment was of little comfort, and contact zones similarly failed to serve.

Oddly enough, Ross's activity level seemed to rise after feeding rather than before feeding. He showed less evidence of discomfort as he became hungrier, and above a certain level his activity actually decreased. It was as though he could tolerate stimulus only below a certain threshold and would then put up a tight barrier to any further encroachment. Hence, when hunger became a definite physiological need, it was not experienced anymore or communicated to the environment. With this in mind, if adults did not know that babies must be fed at certain intervals, it seemed as if Ross would allow himself to starve to death.

While it appeared that he slept uninterruptedly through any and all stimulation, this was contradicted by the lack of peace in his expression. His face twitched and grimaced, and he frequently whimpered. Sleep for Ross was not a relaxing experience but a desperate escape if the environment became intolerable. It became a substitute for tension-discharge patterns which could adequately prepare for action, for communication, and for gratification.

This being the case, whatever the personality of his mother, she would at least have to learn to understand these reactions; that for Ross the climax of hunger and the peak of disturbance led to sleep rather than to action. It was conjectured that such a pattern might well lead to deficient contact with his environment and to an unsatisfactory response from the most important objects of his environment, namely the human partners.

While in the hospital, Mrs. Fallon was gratified by the attention she received from her entire family and their intentions to help her when she returned home. At home she deprecated this help, claiming that her family actually made more work for her because "they never put things where they belonged."

The five-room apartment where the Fallons lived was on the first floor of a two-family home in the old part of the city on a street with heavy traffic. The houses were built close to the street, without a yard but with a front porch. Despite Mrs. Fallon's expressed dislike for housekeeping, the apartment was kept clean, shiny, and extremely orderly.

Mr. Fallon worked a night shift from 11 P.M. to 7 A.M. During the day he slept or was around the house watching television. This restricted Mrs. Fallon from having friends visit, and Mr. Fallon urged his wife to learn to drive so that she could get out when she liked. However, she was afraid she might kill or hurt someone and refused to learn.

Mr. Fallon was reported as being overjoyed with having a boy. In fact, he took a whole week off to celebrate. The home interviewer found him rather crude and rough in his way of talking. During the home visit he chided, contradicted, embarrassed, and then hurt his wife with a cutting remark about her harelip and its effect on the child.

During the first month Mrs. Fallon found that caring for her baby was not as overwhelming as she had expected. Her main difficulty was in following directions about the care of the cord, which she seemed unable to do and avoided. But then other difficulties began to appear. She became concerned about various aspects of Ross — his behavior, growth, some slight pigmentation and body hair — but she was unable to discuss or give a coherent account of any particular. She related everything as stories to be told for amusement but did not ask whether Ross's behavior was normal. She seemed unable to act on various of the pediatrician's suggestions.

Her indecisiveness began to play a large role. Should she break her schedule, a thing so all-important to her, and feed him? What should he wear? How long and in what manner should she play with him? Whose advice should she follow? The neighbor's, the book's, or the pediatrician's? She couldn't explain her rituals of wrapping Ross in a receiving blanket for feeding (despite the heat), or of disrupting feeding with a bath between juice and formula, or of placing him for 1 hour in a supine position although he slept only in prone.

At each home visit she "demonstrated" something to her visitor: the bath (a slap-dash affair), how she talked to him, how she "played" with him. She did not enjoy the latter, she admitted, but did so only at the pediatrician's prescription. The interviewer described Mrs. Fallon as "close to the breaking point in her ability to handle reality situations with Ross."

In Ross's twelfth week the Fallons had a "blow-up." Mr. Fallon wanted the two of them to go off for a holiday weekend and leave Ross with his grandmother. Mrs. Fallon was reluctant to impose Ross on her mother. The following Monday the interviewer found her depressed, disgruntled "with being tied down," and admitting that the baby was "too much for her to manage," especially the responsibility for decisions. She was hostile to her husband, who insisted that the baby was her problem, that "she wanted the kid, not him."

Mrs. Fallon said she felt "different from others, inadequate, always dissatisfied," and repeated that she had wanted the baby *so* much and now found him such a problem. "Why should it be this way? Is it because I'm emotionally disturbed?"

During that same week Mrs. Fallon reported that Ross had been sick over the long holiday weekend. There were no symptoms beyond his crying and irritability. She described her fear and dread of taking a rectal temperature but succeeded with the help of her neighbor. She blamed herself for his illness and associated it with the "blow-up" between herself and her husband.

Feeding reports began to be confused and contradictory. From Ross's second week on, Mrs. Fallon had been concerned about his growth, how little he ate, and irritated with his irregular schedule. She had hoped he would soon give up night bottles and take solids. Although she reported that she woke him every three to four hours for feeding as suggested in the hospital, she also revealed that it was sometimes six to eight hours between feedings. She kept a chart of his routine, but it seemed to have little meaning for her.

When Ross was about two months old and when solids were first introduced, Mrs. Fallon reported the first signs of pleasure and interest on Ross's part. Thereafter, the pediatrician had to restrain her gently from force-feeding of solids. During home visits it was observed that Mrs. Fallon paid little attention to Ross during feeding. There was no cuddling nor any attempt to keep him awake. After a few ounces he would fall asleep.

Sleeping was also a matter of concern from the beginning. Mrs. Fallon was irritated that Ross fell asleep at the bottle and stayed awake during the day only about an hour at a time. She worried that he slept so much, but she gave him no stimulation to make his waking periods worthwhile. She preferred leaving him in his crib because "he gives me so much trouble when he's picked up." Although she said he slept only in prone, she would put him down in supine. After an hour's crying she would turn him over, whereupon he went to sleep. Determined to establish a regular sleeping schedule, Mrs. Fallon decided "he just has to cry himself to sleep" and refused to pick him up or give him any attention once he was put down in the crib.

There was no real problem regarding elimination, and Ross did not seem to fuss over soiled or wet diapers. When occasionally there were softer stools, Mrs. Fallon mentioned the additional unpleasantness and difficulty in washing diapers and became defensive about not boiling them. She said that Ross never had any diaper rash.

His mother attributed a quality of indifference to Ross, saying that he was not particularly interested in things, didn't object much, protested weakly if at all, and didn't seem to particularly enjoy anything either. She was also aware at this point that he did not smile, coo, or babble, vocalized very little, and was not particularly responsive to the human voice.

This was corroborated at the well-baby clinic observation in Ross's third month. He still looked strikingly "unfinished" for a child this age and there was a marked facial asymmetry, possibly due to the blandness of expression. No smile was recorded in response to the adult's face or voice, and his activity actually diminished if an adult was present. The eyes were attracted by the human face, but there was not yet any response which went beyond this generalized reaction to the human being. As in much younger children, Ross's body position was predominantly a flexion of all extremities, especially the legs.

His interest in inanimate objects was unusually low. He never reached for an object even if it was put next to his hand. With the possible exception of the dangling ring, he did not look at any toy. Mastery of his body showed an uneven picture as well. "As he is lifted to a sitting position his head lags so completely that he appears to be either resisting change, or else watching the light on the ceiling. When his back is about vertical, the line of his face is still completely horizontal."

The lack of response to his inanimate environment was not compensated by constant and energetic movement. On the contrary, he moved very little. "There are some waving movements of arms and legs which do not give the impression of much activity and do not change the position." Rather there was the impression of sluggishness. One did not know whether he had any energy, and if he had, where it went.

Mrs. Fallon seemed to be aware of Ross's depressed energy level and constantly tried to stir him up. She talked loudly, made clucking noises which she urged him to imitate, frowned frequently, and rarely smiled. With unmistakable anxiety she asked whether his penis was sore or "just the way it is made?" She wistfully stated, "Even though he does not seem to want to sit, he is growing anyway." She appeared vague about the child's exact age, "three months and maybe a week or two, I guess."

At a home visit during Ross's fifth month Mrs. Fallon appeared cheerful, but evidenced considerable nervous pressure with a steady barrage of reports on family matters. She spoke of her "disagreeable" younger brother, of feeling guilty for not visiting her father in the convalescent home. She complained that Mr. Fallon didn't drive her to see him, although she hadn't asked him to. She also felt guilty for not having visited her sister, "but after all my sister could just as easily have visited me." She was thinking of taking driving lessons because she wanted to be "completely independent" of her husband with whom she "had very little in common." She jumped from one thing to another.

In his sixth month Ross had a cold, and Mrs. Fallon reported coughing and "wheezing." The pediatrician noted that the air in the apartment was very dry and that despite the room temperature of 65-70 degrees Ross was enclosed by several blankets, sleeper, diaper, shirt, and rubber pants. Apropos of Ross's illness, Mrs. Fallon told of the death recently of a young relative who had had "a weakened heart from severe spells of asthma when he was young." She appeared quite anxious.

Ross was now reported to take three meals a day and an occasional small amount of milk to help him get to sleep in the evening. Mrs. Fallon said that he seemed anxious to eat and she felt he was eating better. She attributed this to the fact that she didn't feed him when he first cried but "waited until he really began to scream and then he didn't play around, but ate."

He slept well through the night and usually took three naps during the day. Although he slept mostly in prone, his mother still placed him in supine, where he fussed until she would turn him over and let him go to sleep. She gave the impression that she didn't know what to do with him if he wasn't in the process of eating or having some physical care attended to.

At the well-baby clinic evaluation at the age of six months (26 weeks) Ross was seen to be neither especially underweight nor especially unattractive, but his face still gave an "unfinished" impression. His vocalization was a kind of whining and laughter mixture, without too much conviction. His reaction to stimulus was through heavy breathing, whimpering, and a kicking movement of his legs which went in the direction of a presented object.

On the Gesell test, as on previous occasions, there were some interesting discrepancies on the testing scores. He was as likely to have failures well below his age as successes at his age and some above. On the Viennese test he was below his chronological age in everything except use of materials.

His smile was quite rare and not specifically directed. He appeared really relaxed only when a diaper was put on his head, from which he emerged smiling from the dark. When put in feeding position his hand moved until it landed at his genital region and then he relaxed into a sleep-like stupor, seeming to have fallen asleep at the bottle. Nevertheless the bottle was emptied gradually and sluggishly, with no observable sucking movements.

During the Christmas holidays the Fallons did some visiting and entertaining. A seven-year-old niece visited for three days, and Ross seemed to enjoy her constant attention and care immensely. After she had left he appeared to want the same attention from his mother. She reported that "he was much more difficult."

In the ninth month of Ross's life a toy was seen for the first time in the household, a ragged-looking stuffed animal. A month later another toy was noticed, a huge balloon-type ball almost as large as Ross, which he ignored because it was too much to manage. Also, the Fallons had acquired a five-week-old puppy, which Mr. Fallon had insisted on bringing home. Mrs. Fallon allowed the dog to stay only because Ross responded so much to it.

"Things are coming along much better," Mrs. Fallon reported at the start of this period. She claimed she was trying to find a "middle way" with Ross and to be more relaxed with him. She complained mostly about being tied down and having no social life because Mr. Fallon commuted at night to a city 40 miles away as part of a training program.

But at a subsequent visit Mrs. Fallon appeared to be in a new slump. She centered the majority of her complaints and difficulties on Ross. She was impatient, angry, and almost out of control with him during the visit. She deeply resented other people's comments and implied criticisms of her handling of Ross. In self-justification she referred to the visit of her niece: "You see, I really do like children. . . . I got along fine with her. . . . We had so much in common."

She hoped after Ross was a year old that he would expect less of her and things would be better. Though she claimed that he made her nervous, there seemed to be some recognition of his progress. She still complained of boredom and thought she would like another child. She rejected the idea that this might increase her problems and emphasized only that she could handle her routine efficiently.

To relieve her boredom she undertook to earn some money by selling mail-order greeting cards to her friends. After a month she abandoned it as a failure since she had cleared only two dollars. She also reported with some excitement that she had had a few drinks with a sixty-year-old man upstairs on several occasions when his wife wasn't home. She was obviously annoyed that her husband regarded it as a big joke.

In the developmental evaluation when Ross was 34 weeks old (7 months and 25 days) he earned a developmental quotient of 102 and a general maturity level of 35 weeks on the Gesell. On the Viennese test he had a developmental quotient of 99.

Ross had some episodes of coughing and wheezing during this interim, plus a skin rash which appeared consistently on his cheeks and at times on his buttocks and thighs. At first Mrs. Fallon attributed it to his drooling and chewing on bed clothes but later felt it was due to certain offending foods.

It appeared to the interviewer that the rash was exacerbated when Ross cried or screamed, at which time his cheeks became fiery red and the rash spread to the temples with a dark red streak running up to the left forehead. According to Mrs. Fallon, it became irritated because he rubbed or scratched, then there was some weeping and occasionally some drops of blood. Finally it would become dry and scaly. She believed that there was a definite cycle through which it must pass and that "it would probably go away in time."

The pediatrician suggested that perhaps Ross shouldn't be allowed to get so hungry that he must scream and cry. For some reason it was very important to Mrs. Fallon that he should have just three meals and three bottles a day and be as regular as clockwork. She persisted in this scheduling even though she knew that he was far less fussy if given extra milk.

Ross ate practically everything that was offered, would take juice from a cup, and occasionally held the bottle himself in the crib. But Mrs. Fallon preferred to feed it to him because "he just plays with it unless he's very hungry." She complained that he tried to get his hands in the bowl when she fed him, but she didn't allow it. Instead she distracted him with a large plastic cup with which she permitted him to play.

Although previously Mrs. Fallon had been concerned about Ross's great amount of sleeping, she was now concerned at his resistance to sleep and a constant fight had developed over this. It was illustrated during a home visit when Mrs. Fallon suddenly decided that Ross must go to sleep although he was playing by himself. He protested vehemently, whereupon she violently rocked his carriage, then picked him up and gave him a very hard spank, saying angrily, "This is how it always is . . . sometimes I could spank the living daylights out of him." At this time she also related that once she had let him scream for over an hour, whereupon he became "almost hysterical" and couldn't quiet down even when picked up.

Ross was given prunes twice a week to keep him from being constipated, although there was no evidence of a need for laxative foods. In talking about cleaning his diaper after a bowel movement, Mrs. Fallon also talked about training the puppy. She said she had made no real effort to start Ross's training other than to secure a toilet seat for him, but he didn't give her any clue when he needed a bowel movement.

By his tenth month Ross was able to sit well, creep rapidly, pull to his feet, and support his entire weight. He could walk with one hand held. His fine motor ability lagged behind his gross motor activity, and the pincer grasp was still quite inferior. The quality of his performance generally was poor and his interest short. Language was also poor, although he responded to his name, to "no-no," and understood "bye-bye."

At the well-baby clinic observation towards the end of his tenth month Ross was still considered an odd-looking child with an "unfinished" quality to his face. While he seemed lively, friendly, and active on the whole, there was a kind of superficial quality which suggested no real interest or investment in people or environment. There was no discrimination between his mother, the examiner, or complete strangers, all of whom received the same giggling smile or were ignored completely.

His attention span was short and it took him amazingly long to respond to material offered or to become engaged with it on any level. He was not only disinterested in handling small objects but lacked skill in handling them. He seemed not to differentiate between the specific properties of various objects. In scribbling, he moved the paper instead of the pencil, or tried to use the ball instead of the table as a support for standing up. Ross vocalized almost constantly, but without any consonants, and there were no understandable words.

The summation of this evaluation showed that Ross was a child with a low degree of interest in his inanimate environment. His developmental quotient on the Viennese scale was 104 and on the Gesell 98. He did not respond to the clues of his human environment and communicated poorly with it. His body integration and coordination were also below par. While he could not be designated as organically damaged or mentally retarded, neither could he be deemed unqualifiedly "normal."

As Ross's first year neared a close, Mr. Fallon was transferred to a plant closer to home and worked the day shift, which suited his wife better. They bought a small plastic pool for Ross because he seemed so frightened of the water at the beach. After his father gradually helped him to get over his initial fear of the pool, Ross seemed to enjoy it. The small niece paid a repeat visit, but this time Mrs. Fallon said she was "fresh and stubborn." Mrs. Fallon was relieved and worn out when her niece finally left.

Ross and his mother often visited both grandmothers, but Mrs. Fallon preferred the paternal grandmother, with whom she felt more comfortable and accepted. In her own mother's home she found her brother's fussiness and prohibitions towards Ross objectionable. Mrs. Fallon seemed to depend a great deal on a neighbor who was quite fond of Ross and managed him much more successfully than she did. The neighbor gave much advice to her and often told her not to let him cry so much. Mrs. Fallon frequently counted on her to take him for a walk or to her house for a few hours relief.

Mr. Fallon refused to take his wife seriously about having another baby and consistently repeated that he wanted no more children. He kept a very careful count of her "safe periods" so that "she could not fool him." Nevertheless, the previous month she had thought she was pregnant, and they were both very excited. She would like to have another baby now, she said, rather than when Ross was four or five years old. The experience with her niece had now convinced her that there was extra work in dressing a girl, so at this point she preferred a boy, though she had always thought a girl would be nicer.

At this time, also, Mrs. Fallon felt that the apartment looked dingy and that the wallpaper needed replacing. She suggested to her husband that he do the work, but he vehemently refused and the matter was dropped. To her surprise, however, he arranged to have the job done and had picked out the wallpaper without consulting her. She was quite dissatisfied with the patterns selected, but no change was made. While the paper-hangers were at work, Mrs. Fallon and Ross spent a week with her family. When the job was done she became very vigilant lest her son damage his father's new wallpaper.

Mrs. Fallon found no surcease from her constant battles with

Ross and her inability to get along with him. She was aware that almost everyone else managed him better than she did. She didn't enjoy being with him and suffered from boredom at home. She toyed with the idea of going back to work and revealed that a job had opened up with her old company. The arrangement would be for Ross to stay with the neighbor who was so fond of him, or possibly with another woman several blocks away. Mr. Fallon agreed only on condition that expenses for Ross's care would come from her salary and that she would bank the rest as a "nest egg."

Soon after this discussion the pediatrician was called early in the morning with a report that Ross had a temperature of 104.4 degrees. He had been fretful during the previous day and felt warm when put to bed, but Mrs. Fallon had not thought anything of it. He cried during the night, and finally she had decided to take his temperature. She thought it was "pretty high" but felt that she could wait until the next morning. Her husband, on the other hand, kept insisting that she should call a doctor immediately. He had said, "My God, people die at 105 degrees."

When the pediatrician arrived, she found that the recommended alcohol sponge bath had been given but not the aspirin. Mr. Fallon left the room so as not to witness the shot of penicillin, but then returned and comforted Ross, who quieted very quickly in his father's arms.

Ross had several other episodes of illness as time went on, plus a fall at thirteen months which caused a scalp laceration. The rash appeared more consistently related to crying episodes and became quite red, weepy, and irritated, but Mrs. Fallon believed that it was due to cutting of teeth.

Her response to Ross's illnesses was such that the pediatrician noted, "I'm sure she has a very unclear idea of when he's ill, how ill, how long, or whether or not he has a fever . . . and she wouldn't know this unless he had a great deal of fever." In the course of these developments Mrs. Fallon gave up the idea of a job, concluding, "You have to believe in fate. . . . Things do turn out for the best."

In the early part of his second year Ross was reported to be eating well, and Mrs. Fallon was satisfied with the quantity he consumed. He would take anything given by his father and enjoyed having one meal a day with his parents. But Mrs. Fallon soon discontinued this because it was "too disruptive" of their mealtime. Ross slept fairly well at night and went to bed easily with a bottle. But at times he awakened crying and was allowed to cry for prolonged periods.

Mrs. Fallon still struggled for Ross to take two daytime naps because "with one, he's cross and cranky." But Ross seemed to need much less rest and liked to have company play with him for hours. It both pleased and annoyed his mother that he got along so much easier with visitors than with her. The interviewer summarized, "It is difficult to know whether her great desire for him to have two naps is to have him off her hands, or because his behavior becomes more difficult. Even when he used to sleep most of the time she tried to make him sleep more, beyond what he was willing to tolerate. His abhorrence of the crib began then, and has continued."

Ross's interest in motor activity began to increase actively. He wanted to climb on furniture and move about. He resisted restrictions of his freedom, screamed when put down or while being dressed, and quieted only from exhaustion. Mrs. Fallon reported that he "got into everything" and did a number of things "just for spite," including playing in the toilet.

Developmentally Ross showed more vocalization and greater body mastery as well as more interest in material. His language was still slow, however, and his fine motor development remained crude. At the well-baby clinic observation it was noted that his appearance had not yet lost its badly integrated character and asymmetry. Although his clothes were neither dirty nor shabby, they were put on so that he did not look properly dressed and they hung around him in some odd way. His smile frequently revealed anxiety and bewilderment, but his facial expression remained ambiguous.

This ambiguity carried over to other areas. There were unexplained quick shifts from tension and screaming to placid acceptance of material. For no apparent reason his excellent mastery of walking suddenly reverted to crawling. His performance shifted from one level to another with little relevancy. Generally speaking, he had advanced in the use of his gross motor equipment and showed little of the balance insecurity prevalent with new walkers. But on the other hand, he was not capable of solving an intellectual task at his age level.

On the Viennese test he had a developmental quotient of 102 with a strikingly uneven profile. General maturity level on the Gesell was 14 months, which, when compared to his chronological age of 15 months and 3 days, gave him a developmental quotient of 93. The same unevenness was revealed on the Gesell that showed in the Viennese test, scattering all the way from 9½ months to 18 months.

At most, his level of functioning was uneven and scattered because of a lack of receptivity, interest, or concentrative ability. He was ambivalent in dealing with any object, showing a tendency to destroy what he had and at the same time wishing to keep what he was throwing away. His response was more cooperative with the examiner than with his mother.

One result of Ross's increased activity over the months was that Mrs. Fallon began to feel better about him. This attitude was apparent in the way she handled him. She was more willing to have him close to her and more tolerant of his constant activity. In part, it was his greater ability to respond to her requests that made her feel that at last she could in some way communicate with him. She still complained that his crying was an "attention-getter" and her treatment remained inconsistent. She said that her husband was willing to give Ross anything "when he won't shut up about it" but she refused to "give in to him."

Ross's appetite for solids was very good, but he refused to give up his bottle, which troubled Mrs. Fallon. Because there was difficulty at meals when his father tried to make him "sit and eat like a gentleman," Mrs. Fallon avoided the situation by feeding Ross ahead of time. Then she permitted him to come to the table later and have something with them if he liked.

She reported that Ross slept well at night but also mentioned that they took him into their bed "when he wakes and cries." She felt this was "a bad habit" but it was easier than being up with him for hours. She still tried to get him to take two naps daily and found that it was easier for her husband or even a neighbor to succeed in getting him down. She had discovered that sometimes running the vacuum cleaner would have a soporific effect in putting Ross to sleep. Also, one day, after he had been crying for an hour and finally stopped, she went in and rubbed his back, whereupon he went to sleep. Since then when he had difficulty going to sleep she would say, "Lie down and I'll rub your back."

Mrs. Fallon had not attempted toilet training for the reason that "his BM's are irregular and he doesn't let me know." However, she also reported that Ross himself had been placing the toidy seat on top of the toilet. She found this an annoyance rather than a possible suggestion that he might accept the seat. When he had passed a stool Ross now showed distress and started pulling at his pants. He no longer played with the water in the toilet but occasionally would get a clean diaper and throw it in after watching his mother rinse out a soiled one.

He was described by his mother as constantly moving about and active. She said that he could bring things to her upon request and that he followed her about the house imitating her actions in cleaning. She said he walked in circles and "danced" in response to music on television. He banged a great deal with anything he happened to have in his hand.

At 16½ months Ross was beginning to use some language in what appeared to be a much more normal manner than was characteristic of him earlier. He looked better on the testing and otherwise than at any other point during his life. His general maturity level on the Gesell was 18 months, with a developmental quotient of 109. Whether this was the result of his mother's more positive feelings toward him or whether her more positive feelings came from the change in him, one will probably never know.

The well-baby clinic observation in the eighteenth month found a substantial change in Ross's appearance; he was described as having "handsome boyish looks, careful grooming, and the charm of his irregular features." His expression appeared serious, interested, and alert. The lack of integration which had so concerned observers before seemed to have disappeared. But the transformation was not as radical as surface appearance might indicate.

Ross still manifested transitory contact with objects, giving them little attention or appropriate handling. His speed varied from slow hesitation to quick expedience, and his emotions ran through a quick gamut from anxiety to calm interest, from radiant happiness to annoyed irritation, from aggressive rage to sulking boredom. There was lack of basic relatedness to anything except in seeking contact with the adult.

Interestingly enough, his behavior was less erratic when the adult concentrated on him and gave him full attention. His desire to capture the adult's attention was mainly focused on his mother, who paid little attention to him and continued to talk in an uninterrupted flow. Ross's aggressive outbursts appeared mainly related to this frustration at creating contact with her.

Thus, Ross used toys not for a real interest in them but as a tool to create contact with the human partner. Failing this, the inanimate world became a disappointment and the investment became no longer worthwhile. This disappointment extended to the area of communication as well, because Ross had not found it a way to reach the adult. His language production was still most limited, a matter of so much concern for both his parents that they asked, "Is he mentally retarded?"

Mrs. Fallon said that relatives and even her husband constantly attacked her because Ross "wasn't developing like other children." A more advanced cousin, five weeks younger, was continually compared to Ross. The criticism and the fear of retardation made Mrs. Fallon even more tense and anxious.

She admitted that she had not been very patient with Ross and that his activity irritated her. She was worn out from Christmas festivities and was also disappointed that Ross showed so little response or appreciation of the celebration or toys. The Fallons themselves had not given him any toys "because he never plays with them," but he received many from relatives.

To make matters worse, Mrs. Fallon had become pregnant again and felt "just awful." She explained that they hadn't tried to have another baby but also hadn't tried to avoid pregnancy, since Mr. Fallon had finally agreed to a second child. Now Mrs. Fallon was again set on a girl. She anticipated the rest of pregnancy with pleasure and recalled her first pregnancy as a time when she felt as well as she ever had in her life! The hard part, she noted, "is after the baby arrives." Then her feelings of inadequacy, frustration, and depression came to mind, and she hoped that things would not seem as overwhelming with the second child.

She also hoped that Ross would be less of a problem to her in nine months. Both parents were still concerned about his development and fearful that he was mentally retarded because of delayed speech and the fact that he didn't behave as they would like him to. Mrs. Fallon saw some things in Ross that reassured her that he wasn't "dull," but they weren't enough.

During the interview she tried to show Ross off and make him perform. She became quite upset when he refused. Her expectations for him remained unreasonable for his age, and both parents continued to expect more mature behavior than was warranted.

Mrs. Fallon was disappointed that her pregnancy would prevent her from being matron-of-honor at her sister's wedding in five months' time, and also that this sister's marriage would create family problems. She was the last daughter at home, and her brother had announced that he would move from the house after the marriage. This raised the question of where her mother would live. Mrs. Fallon thought that perhaps her mother ought to live with them but felt guilty because Mr. Fallon absolutely wouldn't permit it.

In the meantime she was also preoccupied with plans to rearrange the house early enough before her confinement so that Ross would become accustomed to it. She planned to convert the present dining room into the master bedroom, with a new set of twin beds. The large bed in their present bedroom would go to Ross, and the new baby's crib would also be in that room. She hoped that Ross would be ready for the big bed and that he wouldn't feel "pushed out by his parents when the baby came."

In speaking of her nausea and the fact that she had a bad cold with low-grade fever, Mrs. Fallon incidentally mentioned that Ross had been sick too. This coincided with the pediatrician's report around this time that Ross "did not look sturdy" and seemed more slender and frail. It was suggested that his vitamin intake be increased and that his milk be fortified. Ross seemed to prefer small amounts of food frequently and often went to the table or refrigerator for small bites during the day. This may have been a way to establish contact with his mother, who usually responded to direct requests for food or drink.

During a home visit at nineteen months Ross wandered slowly from room to room, not interested in much of anything and with a peculiar and very vacant smile. His mother described this as a kind of game he frequently played and called it being "on tour." His only vocalization was a whimper when he lost his shoe. Mrs. Fallon said he became very upset if his shoes were off. When he broke a glass, his mother scolded him sharply, but he sat with the same wide vacant smile and showed no concern, anxiety, or even interest.

He was much better outdoors than indoors and still seemed to prefer company to toys. Some jealousy in relation to his mother was apparent when other children were around. He tended to cry persistently and in a prolonged way for what he wanted, and often banged his head when tired, angry, or frustrated. His language production was still at the one-year level, but his understanding of directions was at the twenty-one month level. He behaved much more maturely when he had the undivided attention of an adult.

At an evaluation when Ross was 20 months and 5 days his general maturity level on the Gesell was 20 months and 7 days with a developmental quotient of 103.5.

Mrs. Fallon reported that she had abandoned efforts at training Ross because he didn't seem interested. She pointed out that this decision had also been made because she hadn't felt like doing anything about it in recent weeks. She had not been well ever since Christmas, and Mr. Fallon took three days off so she could stay in bed.

She reported that she went through a three or four week period of "not being able to think or move" into action, during which she had a sense of unreality as if she were in a dream and knew the things that were happening, but was powerless to control her own actions. Sometimes it seemed as if she would start to think about something, but then would lose track of the thought and not be able to follow through.

She went to a doctor, who prescribed some kind of medicine for a "virus" but it did little good. Then one day she got up feeling much better and "the fogginess was gone." This good period lasted about a week, but then the same foggy feeling returned. Now she was feeling somewhat better again.

Mrs. Fallon said that she found this pregnancy more difficult than the first and wondered whether it was because she must care for Ross or whether it was another kind of problem. She occasionally had some bloody show and also some of the vaginal discharge that was such a problem during her first pregnancy. She had become quite heavy and was very resentful at mention of her weight gain. She claimed that this gain was deliberate, as relatives insisted that Ross was such "an impossible child" because she had starved herself during his pregnancy and "started him out badly."

Mrs. Fallon became more flexible in her insistence that Ross take two naps daily. In fact, she worked hard to make nap time a more happy experience for him and allowed many toys and her large pillow in the crib. Frequently Ross didn't fall asleep but was content with this quiet play time, during which he vocalized and babbled more than when he was up. His mother was now reconciled to one nap a day.

A bedtime ritual had developed wherein Ross asked for things to be put into his crib by pointing and grunting. Then he fussed and pointed to the shades until his mother pulled them down evenly. He complained bitterly until they were just exactly even. Then he settled down with his bottle. The Fallons continued to take him into their bed if he awoke during the night.

By two years Ross had developed some bladder control and permitted himself to be taken to the toilet for urination. But as yet no interest appeared in bowel training. He neither told his mother when he was going to have, or had had, a bowel movement, and he didn't like to be changed. Although Mrs. Fallon felt that the achievement of bowel training would prove to their relatives that he was learning and developing, she nevertheless remained quite inconsistent in her efforts to accomplish it.

Ross enjoyed an identifying game with his mother where he corectly pointed to various parts of her body as she named them. He continued to be extremely active to the point where Mrs. Fallon tied a rope on him when out walking. As noted before, his behavior was more mature and purposeful when he had the attention of an adult. When he was ignored, he was disorganized and often his activity appeared meaningless.

There was still practically no understandable language but frequently he was heard to say a word softly. When asked to repeat a spontaneous sound, he went completely silent. He walked up and down stairs alone and was not in the least fearful. The pediatrician stated, "This is a test profile similar to some of the findings on young autistic children seen in the clinical diagnostic service." The fact that Ross's social responses looked no better than they did when he was eighteen months may have been related, the pediatrician noted, to the progress of Mrs. Fallon's pregnancy and her own increased impatience in handling him.

In the final well-baby clinic evaluation at the age of two years, it was difficult to positively diagnose either the child or the mother. Ross looked well-groomed and well-clad, his dark hair was nicely combed, clean, and fresh despite the heat. The irregularity of his facial features was attractive by now. But there was something disturbing in the overall quality of the child which detracted from his appeal and which engendered no empathy with him.

His mother seemed as well-groomed as her son. She was highly pregnant but wore a nice maternity outfit which looked fresh and attractive. Her face was carefully made up, and the harelip fairly well disguised. Yet there was something in her appearance that impressed as "slipshod," "not coherent," "not well put together," "disorganized." Perhaps her uncontrolled and incessant talking gave this impression, as well as the controlled temper with which she threatened Ross or attacked him.

Ross did not concentrate on any task for any length of time. He started and then discarded, destroyed his own product, and rushed away. Even with help he did not try to solve a task. He forgot what he had started to do and went to something else. While his coordination was good and his movements swift and easy, they lacked a fulfillment and a cognizance of their purpose. It was not the diagnosis of a hyperactive mentally retarded child running around with an empty mind. It was more that his mind was bothered by something which did not simply make him run but made him run away.

On the Gesell test he did not do as well as he had done two months earlier. On the Viennese test he based at the 15- to 18-month level. His profile looked no better than it did at the age of 16½ months.

At the age of two years Ross did not use one single word but vocalized "like a feeble, powerless, and also hopeless animal." When he was whining in this manner, his face was distorted in a terrifying grimace. Other than this, his expression was usually bland. Only if somebody helped him in his task did Ross smile, and when his mother showed him how to manipulate the top, both their faces were lit up by warm and sympathetic smiles. Ross's hands were in the mother's hands that guided him, his body seemed relaxed, and he did not rush away.

Unhappily this picture did not continue long. Ross pointed to this and that, but it was clear that nothing could satisfy him. When his mother prohibited him from the pediatrician's stethoscope and threatened to spank him, he whined and ran to her, his little body seeming literally to merge into hers. It looked as if the mother were his only refuge in this danger, even though it was she who had brought the danger about. When she struggled to undress him, he cried pitifully and kicked her until she slapped him stingingly, while telling the pediatrician how she slaps him at home.

Ross's behavior was not entirely explained by his mother's behavior. It was the result of a vicious circle created by the interaction between this child's personality and that of his mother's. It was the result of combined constitutional and environmental elements that made it difficult for Ross to know what he wanted or to translate his wants into objective terms.

Mrs. Fallon, on the other hand, did not provide him with that guidance or assistance which he needed so desperately. As he became more disoriented, intolerable, and frantic, his mother became more absent-minded and more violent. Even admitting a constitutional handicap, there was no doubt that such interaction with his mother must aggravate Ross's picture. How much so, it was impossible to say. Nor would it contribute much to our understanding to say that Ross was a "deviate" child and his mother a "schizophrenogenic" mother.

On the positive side, one could see an increasing smoothness of relations between parent and child, and some assuaging of the deep inadequacy felt by Hilda Fallon in motherhood. But it could neither be said that she did not love Ross when he was born nor that she no longer rejected him when he was two years old. Mrs. Fallon's ambivalence toward the maternal role was no easier resolved than her ambivalence to other aspects of life.

As we came full circle, Mrs. Fallon was again pregnant, her husband again intolerant, her feelings of depression and inadequacy again rampant. And one might fear, with this mother, that the new baby's experiences might well parallel those of Ross.

The Fallon Family

SUMMARY

A. EXPECTATIONS

1. Maternal Expectations. The expectation of a child did not bring satisfaction to Mrs. Fallon. It brought instead great anxiety about the maternal role and many negative feelings in terms of self-doubts. She wondered how she could ever mother a child and came to see her delivery as a probable defeat rather than an accomplishment. Her deprecation of self as inadequate and unworthy, in combination with forebodings that life conspired against her, created a "gloom and doom" chaos of maternal anticipations.

2. Specificity of Expectations. There were few specific anticipations about the coming child itself, what it would be like, what qualities or character it might have. But there was much concern with matters of self-conduct, such as rooming-in, breast feeding, conflicting information and advice. No detail was too small to require conjecture and analysis, be it a diaper service, help in the home, physical arrangements in the house, or how one should manage. These specific expectations were myriad and constantly threatened the uneasy equilibrium of Mrs. Fallon's life.

3. Motivational Orientation. It seemed that in dealing with her son, Mrs. Fallon found it necessary to involve herself as little as possible. She expected a minimum of intrusion by the baby and a minimum of bother. Her unawareness of the baby's needs was matched by an inflexible desire to adhere to schedule, regardless of the baby's demands. Her routines were mechanical, never mutually pleasurable for mother and child. There was little attempt to adapt to the baby but much effort to make the infant adapt to her preconceived rituals and procedures.

Mrs. Fallon had little tolerance for the ways of an infant and wanted response that could be reasonably expected only from an older child. As Ross grew older, between the eighteen- to twenty-four-month period, Mrs. Fallon showed some relaxation in her strict expectations. At that point there was some increase in response to the child and even some enjoyment of him. Throughout the study, however, she was clearly and consistently mother-centered in her expectations, her conduct, her manner, and her attitude.

4. Role of Child in Fulfilling Mother's Expectations. In one respect Ross fitted into his mother's expectations for a minimum of intrusion, particularly in the earliest months. Because of his extreme passivity in infancy, his lack of social response, and his slow development of communication, he perpetuated for a year and a half the unresponsive, unperceptive management by his mother.

In another respect, too, Ross fulfilled his mother's anxious forebodings. Though she wanted to extend herself as little as possible for him, nevertheless she wanted an attractive, well-developing child, who would be "perfect in every respect." Instead she had reasons for concern over slow development, apathy, lack of speech, and slowness in other developmental landmarks. Her son's smallness and lethargy seemed to her a terrifying further proof of her inadequacy, and this further immobilized her. She felt that she wanted so very much to be a good mother, and now what she had was mostly problems.

It was not until Mrs. Fallon's second pregnancy, when Ross had become more active and had begun to catch up in his development, that his mother began to change to a more friendly and accepting attitude. It would be fruitless to speculate which came first — whether Ross's development was responsible for his mother's beginning change in attitude or whether her greater responsiveness helped Ross in his development. It is certain, however, that for three-quarters of his first two years Ross was not successful in altering the early patterns of mother-child activity.

5. Paternal Expectations. Mr. Fallon on the whole looked forward to having a baby, despite his impatience and intolerance of his wife's complaints. There was reason to believe that "having a baby" was mutually agreed upon, although Mr. Fallon in moments of strife would wash his hands of it with the accusation that "you wanted the baby."

Mr. Fallon expressed hope that the child would be different from himself, and implied that he would make certain the child didn't have bad habits or he'd "beat it out of him." He also believed that religious education was important for a child, despite his own indifference to the Church. Although he was a proud father, he defined child care as his wife's responsibility and tended to discharge his father's role in caustic kibitzing, without abandoning the prerogatives of his own satisfactions and comforts.

B. BEHAVIOR

1. Communication. From the beginning, verbal communication was used by Mrs. Fallon only for direction and control of the child's behavior. She used little language with Ross during the first six months, and when she did, it was a substitute for picking him up and holding him. During the second six months, a period in which her impulsiveness was especially noticed, she alternated between very vigorous use of language mainly for prohibition and not talking to him at all.

The whole matter of language was influenced by Ross's slow development in understanding words at this time. When in the first half of his second year Ross improved considerably in understanding words, though not in using them, it led to his mother's increased use of language to give him orders.

When Ross was about eighteen months old, with the general relaxation and softening of her behavior toward him, Mrs. Fallon began to use words, as other mothers had from the beginning, to comfort, lull him to sleep, or entertain him. Words for Mrs. Fallon were also an occasional substitute for physical punishment, and she used them to scold and berate him vigorously.

Verbal communication became a substitute for physical contact with the child, and until he was eighteen months old, the paucity of physical contact between mother and child was extreme. Far from using physical contact to comfort Ross, his mother put him down if he started to cry while she was holding him or when she picked him up. Later on, the same wide fluctuations which marked her use of language appeared in her physical contact with Ross. She alternately left him alone entirely for long periods or handled him vigorously and frequently for a while.

During his second year there was an increased tolerance for Ross's overtures. As he became more active, Mrs. Fallon permitted him to climb over her, and there was some rough, perhaps caressing, play. When Ross was first crawling, his mother was observed to be very protective in situations where he might be exposed to injury. As he began to get into things, she became irritated. Yet, on the whole, she was relatively permissive of his explorations and rather lenient about his strewing objects on the floor. It was apparent that she took pride in his mobility.

In the first part of his second year Mrs. Fallon made much use of physical control, especially in the struggle over dressing. But by the end of the year the physical interaction was much more positive and playfully active, as the relationship began to improve.

Mrs. Fallon was markedly unresponsive to clues from Ross, tending to ignore them entirely. She could not surmise what Ross might want, what his behavior manifested, what indications he was providing, or even what symptoms of illness he was showing. At times Mr. Fallon showed more response to such clues from the baby than did his wife.

2. Regularity and Flexibility of Scheduling. The indecisiveness and impulsiveness that marked Mrs. Fallon's relationship with her son during the first year particularly influenced this aspect of her care.

There were times when she had to be reminded to wake the baby at least every four hours so he could be fed, and she had difficulty in following this schedule at first. Later she developed a rigid timing that better suited herself, and she would not brook any change despite clear evidence that it did not satisfy the child.

In the first half of the second year some slight evidence of flexibility appeared faintly, and Mrs. Fallon was able to make some adaptations in giving Ross his bottles. By the second half of this year the question of regularity was no longer discussed. Instead there were rigid expectations about what quantity of food should be consumed. When she was concerned with Ross's small intake, she tried to force-feed him with solids or lengthened the hours between meals so that he would "eat more supper." At other times she was impervious to his food intake, and unobservant of his peakedness, describing him "as not a big eater."

Regularity in sleep, which was highly desired by his mother, was guaranteed in the first six months by Ross's inordinately long periods of sleep and generally apathetic response to his environment. But by the first half of the second year his sleep was quite irregular despite his mother's considerable efforts to establish a routine. He had considerable difficulty in going to sleep and this was handled in a highly volatile and unpredictable fashion. Sometimes he was left to cry it out, sometimes brought to sleep in his parents' bed, sometimes given a bottle, sometimes not.

When he was about fifteen months old, struggles about taking naps were especially severe, with Mrs. Fallon determined that he would take two naps a day despite his obvious desire for more attention and less sleep. Here again the struggle was handled inconsistently and unpredictably. Sometimes a neighbor helped to get him to sleep, sometimes he was left to cry it out, sometimes he was spanked, sometimes he was given a bottle. By eighteen months, as Mrs. Fallon became more tolerant towards her child, she was able to be more flexible about his naps, even to the point of settling for one a day and allowing Ross the luxury of toys in his crib, sometimes rubbing his back to help him to relax.

To the extent that Mrs. Fallon was able to compromise her rigid expectations for regularity, life became easier for all concerned.

3. Techniques of Management. Mrs. Fallon's techniques of management ran the gamut from substitution to avoidance. Sometimes she tried to distract Ross with clucking noises or brightly colored magazine pictures. Sometimes she just walked out on him, refusing to listen to his crying. Or she diverted him from messing in his food by giving him a cup to hold, or she discovered that the noise of the vacuum cleaner had a soporific effect on him.

Often she used the technique of scolding and threatening, sometimes the technique of withholding by not offering him milk until he had eaten what she considered a satisfactory amount of solid food. She also used avoidance in her failure to remember to feed him, in not taking his temperature when necessary, in her unawareness that he was ill.

Mrs. Fallon was generally inconsistent in her techniques and markedly indecisive about handling her child, especially in the first year. In the second year she showed something of a shift. Her avoidance of direct contact with Ross began to give way to tolerance of such contact, and her prohibitions became less exacting.

During the first year her reports of non-permissive behavior were in far greater proportion to those of permissive behavior. In the second year this was reversed, coinciding with the better rapport between mother and child. In fact, Mrs. Fallon was the only mother in the study for whom the number of non-permissive behavior reports were smaller in the second year than the first. For all the other families, non-permissive reports increased in the second year because of increased development and mobility of their children, which required greater watchfulness.

4. Relation of Expectations to Behavior. Mrs. Fallon took a long time to come to terms with her maternal role and to find any comfort or satisfaction in her child. During the first eighteen months her expectations turned mainly on non-involvement with Ross and were directed toward his behavior in a way that made her involvement minimal. She wanted a child who would leave her alone, and Ross fitted very well into this need. He was a colorless, apathetic child who made few demands and exhibited little interest in his environment.

With her mother-centered values Mrs. Fallon exhibited little adaptive behavior in the first eighteen months with Ross. In fact, she was quite non-adaptive. She refused to comfort him when he cried, at times forgot his feedings, failed to see when he had a fever, and ignored him as best she could. It was as though she had to make her prediction come true that she could not be a good mother.

In the last six months, however, there was considerable change in the mother-child relationship. There was increased physical contact and play, more mutually satisfactory arrangements of feeding and naps, and generally greater tolerance. As Ross's comprehension of language grew, he was more satisfying to his mother, and as he matured in other areas as well, he came closer to his mother's expectations of a satisfying child.

5. Paternal Behavior. Mr. Fallon required stricter conformity to desired modes of behavior than some of the other fathers in this study, and he exhibited the same disparagement toward his son as toward his wife. He judged him to be "a homely baby." Nevertheless he was not wholly demanding and would also occasionally give in when Ross cried. Although he could appear unsympathetic and sarcastic to the child, yet he proved to be very sensitive and responsive to the child's illness at one time. He was able to comfort the child and was often more successful than his wife in getting him to cooperate. Ross, in fact, responded better in many respects to his father.

Mr. Fallon was father-centered in terms of satisfactions to be derived from the child and adult-oriented in his concern for achievement normally associated with a later age. He was quite upset about Ross's slowness in learning to talk and raised questions about mental retardation. In some ways he attempted to provide satisfaction for the child — by the purchase of a puppy, or in gradually helping Ross to overcome his fear of water. His expectations, however, were of conformity to standards that represented his adult satisfactions rather than those of the child.

Although he gave observers the impression of being indifferent to the child, he did show some interest in Ross. During the period when Mrs. Fallon was having her worst struggles with Ross over going to sleep, Mr. Fallon could accomplish this. When his wife was ill, Mr. Fallon fed and took care of the child quite successfully. Ross's affection for his father was apparent. The observation was made, during the second year, that Ross received more warmth from his father than from his mother, and that Mr. Fallon's demands for conformity were not so consistent as his wife's.

C. SOCIO-CULTURAL INFLUENCES

1. Socio-economic Status and Values. The Fallons could be characterized as having equivocal mobility aspirations. The desire for achievement was never intensely dominant, but there was a certain amount of concentration on job improvement, higher earnings, and security values. The socio-economic aspirations of both the Fallons were ambiguous and contradictory. Mr. Fallon liked to give the impression of being a "high-earner," but he was quite fearful of attempting new jobs or testing his mettle on a higher rung. Hilda Fallon's contradictory and ambivalent social strivings fitted in with her personality difficulties. On the one hand, she denied ambitions for social achievement, but on the other, entertained hopes that her social position might be raised.

She was instrumental in "working on" her husband to take tests and seek employment which would bring more security and benefits to them. She felt she had a right to dream of owning her own home and that it would some day be possible. But her emphasis was more upon higher pay for her husband than upon white-collar or higher-prestige work. To her, a rise in social position was associated with income and the things that money could buy.

Money played a serious role for Mrs. Fallon. As part of her personality difficulties, she could neither accept nor condone her husband's carelessness with money and countered it with a structured handling of their funds which helped her feel more secure. She wanted to appear generous and comfortable in their financial status but tended to act frugally and conservatively. Consequently she felt imposed upon and sensitive that she might be considered "cheap" or "stingy." In attempting to overcome her feelings of inadequacy and self-depreciation, earning money became an important way in which Mrs. Fallon could psychologically accept herself as a worthwhile and contributing person. The fact that she could get a job when necessary often cropped up in her mind as a solution to other difficulties.

The Fallons seemed able to buy what they needed, and Mr. Fallon did take an additional job to earn more money when he felt it necessary. Mrs. Fallon conserved their resources but felt little rewarded at the outcome of her efforts. The economy of using "hand-me-downs" for the baby resulted in jealousy of her sister-in-law for using all new things.

Socially Mrs. Fallon felt somewhat isolated but was not impelled to overcome it by learning to drive. She relished having friends and relied on them a great deal for the exchange of conversation, ideas, advice, and commiseration. She appeared sensitive to her husband's crude behavior, which was socially embarrassing and humiliating to her.

The Fallons had a common religious affiliation, although Mrs. Fallon was more of a church-goer than her husband. Both believed that religious education was important for children. On the whole, there were no basic differences in values or cultural beliefs between them, although there were, indeed, differences in implementation.

2. *Extended Family.* The Fallons established their own home a year before Ross was born, having lived with the maternal grandparents immediately after marriage. Mrs. Fallon felt a strong obligation to her mother but had found it hard to live with her. The relationship with her mother improved somewhat after the death of her father. Although her mother provided some help after Ross's birth, Mrs. Fallon was critical of the kind of help she had received and deprecated its usefulness. Also, she was criticized by her mother for her handling of Ross and deeply resented it.

There were times when the paternal grandmother gave Mrs. Fallon more satisfaction than her own mother, and she felt that her mother-in-law liked her better than did her own mother. But when the paternal grandmother found Ross "impossible" to manage and commented about his developmental lag, it became a source of anxiety and tension for Mrs. Fallon. Thus there was conflict with both sides of the family, which became accentuated when Ross served as the focus for criticism.

Mr. Fallon was ambivalent toward his own and his wife's families. Neither of the Fallons received the unilateral approval or support from their families which their personalities craved.

3. *Spatial Arrangements and Values.* Mrs. Fallon gave much consideration to the details of arrangements and plans for the baby, but it was in terms of her own desires rather than the baby's comfort. An original plan to convert the dining area to a nursery was abandoned, and the baby was placed in a small area adjacent to the Fallons' bedroom because it was more convenient for her. In her second pregnancy Mrs. Fallon again planned specific changes.

She was diligent to keep the apartment free of the clutter of an infant's paraphernalia which was annoying to her husband, and observers found the home clean to "the point of barrenness." Mrs. Fallon did not object to Ross playing with pots and pans or using household objects, and she was even more lenient in the later period. Mr. Fallon was less tolerant of any "messiness," and his wife was quite careful to keep things "picked up."

Her sense of values was weighted more towards doing the right things "practically and sensibly" than from providing the child with comforts for the sheer joy of it. Thus there were few, if any, toys in the Fallon home because Ross wasn't "very interested" in them. And the child, who tended to be inert, withdrawn, and unresponsive, was subjected to fewer social stimuli than most infants.

D. FAMILY RELATIONSHIPS

1. Marital. Mrs. Fallon thought she would never obtain a husband, home, and children because she felt no one would ever marry her. As much as she could recall, her life was characterized by pronounced mood swings ranging from depression and self-derogation to moderate feelings of pleasure. The one bright spark in her life prior to marriage was a sense of achievement in work. Her ability to earn money gave her some sense of personal worth, and she had resigned herself to this satisfaction before she met Charlie Fallon.

The marriage was characterized by volatility and wide mood swings which presented an ever-changing emotional environment. Mr. Fallon was not an adequate antidote for his wife's insecurity. At times he seemed to be concerned about her and sympathetic; at these times she felt some moderate satisfaction and pleasure. At other times he joked with her in a thinly veiled sarcastic way. He was frequently impatient, and his pointed barbs increased his wife's feelings of inadequacy and self-derogation.

Mr. Fallon's early life was characterized by economic insecurity and much emotional deprivation. We have seen that his prolonged separation from his family in childhood affected him. His struggle to find his place in the family took the form of demanding attention and a need to be considered the "favorite child." His lifelong quest for security was not wholly successful, and the remnants of childhood feelings of failure were seen in his later feeling of inferiority and the tendency toward hypochrondriasis. These feelings of inferiority lay behind the arbitrariness and crudeness which at times characterized his behavior toward his wife.

He assumed the dominant position of the two and made the major decisions, freely criticizing his wife, often on her most sensitive points. The only predictable features of their relationship were the ever-changing emotional upheavals and the relative calms.

2. Mother-Child. Mrs. Fallon did not find emotional or psychological satisfaction in her relationship with the child. Her self-devaluation, depressive tendencies, and volatile emotional states made it difficult for her to assume a positive and protective mothering role. It has been indicated, too, that the passivity and slowness of the child's development reinforced his mother's isolation from him. Not only was there absence of pleasurable interplay between them but it was often difficult for Mrs. Fallon even to fulfill the minimum demands of the helpless and unresponsive infant.

This almost wholly negative relationship was modified when two changes occurred: Ross began to catch up developmentally by his eighteenth month, so that more meaningful verbal communication was possible between mother and son, and Mrs. Fallon became pregnant again. However, we do not know what the latter change actually meant to her in terms of increased satisfactions. In some respects Ross did not develop according to the growth norms appropriate to his age, and the observers were concerned that his basic physical or emotional needs would not be met. Yet by the time he was two there was an apparent restoration to minimally adequate functioning.

3. Father-Child. The relationship between Mr. Fallon and Ross was marked by the same derisive devaluation that Mr. Fallon directed towards his wife. It was also marked by adult-oriented values and a wish not to be disturbed by the child. With all his criticism of Ross, Mr. Fallon did assume some responsibility for the child's needs, and was better able to meet these needs than his wife. At times he was even prompted to give some extra satisfaction to the child.

E. PERSONALITY CHARACTERISTICS

1. Handling of Anxiety and Hostility. Mrs. Fallon's considerable anxiety presented a picture of extreme emotional lability. Her self-devaluing tendencies made her feel unfeminine, and she expected a lack of interest from all who met her. Her courtship with Charlie Fallon was an "up and down" kind of dating pattern. In her marriage she achieved things she thought she would never have. But still her doubts and fears were unallayed. The premonition that "something might happen" always remained to haunt her.

Her feelings of anger were associated with her severe mood swings. When she felt euphoric, she denied the existence of anxiety with light bantering and a smiling demeanor. During the depressed phase of the cycle she verbalized the welling-up anxiety by complaints over relatively minor issues. However, even these complaints were accompanied by ambivalence because she felt she had less to complain about than did others. The lability of emotion and the alternation of modes of handling her feelings provided an unstable atmosphere in which to rear a child. This instability resulted in an inadequate meeting of the child's needs and a lack of gratification for Mrs. Fallon in her relationship with Ross as well as in her adult relationships. Ross clearly became one of many sources of dissatisfaction to his mother.

2. Dependency and the Sense of Security. Mrs. Fallon's difficulty in assuming maternal responsibility was a reflection of her general difficulty in establishing an adequate balance between giving and receiving support. Ambivalently, she had a need to be with other people and to be reassured by them, and at the same time, she resented it when they told her what to do. Mr. Fallon was a rather nervous, hypochondriacal husband, who compensated for his inferiority feelings by trying to be the center of attention and speaking to his wife with barbed sarcasm. Mrs. Fallon did not want to be so dependent upon her husband, and yet she was unable to find dependent satisfactions with other relatives or with friends.

The incompleteness of the resolution of this conflict was accentuated by other personality difficulties. Her methods of dealing with her dependency needs, as well as with anxiety and tension, intruded upon family functioning and integration.

3. Feelings of Adequacy or Inadequacy. Mrs. Fallon feared inadequacy, and characterized herself as "nervous and worrying."

She tended to devalue her own role as a person and as a mother. Without doubt, past experiences associated with her harelip had influenced her present feelings. New experiences, such as pregnancy and care of the firstborn, were difficult for her. Any new social demand brought much indecision and uncertainty. Always her reports of behavior with the child were given in an apologetic tone. One of her strongest needs was to have everyone like and approve of her. She could not bear to have anyone even potentially harbor critical feelings toward her.

4. Planning and Impulsiveness. Mrs. Fallon characterized herself as a poor housekeeper with a minimum of planning. Yet her meticulously ordered house was extraordinarily clean whenever the staff visited, which was fairly frequently. However, her effective housekeeping ability did not provide gratification. Planning assumed the dimensions of a problem in Mrs. Fallon's mind, and she thought of herself as impulsive in many ways; yet her housekeeping activities and practical planning belied this view. The problem, then, was one of how she regarded herself, rather than one of actual behavior. Like the other personality characteristics that we have discussed, Mrs. Fallon's concept of herself is important in understanding her general way of dealing with anxiety and her inability to find satisfaction in the mother role.

5. Self-Assertion. This was a problem to Mrs. Fallon. She was unable to ask others directly to do things for her and yet was hurt and resentful when they failed her. She expected her husband to offer help in a number of ways but did not make specific requests of him. She had always thought that it would be an imposition to ask for help. When combined with inadequacy feelings and stress in the marital relationship, this lack of self-assertiveness contributed toward a segmental family organization.

6. Recapitulation of Past Experiences. There was no evidence about the prominence of past experiences as it related to child care routines. But we do know that Mrs. Fallon often made reference to her unhappy childhood, the effects of her harelip, her morose, withdrawn father, and her dominating and suspicious mother. Her own attitude and behavior with Ross had elements of these same characteristics. As for Mr. Fallon, we know that his expressed wish was for the baby to be different from himself, which may be related to his own past experiences.

F. EMERGENCE OF FAMILY INTEGRATION PATTERN

1. Family Structure. The personality difficulties of both the mother and father were sufficient to cast doubt on the possibility of their establishing a strong unitary family organization. The slow development of their child contributed further to the unlikelihood of such organization. Not only was there no firm triadic structure; there were relatively weak diadic relationships between the child and either parent.

Throughout the two year period the Fallons gave the impression of unitary organization only on such occasions as mealtimes and family outings. In contrast to this superficial behavior, however, was underlying emotional turmoil and anxiety in the relationships of the parents with each other and with Ross. We have seen that the marital relationship was characterized by volatility, unpredictability, and ever-changing moods.

For this family, unitary organization was achieved only in terms of physical arrangements. There was little emotional and psychological togetherness. The family was, therefore, characterized as segmental and parent-centered.

2. Division of Labor and Balance of Power. Mrs. Fallon assumed responsibility for management of the child and the home. Mr. Fallon served as caustic critic and commentator when he was dissatisfied with his wife's management. He assumed the role of provider, but allowed his wife to share some of the thinking and decisions in regard to his job and earnings. He also allowed her to manage the household finances. Mr. Fallon was the dominant member of the household because his wife's own sense of inadequacy and self-doubt served to immobilize her. Because the personality characteristics of each could not provide a supportive relationship to the other, there was little emotional sharing.

3. Development, Achievement, and Social Behavior of Child. This was a problem area for both Ross and his parents. Both Mr. and Mrs. Fallon had high growth and achievement expectations, which were more reasonably to be expected from an older child. In the face of this, they were confronted by a child whose development, achievement, and social behavior were slow and even below par in a number of respects. Nor were the parents geared or motivated to provide the kind of stimulus or environment conducive to maximum developmental potential. There was real concern at times about the possibility that Ross was mentally retarded because of his delayed speech. In any event, the child's development, achievement, and social behavior did not prove satisfactory to his parents.

4. Prospect of Siblings. Mr. Fallon laughed at and ridiculed his wife's wish for a second child, but when Ross was eighteen months old, a second pregnancy did indeed occur. Ross's uncontrollability at this time served to accentuate the physical discomforts of the second pregnancy, Mrs. Fallon's fears and anxieties returned, and Mr. Fallon was once again impatient with his wife's complaints.

5. Status of Family in Community. Neither the maternal nor the paternal grandparents provided a comfortable nexus to the community. Mrs. Fallon's father was a source of shame, humiliation, and even guilt to her, and Mr. Fallon's relationship with his own family was tenuous from childhood. While there was visiting with both families, and with siblings and their families, there were also considerable criticisms and differences from time to time.

There was no indication that the Fallons engaged in community activity, and their social life revolved mainly about a coterie of couples and friends from Mrs. Fallon's girlhood, with whom she found pleasant social relations. Mr. Fallon preferred his evenings at home to social or community activity, but his wife chafed somewhat at her relative isolation.

6. Types of Parent-Child Adaptation. The Fallons were clearly parent-centered and non-permissive in their orientation. Although there was some shift in the second year towards greater permissiveness, it was not sufficient to characterize them as other than non-permissive in orientation toward the child. The family relationships did not provide mutually satisfying qualities to engender a "togetherness." The Fallon family emerged as a segmental, parent-centered, non-permissive family organization.

POSTSCRIPT

Contact with the Fallon family was maintained for approximately ten more months. The ambiguities in Mrs. Fallon's personality continued to impair the maternal role and to perpetuate the difficulties in the mother-child relationship. In her second pregnancy Mrs. Fallon suffered physical and emotional ups-and-downs similar to those in her first pregnancy. Matters were further complicated by her need to care for Ross, whose demands for attention she found particularly intolerable. As her iritation increased, Ross's behavior deteriorated.

Somewhat prematurely Mrs. Fallon gave birth to the female infant for whom she had fervently hoped. This gave her much satisfaction and a sense of achievement. Immediately her attitude to the new baby was impressively different from what it had been with Ross. She reacted positively and favorably to everything about the baby. Despite the fact that the infant showed signs of prematurity and lacked vigor, Mrs. Fallon found her perfect. Regretfully she admitted that she had never accepted the idea of a male child and it had influenced her attitude toward Ross.

Although Mrs. Fallon was aware that she had failed Ross in terms of warmth and attention, her interaction with him remained disapproving. On the one hand, she felt unsuccessful in her efforts to train him properly, and on the other, she felt guilt and responsibility for "the kind of child he is." In despair she wondered whether she had irreparably "ruined his life."

In point of fact, Ross was not an easy child to manage and did have problems of realistic concern. The pediatrician characterized him as a child whose development was deviant from the beginning through a combination of equipment factors and the very unfavorable home situation. Often he was whiney, negative, and excitable to the point where he was out of control. At times he was seen to hit himself or flail out at others. He had a number of ritualistic and compulsive patterns. His unhappiness was apparent in moods of vacancy or purposeless activity.

In spite of Mrs. Fallon's considerable satisfaction with her daughter, Karen, which enabled her to be more giving, the basic maternal patterns were not substantially altered. Routines with Karen began to take on the same overtones as with Ross. Although Mrs. Fallon was worried about the flattened right occiput of the baby's head, she seemed unable to follow advice about changing the infant's position. As ever, she was unperceptive to the baby's clues and clung to regimes which hardly satisfied the baby. At the same time she worried about inadequate milk consumption, feeding, and other problems. Then she blamed Ross because his demands took time away from the care she preferred to give to Karen.

In the well-baby clinics Karen was seen as a nice-looking baby who lacked activity and gave evidence of depression and insufficient stimulation. As with Ross, Mrs. Fallon found it preferable for Karen to sleep as much as possible and be "out of the way." Karen was somewhat slow in motor action and by ten months of age still did not crawl although she made rolling movements.

Notwithstanding his obvious displacement, Ross took the new baby rather better than one would expect. At the beginning he was eager to help and proud to display his sister. Actually his development was seen to accelerate with the advent of Karen. Occasionally Mrs. Fallon complained that he was "jealous." Once she gave him the "spanking of his life" because she saw him poke a finger at Karen's eye. The favored status of Karen was not lost upon Ross. While his mother fondly ministered to the baby, Ross dejectedly removed himself from witnessing it.

He had numerous episodes of respiratory infections, complicated by asthmatic wheezing. Both parents were exceedingly distressed and anxious over this condition. Mr. Fallon was particularly unreconciled that "an innocent child should suffer such an illness." He insisted that no stone be left unturned to overcome the disorder.

Riddled with guilt that she had been unable to give more to Ross, Mrs. Fallon castigated herself as a "bad mother" who was unable to do right by either child. Determinedly she made efforts to be patient and indulgent with Ross, only to suddenly erupt in anger as her tolerance reached the breaking point. Then Ross was spanked, scolded, berated, and threatened. Quite as suddenly thereafter he was comforted, cajoled, and accommodated. The same inconsistency prevailed in toilet training and by the end of this period it had not yet been achieved.

In nursery school Ross did quite well, seeming to enjoy play with other children and the activities offered. He was considered quite adept in manipulative skill and use of body. Although sometimes negative, on the whole he adjusted well. His speech became more distinct and he began to speak in sentences. It was characteristic of Ross that he responded better and more reasonably to any one other than his mother. As Ross matured, his father seemed to enjoy and appreciate him more readily. In fact, Mr. Fallon was reported to consider both his children "wonderful."

With the passing of time Ross's ritualistic patterns disappeared, and he appeared more purposeful and better organized. In searching self-appraisal, Mrs. Fallon wistfully commented that the traits she most deplored in Ross were the very ones that she herself had. In the resolution of accepting and liking herself, Hilda Fallon may perhaps find the prerequisite to enjoy and cherish Ross. It may well prove to be the crux of Ross's potential to provide satisfaction as a likable and attractive child.

The Bjornson Family

TOWARD THE AMERICAN DREAM

For Edna and Carl Bjornson the American dream of a fine home, a secure professional position, and acceptance in the social circles of their suburban community was well on the way toward fulfillment. But there is always a price for the substance of dreams, and for Edna Bjornson, at least, the toll was high.

If ever the integration of a firstborn child into a family had a difficult beginning, it would seem that it was so in the case of the Bjornsons. Perhaps it started in the joyless recollections of Edna's own childhood, which she was loathe to dwell upon, and the resolute determination that for her own child it had to be different.

Edna was an only child of hard-working Danish parents, whose years in America did not erase memories of the old world. Carl, too, was an only child, with identical origins. In fact, Carl and Edna had met each other at a gathering of their parents' Danish friends.

Although Mr. and Mrs. Bjornson had successfully risen in American society, the clash of American ways with ancestral values was omnipresent. Thus, Edna felt that it was very important to do things correctly and to have continuing advice lest she fail. And even as she attained her aspirations, she still felt a lack of fulfillment, both past and present. "I can't understand why it is that when I get something I've wanted, I'm never satisfied with it."

Edna could never speak ill of her parents, but she often mentioned the restricted atmosphere of her youth. She had no playmates, and her mother tied her down to the house. Both parents worked, and she was cared for by a grandmother who enforced strict discipline. Above all, the economic hardships at home fostered an intense desire for the better things of life.

Edna's feelings about money were so strong that she felt it worth sacrificing other goals to gain and keep it. Although she liked school, she took a commercial course in order to earn money more quickly. Ever since, she bitterly regretted that decision and blamed her parents for not helping to plan her future. It just had to be different for her own baby — but how could one be sure?

In her quest for answers, Mrs. Bjornson was most eager to join the study. "It will be such a help. A young mother needs an authority to help her. There is so much to learn and you certainly need somebody to tell you what to do."

The blond, blue-eyed, well-dressed young woman in her fifth month of pregnancy was friendly, talkative, and smiling. She immediately revealed her difficulties. From the onset of pregnancy she was nauseated and began to vomit. By the third month it was so bad that the doctor suggested she be hospitalized. From 145 pounds at the beginning of pregnancy Mrs. Bjornson had fallen to 136 pounds. "I was first fed intravenously and then bit by bit they got me on to liquids, then purée and then soft foods. Now I'm finally eating solids." Through all this her husband "had been wonderful" and was so concerned that he insisted she go to the hospital.

Actually Mrs. Bjornson looked quite well. She said she carried "just the way our mothers on both sides carried us, all around and high up." Her husband had commented, "I can't believe you're pregnant, honey. I'll bet you're just fooling me."

It hardly seemed possible to Mrs. Bjornson that it was already four years since she had first met Carl at a party for his thirtieth birthday. Edna was twenty years old at the time. On Carl's weekend trips home they became "pretty much sold on each other." Two years later they were married. Of Carl, Edna said that he had been made to "toe the mark" even more strictly than she. He was not allowed to engage in sports and often felt "left out." Nevertheless, he was successful in college, and now in his professional life he could use his success and affluence in the cultivation of friends. He had bought a sailboat and had joined a yachting club.

They had already been married two years, and their friends thought they should have had a baby sooner, but "we thought we might resent it if it came too soon." Mrs. Bjornson hoped to have at least three children. "I think three is a good number. . . .

I would have more if I could give them an education and we had enough money. . . . The minute this baby is born we will get an insurance policy for his education." About names for the baby she said, "I like fancy names like Roxanne or Deborah, but with our last name we have to have something simple. So we'll call it after both grandfathers if it's a boy and both grandmothers if it's a girl." She had no sex preference for the baby. "We just want it to be healthy. Oh, I do hope it will be all right, because I've been so sick and can't help worrying whether I've been able to nourish the baby properly."

Mrs. Bjornson was susceptible to other worries as well, even the most unlikely ones. A family friend, an older woman of about sixty-five, had asked her to go on a shopping expedition. When she refused, the woman had said, "The baby could turn out to be a nitwit if you stay home and don't do things." Mrs. Bjornson stayed home and cried all afternoon in dread that the baby was going to be a "nitwit." She was especially concerned that her lack of appetite might make the baby small, although she drank a very special and expensive kind of milk.

The interviewer assured her that there was no relation between the mother's weight gain and the baby's size. Then Mrs. Bjornson said, "Yes, I know, but this woman told me about Pearl Buck's baby, which looked just perfect when it was born but turned out to be feeble-minded." She was also reluctant to buy things for the baby at this point because she "wouldn't want the clothes around if anything should happen."

Mrs. Bjornson found it hard to recall her first menstrual period and said she'd have to ask her mother. Her mother had never spoken to her about menstruation. "In the old country women just don't talk about this kind of thing." Actually she had learned about menstruation from girl friends and had envied her best friend, who started before she did. They bought magazines at the drugstore and talked "the way girls do when they get together." They had a lot of funny ideas, she said, and thought that "if you were kissed, you could get pregnant." When asked if she had been surprised after marriage, Mrs. Bjornson answered rather coyly, "I was and I wasn't." She didn't seem the least inclined to discuss her marital or sexual relationship.

In the seventh month she commented, "The baby is just kicking me — kicking me everywhere." She wondered how much worse it would be toward the end of pregnancy. Her mother planned to help immediately after delivery and then her mother-in-law would come to help out a little later. Mrs. Bjornson was pleased at these offers of help because "you're not as strong as you think you are in the hospital" and the responsibilities with a new baby at home would be overwhelming.

Mrs. Bjornson had not considered having diaper service because her husband had given her a washing machine. She said she had tried to do his shirts but had given up because they were too difficult to iron. However, she felt that the least she ought to do was the diapers. She reported that Mr. Bjornson was working very hard on their new home in order to get most of the carpentry done before the baby arrived, as the noise might be disturbing. As for herself, she was taking things easier than usual and felt a great deal better than before.

During this month the interviewer happened to speak to Mrs. Bjornson's obstetrician, who commented that she was having a lot of trouble and usually vomited when her husband was at home. It was the doctor's opinion that in cases of continued vomiting, "ninety percent of it is psychological."

At the interview with the pediatrician Mrs. Bjornson reiterated how wonderful it was to have such an opportunity to participate in the study and to have this kind of service. She explained that she had deliberately come to the hospital's obstetrical unit because her husband had taken a psychology course in his bachelor days and had heard much about natural childbirth. He said it was something she should try. She had also read articles about rooming-in and wanted to take advantage of the opportunity. It was the pediatrician's impression that by making sure she had the very best, Mrs. Bjornson felt assured that everything would go all right. Mrs. Bjornson thought it would be nice for the oldest child to be a boy, but "I'll be just as satisfied with a girl and I think I've convinced my husband too." With great pleasure she described how pleased the grandparents on both sides were about the coming baby.

Mrs. Bjornson had no specific child-care questions to ask of the pediatrician, only what additional books she might read. Since she had already done considerable reading about pregnancy and childbirth, the pediatrician had nothing more to suggest. As they went to the laboratory where Mrs. Bjornson was to have a blood count, she suddenly asked, "Does it hurt?" and looked obviously relieved to hear that it was just a finger prick.

In the ninth month Mrs. Bjornson looked particularly attractive and exceedingly well groomed. "Her hair was nicely fixed, and her face was clear and quite beautiful," according to the report. With termination of the nausea Mrs. Bjornson found the end of pregnancy very enjoyable. Her appetite was still not entirely back but her diet became "more sensible." She ate fruits and vegetables almost exclusively, complaining that "spending so much money for them is knocking my budget all out, but it's worth it." In the Bjornson home Mr. Bjornson turned over his check to his wife to manage all household finances. She said that this was in the tradition of both their families, "where the father gives the mother his checks."

Mrs. Bjornson had heard from other mothers that time dragged at the end of pregnancy, but for her it had dragged only in the early months when she had been so sick. "Now the days just seem to fly away." She had also heard that if the early months were difficult, the labor would be easy. However, she continued to worry "about what has happened to the baby because of all the vomiting." Preparations for the baby were well in hand, as the Bjornsons had bought or secured from friends a crib, carriage, bassinet, and stroller.

Mrs. Bjornson was pleased that her own mother would help after the birth because she could talk more freely to her and ask questions which she wouldn't ask of her mother-in-law. Nevertheless, she enjoyed her in-laws "because they get along so well and are happy. Not all families are that happy." She commented that "the very helpful services, prenatal classes and discussions" she was getting were the kind of thing that her mother couldn't possibly have gotten. She often compared her own status with that of her mother, pointing out that her parents came from rather simple circumstances in Denmark, while she was a first-generation American, with all its implicit advantages. She hoped to give her baby a better start in life than she had been given.

At home Mr. Bjornson was busily occupied in renovating the kitchen in order to save the high cost of having it done. His wife commented that without his work they couldn't afford the house at all. She said she always praised his work and was appreciative that he could do it.

At the next visit Mrs. Bjornson asked some questions about who would provide care for the baby during illness and also about the frequency of well-baby clinic visits. She had read Dr. Senn's article on breast feeding and was disappointed that she would not be able to have him as her pediatrician. She said she felt a little silly talking so much about herself, and commented that her husband seemed to think she talked about things that weren't particularly important.

It amazed her that she was feeling so well, and she was thrilled that "it is spring and everything seems to be budding." She felt part of the whole spring scene and hoped that the baby would be born on Mother's Day, although that was unlikely. With her better health and newly found energy, Mrs. Bjornson was getting a lot of housework done and compared it with how she used to feel before her menstrual periods, when she wanted to "neaten up everything."

She reminisced about the many months of nausea and vomiting, which she said began in the very first month of pregnancy at the time her small dog got into a fight with a larger dog. Immediately afterwards, she began to "shiver and shake and vomit." She continued to vomit for the next seven months and imagined that there might be some relation between the nausea and the dog fight.

Mrs. Bjornson had become pregnant in the midst of moving to their new home, just after her mother had left to go back to Boston. She said that it would have been better "to just sit in the apartment and be pregnant" instead of going to the topsy-turvy atmosphere of a new home, where nothing was in its place and she could never find anything. Furthermore, her mother was no longer around to talk over various problems. Mrs. Bjornson commented that her husband was unsympathetic, that he wanted to do things for her but just didn't understand how bad she felt and what it meant to her.

She stated that she felt "the baby hiccups all the time," and she hoped it would not be a baby that spits up a great deal because "I've been through so much nausea." She said that their dog heaved and vomited easily, she herself vomits, and she "couldn't stand another person spitting up in the house." Mr. Bjornson was the only one in the house that seemed to have a steady stomach.

The layette for the baby was bought by her mother. Mrs. Bjornson was surprised at "the terrific expense of the clothes. Why, just a little shirt costs $1.95!" She herself had not bought any "fancy things" for the baby and expected that her friends would provide them. She asked if it would be safe to travel with the baby to Boston for the christening.

Caring for the baby was now prominent in Mrs. Bjornson's thoughts. She expected to be "scared to death by the slightest sneeze and not know what to do." She said that she was in no particular hurry to have the baby born. While she was well pleased by the prospect of a baby, she found it an agonizing experience because of her anxiety, and she searched everywhere for comfort and advice. Her obstetrician found her excessively dependent upon him, and the study staff soon found that her need for help and reassurance could scarcely be satisfied.

Interestingly, however, she raised few specific inquiries about the details of caring for the child but spoke only of general fears and questions. She raised no discussion about breast or bottle feeding other than that she had read Dr. Senn's article. Except for worrying, she seemed to rely on others, including her mother, to give the support and authoritative answers. Throughout, she dreaded the inevitable day when she would be called upon to play the role of mother.

Certain changes in her own attitude came as a surprise to her. Formerly she wouldn't have considered going to church on Easter without a completely new outfit. Now she wanted to spend the money on the baby's things instead, and said she felt "different now about the kinds of things I want from life."

Mrs. Bjornson's mother matched her daughter's capacity to worry. She wrote that she would like to have the baby for her. However, Mrs. Bjornson was relieved that she wasn't around because "she would just tell me of all the hard times she had had, and how difficult it is to have a baby." Mrs. Bjornson said, "I'm just putting those thoughts out of my mind." She was certain that she wouldn't let her mother bathe the baby because "it's been so long since she cared for a baby and besides my grandmother used to do the bathing. She had had four children and knew what to do."

Mrs. Bjornson's only pleasant memory of childhood was of walks in the forest with her father to select and cut a tree for Christmas. She had loved to be outdoors and would have enjoyed participation in sports but she was denied the opportunity. Also, she had never had the chance to know children her own age but had to "sit close" by her parents. This was somewhat relieved in the small high school, where "everyone got to know each other."

The next week Mrs. Bjornson said that her husband had been driving her to appointments because it was past her due date and they didn't want anything to happen in the bus. She reported that she had gardened the day before and done as much heavy work as she could "so that the baby might be born." She looked well and did not appear to be under strain or overly impatient. She was resentful when people asked on the phone, "Are you still home?" But, on the whole, she seemed less upset by the delay than one would suspect from knowing her.

Eleven days later Mrs. Bjornson was admitted to the hospital after the membrane had ruptured spontaneously and she had had a bloody "show." During the next thirteen and a half hours of slow labor she was given Demerol on several occasions to help her sleep. A good part of the time she was awake worrying and complained of "restlessness, insomnia, and backache." She alternated between discouragement, crying, and cheerfulness.

It was apparent that she desperately wanted to keep up a good front, not forget her manners, and maintain standards to satisfy other people. She intensely wanted to succeed in natural childbirth and asked, "If you have Demerol during labor can you still say that you had natural childbirth?" The doctor emphasized that Demerol did not alter the fact that she did most of the work herself and that the important thing was to have a satisfactory experience during labor, regardless of what it was called.

Mr. Bjornson looked somewhat haggard and unsmiling. He tried to comfort his wife by rubbing her back but she was critical of his efforts. "His fingers dig into me somehow. He doesn't know how to do it very well." Although Mrs. Bjornson tried to follow instructions to relax the perineal muscles during contractions, she seemed afraid to push down for fear that she would break or tear something. The obstetrician reassured her, but again she lapsed back to a tightening of the outlet, although continually expressing the wish to do it "right" and the hope that she "was not being a bad girl."

Several times during contractions she yelled with pain, not extremely hard but definitely. Each time she apologized for it. Whenever the doctor inserted his fingers into the vagina for examination she asked him, "What are you doing? It feels terrible and I don't like it." As little progress was being made, and Mrs. Bjornson was becoming exhausted, it was decided to do an outlet forceps delivery. A low spinal anesthetic was administered.

Mrs. Bjornson was quite aware of everything and wanted explanations about efforts to stabilize her blood pressure, which had fallen somewhat precipitously following the spinal. An infusion of glucose was started and she asked about this. She accepted all the explanations and appeared relieved that things had been taken out of her hands and that she was no longer expected to do any of the work. Through the rest of the proceedings, which lasted about an hour, she was quite cheerful.

When she was a bit drowsy from gas, someone asked what sex baby she wanted. Her immediate answer was, "Why, a girl!" It appeared to the pediatrician that Mrs. Bjornson felt obliged to prefer a boy in deference to her husband's desires, but in less inhibited moments she could acknowledge her own wish for a girl. Near the end of delivery Mrs. Bjornson was able to bear down enough on request to assist in the delivery of the baby. The doctor wisely pointed out that she "was helping, after all."

Mrs. Bjornson was enormously pleased with her baby girl, who cried vigorously upon delivery. She seemed in complete accord with the various comments that the baby was cute and attractive. As she watched its movements she said, "Isn't it wonderful — the baby starts out as such a little thing and even when it's born it can already do many things."

She checked whether the baby had all its fingers and toes, and whether it had any birthmarks. Then she profusely thanked all the doctors and staff, individually and collectively, for "having been so patient with me." "I'm sorry I made so much noise," she said. When reassured about her behavior, she added, "You're just trying to make me feel better."

The baby was well formed, with good color, and moderately active. She cried lustily but did not scream. She kept her eyes open almost constantly, and reacted to the light by squeezing her eyes down tightly. It was noted during the crying that she seemed to be a baby who used the whole face and forehead.

The psychological observer described the newborn as "fair enough, with regular features, blond hair, blue eyes, even round and rosy, but with an expression of suffering that was painful to look at." The deep frown on her forehead and the drawn down corner of her mouth was "like an antique mask personifying tragedy." The tenseness of her little hands gave the impression that she was overwhelmed by herself and by the world around her. At no point of the detailed observations did Lorna, as she came to be named, seem relaxed or at rest with herself or the world around her. Even when most of her body seemed in repose, there was still one hand or one foot which remained extremely tense. The impression of constant tenseness was shared by all observers.

For most newborns motor action usually seems to discharge tension or disturbance. It did not seem to serve this purpose for Lorna. Her movements seemed to accentuate a helplessness against outside forces. In the face of stimulation there were three distinct kinds of responses from Lorna. The most frequent was a startle, fourteen of which were observed in the course of a few minutes. They were rarely expressed in one single push, but repeated themselves as reverberations of the original stimulation.

A second type of reaction was "a quivering and trembling, more or less over her whole body," which did not result in relaxation. The third reaction was one of increased passivity, where her mouth fell open and it looked to the observers like something resembling a seizure. In any case, none of these actions served to rid Lorna of the excess tension which she seemed to have. She could be called a hypersensitive child.

This "over-sensitivity" appeared with the lightest stimulation, such as the mere touch of the crib or the cautious turning of a page. Any stimulation seemed to overwhelm her and to lead to a decidedly negative response The acoustic stimulus most often provoked the startle; disturbance of equilibrium, combined possibly with tactile stimulation and with temperature changes, resulted mostly in trembling. It was not easy to pick Lorna up skillfully. She did not cuddle at all, usually screamed, and was never comforted by being held. Every observer was afraid of changing her position because they knew that even when relatively quiet, Lorna would break into desperate sobs if lifted. For most newborns being held seems like security, but for Lorna such refuge seemed to represent the utmost threat.

Lorna found no peace in hand-to-mouth movements and sucking. Mostly there was a pushing-out movement of the tongue rather than sucking. If she did achieve hand-mouth contact, it involved rather large and complicated movements which tended to overwhelm and disorganize her so that the search for peace ended in new catastrophe.

Even food seemed to provide no comfort, particularly with the mother's clumsiness in feeding which is typical with a first child. The pediatrician also tried to give Lorna the bottle. She sucked regularly for a very short time, and then the sucking became irregular and remained so even though the bottle was removed and reinserted. Sometimes there was severe hiccoughing, which seemed to shake Lorna's whole body. Only by giving the bottle in fragmentary doses could the feeding be accomplished, and Lorna looked far from relaxed. The frown did not disappear from her forehead, the hands were tensely fisted, the legs were "knotted" into each other. Her position looked so strained that one wondered how well she could digest, and indeed vomiting after feeding did start a few weeks later. Lorna did not fall asleep during or after feeding as most infants do. Instead, she continued to mouth her own hand, which babies usually do before rather than after feeding.

Sleep also did not prove restful to Lorna. If anything, she reacted even more to outside stimulation than when awake. Like everything else, sleep seemed to overwhelm Lorna, to paralyze the few spontaneous movements of her little body, and to suddenly change the rhythm of her respiratory system without forewarning. The surprised observer stated that "she was awake a split second ago, but is now asleep."

Lorna's organism seemed entirely too vulnerable to outside stimulations, with too low a threshold for warding them off. Thus, she went from the startle, quiver, tremble reaction to the "catastrophe reaction," which resembled the "seizure" picture mentioned above. These seemed to be her "adapting" patterns, but they only appeared to emphasize the trauma.

At one time during the observations, an island of relief was noted in the misery of Lorna's earliest period. She was tense as usual, but her mouth was wide open this time and her legs extended in an energetic kick. One first heard gases, then grunts, and then saw the stool coming out from the diaper. After this she seemed to quiet and relax for more than a minute. The change was so dramatic that the observer wrote, "One could appreciate that her features were soft and round, and suddenly she had the peaceful face of a pretty little baby girl."

The psychological observer summarized that "Lorna is an overly sensitive child who cannot use adequate channels of discharge and relaxation." The observer speculated, "how can poor, timid Mrs. Bjornson intrude in Lorna's life, when Lorna can brook no intrusion?" The pediatrician viewed Lorna as a "fidgety, irritable, jerky baby, hard to hold and hard to quiet." Although there was nothing definitely pathological in her reflex picture, the pediatrician conjectured "whether the type and character of the movements is due to a general irritability of the central nervous system, possibly caused by some degree of cerebral injury, or whether this simply represents an immaturity of the central nervous system. She does not look as good at this point as I would like her to."

Two days later the pediatrician said, "She looks somewhat better but still a little knocked out." Six days after birth the pediatrician's general impression was, "An attractive, well-formed infant, active and somewhat immature in respect to the central nervous system."

In the hospital Mrs. Bjornson was somewhat uneasy and disturbed that Lorna fussed, did not nurse very well, and was not easily relieved or satisfied with feeding. But she was happy to "leave it to the doctors" and seemed to relish the security of the hospital. She expressed considerable pleasure in how the baby looked and agreed with everyone that Lorna was really very pretty.

To the social worker Mrs. Bjornson said, "I just can't take my eyes off of her." At first she commented that nursing went very well, and then she added that the baby had quite a bit of mucus and she was worried about coughing and choking. She reported that the baby had hiccoughed all through her pregnancy and that now it also hiccoughed. She had read of people hiccoughing for weeks and wondered if the baby's hiccoughs were significant or dangerous. She wondered how thoroughly she was "observed" during delivery and said she didn't feel that she had done well enough in the natural childbirth. She expressed the desire "to have two more babies very soon."

When the baby was brought for feeding she nursed for a minute or so but then went sound asleep and would not be aroused. Mrs. Bjornson handled the baby gingerly and didn't seem to know how to hold her. There was no question but that she was extremely nervous and anxious about the baby but also caught on quickly.

Before leaving the hospital she asked the pediatrician for a special instruction sheet and inquired "if it would be all right to make a formula" so she could occasionally be absent at feeding time.

She was very anxious to have everything written down in one-two-three-four order so that she could follow it to the letter. She asked about the type of sterilizer to use, about special kits for bottle, brushes, tongs, spoons, cotton-ball jars, etc. She asked about diaper washing and was surprised that a soiled diaper could first be washed and rinsed in the toilet. Wide-eyed, she said, "Oh, I hadn't thought of that." She also asked about the character of the baby's bowel movements, about "the little white lumps." The difference in appearance of breast-milk stool and cow's-milk stool was explained. She said she would "probably have a lot of other questions" about which she would call the pediatrician.

The pediatrician visited the home when the baby was a little over two weeks old. The house was still being renovated and things were considerably unsettled. Lorna was lying in her bassinet yelling at the top of her lungs. Mrs. Bjornson said that she couldn't seem to do anything to quiet her and wondered what was wrong. The pediatrician talked about the difficulties in adjusting to a new baby, and Mrs. Bjornson said, "There are so many things I don't know about her, or how to do for her, that I've just lost all confidence in myself." Advice from her mother and neighbors about the baby's care had further unnerved her. She spoke with feeling about this. "I want to raise her in the right way and I'd rather talk to you about it, and what to do for her, and not be bothered by the neighbors."

Mrs. Bjornson asked so many small questions that the pediatrician noted, "I was a little surprised that many of the questions were things that one might ordinarily consider unimportant, while areas in which she might quite legitimately have asked questions were overlooked, such as about a slight rash and about the cord, which at that point looked unsightly. It was all suggestive of a diffuse anxiety."

In an offhand manner Mrs. Bjornson brought up the question of continuing to breast feed. One of the reasons she seemed to want to continue was that she had heard that breast-fed babies were less constipated than bottle-fed babies. "I would hate for her to be constipated because I know how uncomfortable that is." The pediatrician felt that Mrs. Bjornson might be considerably preoccupied with bowel functioning in the baby.

A month later the interviewer visited and described the Bjornsons' home. It was in a comfortable middle-class neighborhood surrounded by trees, shrubs, and a beautiful garden. Both the living room and dining room were large, with wall-to-wall carpeting, fresh paint, and wallpaper. The furnishings were attractive and in good taste, with a large television set on one side of the living room. Mrs. Bjornson looked well groomed and cool despite the hot weather. She carried Lorna in her arms, and her first comment was that the baby had been awake since 8 A.M. and refused to go to sleep. This had also happened the day before. Since she was awake most of the day, it was impossible for Mrs. Bjornson to get her work done.

Mrs. Bjornson could not clearly remember exactly when feedings took place but said she fed the baby whenever she was hungry. She found that Lorna spit up more from breast feeding than from the bottle and did not seem to be contented after a feeding. She commented that Lorna lost interest in the breast and seemed to fall off to sleep and did not try to suck. When she switched to the bottle, Lorna reacted in the same manner. The interviewer successfully gave Lorna some water from a bottle and it was her impression that the baby sucked vigorously.

Mrs. Bjornson still seemed to handle the baby gingerly and with not too much confidence. Once when the baby cooed quite distinctly and the interviewer commented, her mother said, "Yes, she is saying something. I guess I don't appreciate her." When she changed the baby's diaper, she noted that the night before she had washed thirty-six diapers and she really needed four dozen.

As soon as the baby was asleep, Mrs. Bjornson took the interviewer for a tour of the house. It seemed to the interviewer that Mrs. Bjornson was more at ease showing off her house and garden than her squirming baby. From time to time she commented on the amount of money they had saved by Mr. Bjornson's doing the work. They needed to buy a great deal more furniture and had already bought some period pieces at an auction. The large and beautiful garden was surrounded by a fence so that the dog could not run away.

Mrs. Bjornson's appetite had returned while her mother and mother-in-law had done the cooking, but now that they were gone she wasn't eating as much because it was trouble to fix the food. They frequently had company and weekend guests, which was tiring, but she nevertheless enjoyed it. When asked how Mr. Bjornson reacted to the baby, she said that he gave her a bottle occasionally as he viewed television and it was rather surprising that the baby quieted down better with him than with her. Both parents had noted this.

The interviewer noticed that the baby startled frequently in her sleep. The startles were even more frequent when she was awake and fussy. There were also rasping noises in her sleep, which Mrs. Bjornson defined as a "light snoring." She reported that the baby still hiccoughs too. The overall impression was that Mrs. Bjornson handled the baby "with little softness and ease" and that her behavior was "anxious and brusque."

At the first well-baby clinic at six weeks, Mrs. Bjornson discussed the question of breast feeding at some length. Since the baby spit up so much, she wondered whether to continue. She herself was more tense since both grandmothers had gone and she had to do her own work. With relief she accepted the pediatrician's recommendation to terminate breast feeding.

Both Mr. and Mrs. Bjornson were somewhat concerned about the raspy, crowing sound that Lorna continued to make but did not seem concerned that she was quite trembly and jittery. Mrs. Bjornson asked why Lorna's head was flat on the right side. In the bassinet the baby's head was constantly turned to the right because the paternal grandmother thought there was less chance of suffocation. Mr. Bjornson was also present at this examination but said very little. At one time he corrected his wife on a point of information and later asked a question about the research project. He watched the examination carefully, with a sober and unsmiling expression.

Lorna weighed nine pounds, four ounces and was twenty-two inches in length. She looked a bit scrawny but was not an unattractive baby. Because of her jitteriness and the tendency to startle, she was more difficult to hold than some babies. Although the pediatrician found no definite clinical signs to account for the trembling or startling, she placed her on calcium to see if it would have a general toning-down effect on the central nervous system. It was apparent that Mrs. Bjornson was still fairly inept in handling the baby. In turn, this was not the easiest baby to handle. The introduction of solids was recommended, which seemed to please Mrs. Bjornson.

About six weeks later Carl Bjornson was taken to the hospital for an appendectomy. There was no difficulty in the surgery and he was reported to be doing well. While he was in the hospital, Lorna was examined at the age of three months. Her weight was now eleven pounds, eight ounces, and she was twenty-five inches long. Fruit and cereal were part of her diet. She was happy with the fruit but did not seem to like the cereal and cried a lot while eating it. But Mrs. Bjornson said, "We get it down." Lorna slept from about 10 P.M. until 8 A.M., when she took her first bottle of the day. One good bowel movement daily was reported, sometimes more.

Mrs. Bjornson was still disconcerted that Lorna spit up a mouthful or two of formula several times a day, that the laryngeal stridor had not disappeared, and that the flattened head area was still noticeable. The pediatrician had the impression that "Lorna was far from being Mrs. Bjornson's idea of a satisfactory baby." She remained tremendously concerned about her role as a mother and needed to be told repeatedly that the baby was all right and doing well.

Lorna herself appeared to be a rather colorless infant, and one might wonder about her development. But after watching, handling, and stimulating her for several minutes, one realized that she actually did very well. At the age of 3 months and 2 days her general maturity level on the Gesell was close to 16 weeks, and on the Viennese test she did some items at the 4-month level. She showed interest in the materials first with her eyes and later reached out for the rattle on the dangling ring when it was placed near her. In general, she was somewhat less hypertonic than before. She vocalized and smiled in a rather quiet way when the examiner talked to her, and vocalized at her own mirror image. She had sufficiently good body control in prone to raise her head up high, with the chest off the platform, and in this position followed a toy from side to side with her eyes. According to the pediatrician, "One might say she is better than she looks, although she lacks the drive and sparkle which would make her a more interesting infant."

The uncertainty of this mother and the almost paralytic lack of confidence in herself "to do the right thing" led the staff to consider offering psychiatric help. With this in mind, the interviewer paid a home visit when Lorna was three and one-half months. As usual, the house was extremely neat and attractive, and the kitchen remodeling had been completed.

The baby was asleep, for which Mrs. Bjornson was grateful because it was most difficult to get Lorna to sleep. In the evening the only thing that helped was to hold Lorna and sing to her. It surprised Mrs. Bjornson that the baby "likes my voice." Each feeding took about an hour, what with burping Lorna three times for each ounce — and then she still vomited. Mrs. Bjornson wondered whether her feeling about the vomiting might be communicating itself to the baby.

At this point, Mrs. Bjornson said, "The first three months with Lorna were the worst three months in my life." She didn't know how she "ever lived through it." The most upsetting thing was Lorna's crying. She just didn't know what to do to make her comfortable. The crying upset Mrs. Bjornson so much that she herself would stand by the crib and cry for long periods of time. Wistfully she said, "I read everything, went to all the classes, and nothing I learned or heard about helped me care for Lorna."

Again Mrs. Bjornson asked whether she would be told if she were "doing something wrong." The interviewer asked what kind of things she thought she might be doing wrong. For one, Mrs. Bjornson felt she fussed too much over Lorna. Whenever she heard her crying, she dropped whatever she was doing. For another, she believed she expected too much from Lorna and tried to push her too fast. For example, she had tried to teach her how to grasp a toy when she lay on her back. She despised herself that in giving Lorna vegetables, "I was so stupid I gave them cold and hadn't even thought of heating them until the pediatrician suggested it."

Mrs. Bjornson commented, "I've lost all my self-confidence, am depressed, and just have no faith in any of my own decisions."

Then she said that "the outside things don't matter so much as what's inside." She wondered if she would be "told the truth" about the baby's development. The interviewer suggested that possibly Pearl Buck's article on her retarded child must have frightened Mrs. Bjornson considerably. Mrs. Bjornson agreed that it certainly had and that she didn't think such an article should have been published. She asked if the staff could tell "whether the baby was really normal."

The baby awoke and started to fret. Mrs. Bjornson went to prepare a bottle and applesauce. The interviewer failed to elicit any smile from Lorna and "had the feeling of weakness, smallness, and lack of responsiveness." As the interviewer prepared to leave, Mrs. Bjornson said she hoped Lorna would learn to go to sleep at night, because it angered her husband that most of their evening was taken up rocking the baby to sleep. Her final comment was, "It's the unknown about Lorna that is so disturbing. Carl and I have to work everything out on paper before we do anything, but here such an approach just doesn't work."

At the well-baby clinic in the fourth month the pediatrician had the opportunity for a meaningful talk with Mrs. Bjornson. It came about when the pediatrician said that Lorna's spitting up and marked sensitivity did not interfere with her development. Mrs. Bjornson wept quietly and berated herself for not being satisfied with anything, for expecting too much of the baby, of her husband, and of herself. The pediatrician suggested that there were people, apart from the study, who could help her handle these feelings, and Mrs. Bjornson asked if this meant she should see a psychiatrist.

The pediatrician replied that it was only in terms of alleviating her own feelings that she might do so, not because there was any question about her failing as a mother. The doctor further added that she was satisfied with the baby's development, and that this was a normal baby who was hard to manage. Mrs. Bjornson then asked what it was like to go to a psychiatrist and, "would he tell me what to do?" The pediatrician explained the role of such a person. There was little doubt that Mrs. Bjornson well understood her need for help and for change within herself.

In this examination the pediatrician found Lorna "much more attractive than before. . . . She had filled out considerably, had a very beautiful fair skin and a sort of peaches-and-cream complexion." It was "quite easy and natural to make comments about Lorna's attractiveness and the way in which she has developed." Although Lorna burst into sudden vigorous crying several times, the pediatrician found her somewhat less sober and high-strung than before. The flattening of the head was also much less marked.

The comments of the psychological observer, however, were not nearly so optimistic. In her view, Lorna's psychological "misery was so strong that it colored her physical impression." The positive evidence for "misery" was seen in frequent whimpers, whines, and desperate crying. The picture of discomfort was aggravated by hiccoughs. There was "nothing joyous about Lorna's movements" and rarely, if ever, did she smile.

The hands were tightly clutched or stiffly extended most of the time. She did not look directly at the examiner or at her mother but concentrated on viewing the periphery of things as if intense stimulation were intolerable for her. The mere touch of the pediatrician caused the baby's body to tense; she cried hard and held her breath, and the skin reddened over the entire body. To the psychological observer this reaction indicated protest against the intrusion of another human being. This impression was heightened by the stiff and uncuddly way that Lorna sat in her mother's lap, with her back held completely erect, arms extended, legs spread, and even her feet turned out. It made cuddling difficult or impossible, and effectively removed tactile contact between her mother and herself.

A month later at the well-baby visit the pediatrician felt that Lorna was beginning to show some stranger apprehension. This was corroborated by her mother. Lorna tended to stiffen and withdraw from an unfamiliar face. The pediatrician found that Lorna again gave "a performance far beyond what one might expect in looking at her." In supine she was rather passive, but in prone she became an extremely different baby, immediately more active. She pushed herself on all fours and moved from one end of the crib to the other after a toy. She was interested in, and exploited, the test materials, while maintaining her interest in the examiner.

At 22 weeks Lorna's general maturity level on the Gesell test, except for maintenance of posture in the sitting position, was roughly at the 26-week level, a full four weeks in advance. She went persistently for toys out of reach and patted, smiled, and vocalized at her mirror image.

While Mrs. Bjornson fed Lorna, the pediatrician had a chance to observe her intense ritualistic way of "bubbling" the baby. Mrs. Bjornson considered "the bubble" the prime reason for all of Lorna's fretfulness, discomfort, or "uncooperative" behavior. She said that when Lorna cried in the night, it was caused by the bubble. The pediatrician asked whether she offered a bottle on those occasions, as the baby might be hungry, but Mrs. Bjornson felt sure that she was not hungry but that "it was just the bubble." Then she said, "I'd rather she be uncomfortable from hunger than from pain." It always took Mrs. Bjornson at least 35-40 minutes for feeding because she waited for precisely three bubbles after each ounce and a half. She insisted that if she gave Lorna four ounces at a time and then bubbled her, there was more spitting up. She added, "Surely something must be wrong," and "Shouldn't some X-ray pictures be taken of Lorna's stomach?"

Since there was no clinical picture for any reasonable suggestion of pathology in the gastrointestinal tract, the doctor assured Mrs. Bjornson that she had nothing to worry about on this score. A recommendation was made to try a solid-food feeding in the evening instead of just a bottle. Also a prescription for phenobarbital was provided if the baby became very fretful. The appearance of Lorna's head was now almost entirely normal. She was well nourished and large enough, even though she did not look plump in any way.

In this fifth month the interviewer paid a home visit and for the first time had "positive feelings" toward Lorna. The baby "responded with vigor, strength, and spontaneity" to play and pulled herself to standing in the crib. Anxiously Mrs. Bjornson asked whether or not she should be standing, because her mother had said that it would give the baby bow legs. For this reason Mrs. Bjornson did not encourage play in an upright position.

Lorna was fed lunch strapped to the bathinette. Mrs. Bjornson said, "You will probably tell me not to put her down on the bathinette to feed her." The interviewer assured her that if it pleased the mother and child, any way was satisfactory. Lorna had no trouble downing almost a whole jar of soup, whereupon Mrs. Bjornson wondered "whether she's getting enough." During the feeding Lorna burped once or twice quite loudly and spit up a little. Her mother said, "This spitting up is not the same as vomiting and it just seems to be a little food on top of the gas bubble." When Lorna spit up, the expression on Mrs. Bjornson's face was one of horrible disgust. In an "I told you so" tone of voice she commented that Lorna was on phenobarbital, as though things were so awful that they had to put her on dope. For the past couple of days Lorna had been on a three-meal schedule, and Mrs. Bjornson fervently hoped that it would continue because it was so much easier for her.

Mr. Bjornson had just bought an electric dryer for his wife as an anniversary and Christmas present. It was evident that his wife derived much pleasure from this gift and from the purchase of all material objects. She expressed concern about her own weight, which was the same as at the end of pregnancy, and also about her menstrual periods, which were irregular since Lorna's birth. At the interviewer's question whether she might be pregnant, she said, "I can bet my last dollar that I'm not."

Two weeks later Lorna ran a slight fever and was uncomfortable. Mrs. Bjornson called the pediatrician and followed her instructions. When the fever continued, a house call was made. The baby was found to have a red throat and a moderate nasal discharge. She was given an injection of penicillin. The pediatrician was surprised at the assurance and composure with which Mrs. Bjornson reported the events and progress of the illness, as if the tangibility of illness liberated her powers as a mother.

Mr. Bjornson arrived during the examination and watched carefully. He disappeared, however, during the injection. He was still busily occupied with much work on the house, currently remodeling the bathroom, and said that he enjoyed these pursuits. In the course of discussion he mentioned that he always had difficulty in going to sleep so the baby's restlessness didn't really bother him. The following day Mrs. Bjornson called to report that Lorna was feeling better, but had developed a rash on her face and body. It proved to be roseola infantum. After about two days the rash disappeared. In the course of this illness the pediatrician felt that Mrs.

Bjornson seemed less concerned whether Lorna was a "normal" infant and somewhat more proud of her.

Just before the Christmas holidays the Bjornsons paid "a very nice and successful visit" to their parents' homes. Lorna seemed afraid when they walked into the grandparents' home, but after a few minutes she adjusted to the strangeness. Mrs. Bjornson's father became her favorite, and Mrs. Bjornson said that "he could do more with her than anyone else."

Mrs. Bjornson came to the next well-baby clinic visit laden with Christmas gifts for staff members. She looked quite like she did in the "good" period of her pregnancy. Lorna, however, was in a poor humor throughout the test, and cried almost constantly. According to the psychological observer, "Her whole face participated in the crying, the ever visible frown deepened, the whole lower part of her face quivered, and she literally went to pieces." The crying was not related to anything specific in terms of stimulation or restriction. The fact that she was sniffly and incubating a cold may have been a contributing factor.

The mother's touch, voice, and comforting seemed to have little influence. When in distress Lorna did not even look at her mother. The calming value of a toy was more effective than that of any social stimulation. Only at one point did Lorna grasp her mother, but even that did not change her emotional discharge. On the contrary, Lorna cried even more intensely in her mother's lap than in the crib.

Mrs. Bjornson did not comfort Lorna in a physically close way. She stood stiffly in front of the crib and verbally tried to interest the baby in objects. When this was unsuccessful, she gave the child a toy and withdrew from the picture. Lorna fleetingly smiled on a couple of occasions, but it did not alter the sad, serious quality of her expression. The observer found this expression a duplicate of the mother's own unsmiling countenance when handling the baby.

Once more the psychological observer commented that the merest physical touch by another human, even that of the hand in passing a toy, produced crying "as if she were hurt." It resembled that of an immature newborn for whom stimulation is so badly tolerated that the reaction takes on the character of shock-producing pain. A head-shaking "no" gesture was also observed in Lorna, possibly in imitation of her mother. In manipulation of objects Lorna seemed to be right-handed. But if she intended to mouth the object, the left hand was used. Lorna more often grasped the softer-noise rattle than the louder sounding one and also showed a preference for small objects over larger ones.

Her test results not only showed a generally advanced behavior but also an amazing lack of scatter. It finally and definitely precluded any assumption of pathology. On the other hand, the lack of emotional relating, resistance to handling, and exaggerated sensitivity suggested some deviate behavior development, partially of environmental and partially of constitutional etiology. There was no basis to decide which of the data had the greater predictive value.

The pediatrician's estimate was that "Lorna gives a performance which is quite good. . . . Once she gets into the situation and begins to exploit the materials, her good development becomes apparent." At 6 months and 29 days she scored solidly on the Gesell tests at the 36-week level, 6 weeks in advance of her chronological age, while body and social levels were at 8 months and 10 days. The pediatrician felt also that there had been a modification in Mrs. Bjornson's attitudes toward Lorna in that she found her a great deal more acceptable than before. Her conclusion was, "I am not prepared to say what has happened over this period, but there is no doubt in my mind that Mrs. Bjornson's feeling about Lorna as a satisfactory infant is quite different than it was during the first few months."

A few days later in a home visit the interviewer commented, "Both Mrs. Bjornson and Lorna looked better than I have ever seen them before." Mrs. Bjornson had a "surprise" for the interviewer, namely Lorna's two front teeth, which had come in a little before Christmas. They had caused her some fretfulness and difficulty. The sleeping problem had worked itself out nicely, which amazed Mrs. Bjornson. Furthermore, Lorna no longer needed to be held and rocked to get her to sleep. When the phenobarbital prescription ran out, Mrs. Bjornson stopped giving it to Lorna. The baby was eating much better, although she continued to dislike cereal.

The interviewer asked Mrs. Bjornson if her menstrual periods had been re-established. The reply was affirmative, and Mrs. Bjornson guessed that she had "miscounted." She didn't plan to have another baby soon but wanted to wait until Lorna was toilet-trained. "I wouldn't want to be so busy with the new baby that I really couldn't appreciate the wonderful things that Lorna would be doing." Mrs. Bjornson recalled, "How silly I was to worry during pregnancy that the baby wouldn't get enough nourishment because of the nausea." She also recounted that during labor she had been sure the baby had died but was too scared to ask the doctor.

To a question about Mr. Bjornson's response to Lorna, Mrs. Bjornson said that in the first weeks he paid little attention to her, "but now that she has really gotten to be somebody he plays with her after supper and rough-houses on the large bed." This gave his wife a chance to get the dinner dishes cleaned up.

Mrs. Bjornson proudly displayed her husband's remodeling of the breakfast nook and also the bathroom. The interviewer was impressed with how much had been done to enhance the attractiveness of the house. Mrs. Bjornson mentioned their new Pontiac and the fact that they also had a sailboat. To help clean the house Mrs. Bjornson had a colored maid in occasionally.

During the visit Lorna did not smile at the interviewer but looked at her, played with her bracelet, touched her, and seemed to listen quietly to the conversation. It was apparent that the relationship between mother and daughter had improved and that "there was real enjoyment of Lorna on her mother's part and a sense of pride in Lorna's achievements."

In the sixth well-baby clinic visit, when Lorna was thirty-five weeks old, her general appearance remained as before. Her face was quite serious, particularly with strangers, but it was not immobile. She frowned fairly often and the smiles were rather tentative and small. It was more apparent than ever that Lorna strongly objected to being touched by anyone. Mrs. Bjornson corroborated this with an account of what had happened when she left Lorna with the cleaning woman for about three hours. Everything had gone well until the woman went to pick Lorna up to do something for her. Lorna had burst into such loud and persistent yelling that she was finally comforted with great difficulty by one of the neighbors. The pediatrician was acceptable to Lorna only if she didn't touch her. Lorna herself, however, did considerable touching of both her own and her mother's body.

The sleep pattern remained good at night. Lorna went off to

sleep by playing with a diaper for a few minutes and then slept for twelve hours. She apparently used the diaper as a play object. She took three meals and four bottles daily, and ate well most of the time. Feeding did not seem to be the problem that it had been. Lorna was now interested in taking things from a small glass or cup part of the time, and the pediatrician suggested trying some fruit juice. Mrs. Bjornson had not given this before because she didn't know "whether it would be all right or not." Lorna enjoyed sitting near her parents while they ate dinner, and the pediatrician suggested that she be given a little of the table food and allowed to feed herself. This idea seemed to please Mrs. Bjornson very much, as she had not felt free to give Lorna some table foods such as mashed potatoes, vegetables, and meats. Lorna also enjoyed mouthing zweiback and seemed to get great comfort from it.

A month later at the home visit it appeared that Mrs. Bjornson's need to find answers for all possible questions was again on the upswing. She asked whether the study project was "interested in taking care of second babies" in the families, although she reiterated that she was not planning on another baby before Lorna would be two. Spontaneously she asked whether psychiatric help would help with nausea during pregnancy and specifically "whether nausea after the third month of pregnancy is psychological in origin." She said, "I don't see how I could go through another pregnancy with as much nausea as in the first. . . . If I was that sick I'd have to neglect both Carl and Lorna as much as I neglected Carl during the first pregnancy." Mrs. Bjornson had discussed with her husband the idea of seeing a psychiatrist and he had approved, but she had not yet phoned for an appointment. The interviewer thought that Mrs. Bjornson might begin therapy if she felt that the nausea symptom of pregnancy might be alleviated.

Lorna's reaction to the interviewer was one of cautious observation. Mrs. Bjornson warned that when a stranger rushed at Lorna or suddenly played with her, she was likely to cry. A few moments later, when Mrs. Bjornson left the room for some tea things, Lorna began to scream. Mrs. Bjornson hurried back, saying, "I've never seen such a child. . . . I must be with her constantly or else she screams in fright." At a recent Christmas party Lorna had tenaciously clung to her mother's lap while all the other children played together. Mrs. Bjornson wondered what she had done to cause

Lorna to be "so terribly shy." Mrs. Bjornson's mother had pointed out that this was exactly the way Edna had behaved as a baby. She "had never let her mother out of her sight until she was three or four years old." Mrs. Bjornson did not want Lorna to turn into "a mama's baby" and thought "something should be done about it." Yet the Bjornsons had not gone out for a single evening since Lorna's birth. Mrs. Bjornson said, "It must sound silly, but I hate the idea of Lorna waking up and saying 'why has my Mommy left me.' "

At the next regular visit Mrs. Bjornson was a few minutes later than usual because of difficulty in parking her car. Finally she chose a "no parking" zone rather than pay a 35-cent parking fee, although she was anxious about getting a police ticket. She said they "couldn't afford one right now" because they had just bought a new bathtub and commode.

Mrs. Bjornson brought with her a recently purchased expensive combination walker and stroller. She said that Lorna enjoyed this piece of equipment enormously and followed her around the house in it. From her seat in the stroller Lorna regarded the pediatrician soberly, with her head to one side in a rather coy and shy manner. Mrs. Bjornson reported that Lorna's fearfulness with everyone except her parents had led to considerable embarrassment during a recent trip to the grandparents' home. It was only on the third day that Lorna would agree to being held by any of the grandparents.

Mrs. Bjornson described a visiting nurses' mother's class, which she did not find pleasurable "because women just come and brag about their children." The Bjornsons were not in the habit of bragging about Lorna, she said, and then asked whether it would harm Lorna in some way if they did not brag about her. Mrs. Bjornson reported that Lorna's eating was satisfactory and that she now insisted on holding her own bottle for the first few minutes but then allowed herself to be fed. She also described Lorna as being "more cuddly" and responsive to being held than before.

Lorna regularly had one bowel movement shortly after breakfast and sometimes another in the afternoon or evening. Her mother said that she could tell by the expression on Lorna's face when she was about to have one. They had not yet gotten a toilet seat because of the many other expenses, and Mrs. Bjornson asked if it was all right to wait to train her. Lorna said several words such as "dada," "mama," and "hi," and imitated sounds, including such things as coughing. She pat-a-caked and vocalized in incipient jargon.

The pediatrician described Lorna as "a solid, well-nourished, well-developed infant whose sparse blond hair fit closely to the head like a cap and remained quite short." She looked out at the world through rather large blue eyes and the expression on her face was quizzical and investigative a good part of the time. Because of her apprehensiveness about the crib, she had to be tested on her mother's lap but nevertheless she performed in an advanced manner. When given the material and left alone with it she displayed considerable interest and drive to perform.

At the chronological age of 41 weeks Lorna's general maturity level on the Gesell test was 47 weeks, with a developmental quotient of 115. On the Viennese test her developmental quotient was 132.

At an evening home visit the following month the interviewer described Mr. Bjornson as neatly dressed, strong and healthy, but not particularly handsome. He seemed rather shy but was poised and gracious even in his reticence. Lorna closely clung to her mother as a shield against the interviewer. Mrs. Bjornson commented that "Lorna's heart was going a mile a minute" in her fright at the unfamiliar person.

The interviewer mentioned the nice beach close to the house, and Mr. Bjornson said that he never went in the water but preferred sailing a boat which he had bought some six years before. When the interviewer discussed Lorna's excellent development her father said that he didn't think it was very important for her to be intelligent — that the important thing was for her to be happy. He added that he was glad she was normal and average but didn't expect her to do anything outstanding. Mrs. Bjornson asked her husband if he thought Lorna was a happy baby, and he agreed that she was.

Mrs. Bjornson proudly reported that she had lost seven pounds and hoped to lose more. She said that she did not want to become pregnant again until she lost the weight which had accumulated after Lorna's birth. There was discussion about the considerable work yet to be done on the house and Mrs. Bjornson complained that her husband spent evenings working in the cellar. She said that he was saving $250 in plumbing by doing it himself. Mr. Bjornson asked the interviewer directly if one can pamper a baby too much. He thought it might be good once in a while to "just let her cry it out."

Lorna could almost walk alone by hanging on to low pieces of furniture. She grabbed at the newspaper on the sofa and had a fine time tearing it up. Mrs. Bjornson said that she "didn't like to see such destructive behavior." Her husband countered with the remark, "You can't make her into a lady until she is older and more intelligent, and it's silly to try." When the interviewer suggested that such rougher play might be good for Lorna to help overcome some of her timidity, Mrs. Bjornson remarked to her husband, "Dr. —says we should make Lorna destructive."

Lorna was next seen at the age of ten months and twenty days. Mrs. Bjornson had lost some weight and looked much better. Her main concern at this time was "Lorna's lack of friendliness," which she interpreted as a possible sign of social retardation. Mrs. Bjornson reported that Lorna cruised about the house from one piece of furniture to another and was eager to explore her surroundings. There was a period when she cut down on her milk consumption, which led her mother to experiment with the cup. This did not prove successful, so she resumed with the bottle. To the pediatrician it seemed a significant development that Mrs. Bjornson made an interpretation of Lorna's behavior on her own and dared to experiment a bit without being overly concerned when it failed.

Lorna's verbal development and incipient jargon was demonstrated during the visit. She also was able to understand simple directions. The characteristic soberness was still quite prominent. Most of her smiling was in response to her own image in the mirror or the pictures which she called "baby." At those times she was quite animated and less apprehensive about danger from the environment. It took several minutes before she warmed up to the test materials and the examiner. Once she did, however, her performance was excellent.

On the Gesell test at the age of 46 weeks she was in the 52-week range in all areas. She had a general maturity level of 14 months, a developmental quotient of 132. On the Viennese tests her intelligence was at 1 year, 5½ months, with a developmental quotient of 138.

The pediatrician explained the testing process at length to Mrs. Bjornson and felt that it was quite helpful to her. In the course of this, Mrs. Bjornson said, "Well, I really don't have anything to worry about, do I?" Her fear that Lorna might be retarded, of which the staff had long been aware, came out again at this time. Mrs. Bjornson went on to say that she was having more fun with Lorna now and had an increased confidence in herself as a mother. She was also glad that she no longer felt the need to check before making the least decision.

The psychological observer commented that although Lorna was "still a predominantly frowning child, it no longer had the character of sadness." As a matter of fact, Lorna did not appear sad throughout the whole observation, even when she showed signs of annoyance. There was much mouthing of her own hands as well as objects. In mouthing, her facial expression remained stern as if she were thinking about something else. The mouthing of any one object was not prolonged, and she constantly traded the object or its position in her mouth.

This exchange pattern applied also to her manipulation of playing objects. She kept each for only brief periods and then grasped for another, even those out of reach. Mrs. Bjornson remarked, "As soon as she gets something, she wants something else." It was interesting that Lorna did the identical thing with each object for a specific period of time. At the beginning she mouthed everything, then she went through a period of throwing, then of pulling, then of putting things down carefully, and finally a period of "speaking" and pointing. Throughout, Lorna's vocalizations were mainly related to the activity at hand and were rarely meaningless sounds.

When she was frustrated by the disappearance of the dangling ring behind the screen, Lorna became angry and vocalized fretfully. She could not easily grasp around the screen and also had difficulty in dealing with more than one object at a time. One had the impression that if two things were offered at once it raised a question of decision for Lorna which was not well tolerated. On the one hand, the "new" might be experienced as "danger," and on the other, the "new" might be "contaminated by the old."

Lorna still impressed the psychological observer as "a quite colorless child who is far from being brilliant but whose general developmental level is nevertheless four months above her age." This was attributed to the fact that Lorna "interrupted her monotonous periods by sudden short intervals of exceptionally advanced behavior."

A staff research meeting thoroughly discussed the etiology of Lorna Bjornson's behavior. The staff held some tenuous clinical and theoretical impressions about the possibility of either minimal cerebral damage or pre-autistic behavior. The conclusion was that Lorna's overall improvement and excellent development indicated that she was not moving in the direction of autism but that she might become an adult who uses intellectualization as a defense.

A few days after Lorna's first birthday Mrs. Bjornson reported to the pediatrician with much chagrin and shame that lesions on the baby's neck, back, and arm, which had occurred on two occasions, were flea bites. Their dog was the culprit. Needless to say, the dog was banished to the outside and a vigorous campaign was waged on dog, furniture, and house to eradicate the fleas.

Mrs. Bjornson's parents had decided to move near their daughter and had purchased a house close by. She was genuinely delighted and felt that Lorna had been a deciding factor. She thought that her parents would probably spoil Lorna but it did not seem to be of great concern.

Lorna had been walking well for the past few weeks. On occasion she fell, but picked herself up and went about her business. She could also very nicely negotiate the obstacle of a step from the kitchen to the porch. Lorna had a plethora of toys and enjoyed having new ones. The pediatrician thought that she had twice as many toys as any of the other children in the study. Mrs. Bjornson said that Lorna did not mouth as much as before and that she responded to the prohibition of "put it down." Lorna loved music and tried to whistle to the records as a way of participating.

There was no longer a question about Lorna's eating because she liked solids and her food intake was acceptable. She was allowed to finger or spoon-feed herself with bite-sized foods, but Mrs. Bjornson did not encourage this with strained foods because the mess would just be too much.

The pediatrician commented, "Lorna remains the most solemn,

sober-looking little girl I believe I have ever seen." She was husky and robust looking, with very large blue eyes, fair skin, and scanty blond hair. Lorna was especially suspicious of the pediatrician's physical examination and strenuously objected to any touching connected with it. Her crying sounded like a mixture of anxiety, fear, and anger. After the examination she continued to cast suspicious, baleful looks at the pediatrician but finally was comforted by her mother and became interested in a picture book.

The following month during the interviewer's home visit, Mrs. Bjornson's mother-in-law was present. She quietly listened to the conversation, and when she spoke it was with a distinct accent. Once in a while she made a comment which seemed to indicate that she was rather broad-minded as far as child-rearing practices were concerned. Mrs. Bjornson discussed the type of shoes which Lorna should wear, as she was concerned with "flat feet, which run in the two families."

Mrs. Bjornson said that "Lorna is a lady's girl." She was friendly and accepting of both grandmothers, but when faced with a man or woman she seemed to prefer to go to the woman. A toidy seat had been bought, but Mrs. Bjornson felt that she had no success in toilet training. She said that it was impossible to force Lorna to do anything and that toilet training would proceed only when Lorna was ready. In summary, the interviewer said, "There is a striking improvement in Mrs. Bjornson's reaction to Lorna's growth and development . . . and she is really beginning to 'understand' her baby."

Later in the month another interviewer from the study group paid her first visit to the Bjornsons' home. She was impressed with the lovely décor of the house, the spacious uncluttered arrangement of the furniture, and the attractive appearance of Mrs. Bjornson. Lorna was asleep, so there was ample time to talk. Mrs. Bjornson first asked an opinion about purchasing a series of publications by Childcraft. It was rather expensive, but she thought it might be a rich guide for her future years with Lorna. She laughed apologetically, and said, "This is my first baby and I feel as though I need a guide." She was reluctant to ask the pediatrician's opinion about the publication, as she "had called so often about so many things." The interviewer noticed a large pile of publications about infancy and childhood on a lamp table in the living room.

Mrs. Bjornson's main concern at the moment was that Lorna "shied away" from certain adults unless she herself made overtures first. There was considerable discussion around feeding. Mrs. Bjornson asked whether it was correct to allow the baby to hold the bottle in the crib because she felt that "children should be held in close contact with the mother during feeding." Also, she had read that it was not a good thing to prop the bottle during infancy. The interviewer sensed ambivalence about Lorna becoming more independent of her mother. However, Mrs. Bjornson denied that this was a consideration, as she felt that "the baby should become more self-sufficient." A further factor about the bedtime bottle was Mrs. Bjornson's fear that it would delay weaning to the cup.

Mrs. Bjornson acknowledged that she was still uneasy about Lorna despite the pediatrician's assurance that Lorna was developing well. The anxiety still remained that "Lorna might slip back," and she needed to be sure that she was "doing the right thing." To explain this feeling Mrs. Bjornson discussed her own and her husband's backgrounds. Both of them had felt extremely deprived during their childhood. In addition to considerable poverty her parents had experienced a severe language difficulty and were unfamiliar with the American way of doing things. They were always extremely thrifty people, and even in their present, more comfortable, circumstances they frowned upon any extravagance. Mrs. Bjornson herself felt guilty about financial expenditures even though she was not wasteful with money. She said that her husband had even more difficulties in this area than she did. Because of her feeling that she was "always on the outside looking in," Mrs. Bjornson wanted Lorna to have everything that she had been denied.

The interviewer was struck by Mrs. Bjornson's forthright manner and her recognition of considerable anxiety about herself as a mother and her capacity to give to Lorna. She also realized that this was somehow related to her own family experience and feelings of deprivation.

Early in the fall the interviewer noted that Lorna looked extremely pretty but was so sober and lacking in animation or responsiveness that the interviewer "did not find her attractive." Mrs. Bjornson described the summer as enjoyable although extremely busy. As soon as the study pediatrician had left on vacation Lorna became ill, with a temperature of 103. Mrs. Bjornson was referred to another pediatrician, who associated the fever with teething. Mrs. Bjornson did not like this doctor's manner, which conveyed the implication that she was an over-anxious mother. The summer had included much visiting of family and friends, which had been tiring but stimulating.

Mrs. Bjornson believed that Lorna's relationships with other people had vastly improved. She claimed that Lorna played extremely well with other children and showed very little anxiety with new people. This was hardly substantiated by her reception of the interviewer. Mrs. Bjornson had found a high-school girl to take care of Lorna in the mornings. Lorna liked her and looked forward with excitement to their walks. At those times she could separate easily from her mother, but otherwise at home Lorna could not endure separation. Once when Mrs. Bjornson placed Lorna on the porch and closed the door into the kitchen, Lorna cried and screamed so hysterically that it was extremely frightening.

Mrs. Bjornson also commented that Lorna did a good deal of climbing. She was concerned because Lorna had "no notion of the correct way to get down." If she climbed on the sofa, she would attempt to "step off into thin air as though there were no drop between her and the floor." In respect to toilet training Mrs. Bjornson denied any concern and said that the idea of using the toilet already had some meaning for Lorna. She had "tinkled" in the toilet several times and often sat on her own little seat when Mrs. Bjornson was using the toilet. Sometimes Mrs. Bjornson placed Lorna on the seat when she observed a bowel movement in progress but she did not remove the diaper for fear of interrupting the bowel movement. She felt that Lorna had a tendency to constipation and would withhold the stool if interrupted.

Mrs. Bjornson said she planned on having a second child when Lorna was three years old. In fact, she also wanted a third child, but she felt that if she spaced them at three-year intervals, she might be too old by then (thirty years) to run after a baby or sit on the floor to play with it.

Lorna still drank from the bottle, and Mrs. Bjornson said that she was "not going to worry about weaning until someone comments about the fact that at her age Lorna shouldn't be drinking a bottle." She mentioned that it was curious that Lorna drank from the bottle only when she was alone in her crib. For example, she would make no attempt to drink the bottle or settle down to sleep until the grandmother had left the room.

In her interaction with Lorna, Mrs. Bjornson seemed warm, responsive, and alert to every activity. While she talked, she pushed Lorna in the chair swing but immediately recognized when Lorna preferred to get down. Lorna spent considerable time playing in the dirt near the house, a favorite spot for her. From time to time she brought bits of dirt, leaves, or stones to both her mother and the interviewer as "gifts." It was the first direct contact with the interviewer. Mrs. Bjornson did not prohibit Lorna from playing in the dirt, although she lamented the fate of the clean yellow dress. Lorna could not be enticed to play ball with the interviewer and smiled directly at the visitor only when she was about to leave.

At the next well-baby clinic visit it was disappointing to Mrs. Bjornson that Lorna was still apprehensive of the pediatrician, because she had felt that Lorna's attitude to people had improved. Mrs. Bjornson reported that Lorna was very interested in self-feeding and spilled only a moderate amount in the process. She would permit her mother to finish the feeding if something was provided for distraction. "When I'm in a hurry I just give her a magazine and she looks at it while I stuff the food in." Mrs. Bjornson asked whether or not it was all right for Lorna to continue having the bottle, as some of her neighbors and friends had said that she should be weaned by now. When the pediatrician said that Lorna did not need to be weaned now, Mrs. Bjornson responded by saying, "She doesn't need to be grown up all the time."

Mrs. Bjornson was also struggling with conflicting advice about toilet training, whether to concentrate on it or be gradual. She had made some efforts in this direction but wondered if she had been wrong in trying to get training started. Lorna was particularly skillful in the use of language for purposes of communication. She did not use words just for the sound but definitely to communicate. She moved well but was not particularly agile or as graceful in her movements as some other young children. Her relative immobility during the entire time she was in the examining room was characteristic of her. But when she was no longer under scrutiny she moved about the room much more vigorously and freely.

At 15 months and 11 days Lorna's general maturity level on

the Gesell was 18½ months, with a developmental quotient of 122. On the Viennese test she similarly gave a very high performance, not below the 1½-year level in any area, and with a developmental quotient of 148.

Mrs. Bjornson was quite uncomfortable during the testing and very eager for Lorna to do well. She appeared as deeply involved in the testing situation as Lorna. Her facial expression was serious and tense as she watched, with a tendency to draw down the corners of her mouth or to bite on the lower lip. She showed pleasure when Lorna's performance appeared satisfactory, but her pleasure was far outweighed by her anxiety. She expressed great relief when told that Lorna was not supposed to be able to solve the formboard puzzle completely.

During the physical examination Lorna began to protest almost immediately. She cried quite loudly in what sounded like a combination of fear and anger. She did not stop crying until she was safely out of the crib and on the floor again. Although she smiled more frequently than at the time of the last visit, the pediatrician commented, "She remains the most sober little child I have yet seen."

The psychological observer stressed Lorna's "stay at a distance" behavior toward the stranger. "Her smile is still rare, her expression is reserved or serious; there is nothing inviting in the way she glances at people and at objects; her hands are frequently lifted in a stop gesture." But despite her stranger anxiety she did not attempt to get on her mother's lap. Instead, she offered her mother every new toy, looked at her repeatedly, and talked to her a great deal. One had the impression that although Lorna sought either prohibition or encouragement from the mother to classify an experience as positive or negative, she nevertheless reserved her right to doubt or challenge it.

It was obvious that Lorna knew she should not mouth the pellet, but she approached it so close to her mouth that all observers expected her to mouth it. She actually did mouth the crayon. In ball play her teasing behavior was even more evident. When asked to give the ball to her mother, she threw it to the examiner and vice versa. It seemed to surprise her pleasurably that she dared do other than told and that nothing happened. In fact, she smiled radiantly during the game and laughed aloud. The psychologist noted that "it was the first time in 15 months" that she had seen such spontaneous joy in Lorna.

The child showed a tendency to explore her environment and to be interested in any new object. She moved eagerly toward objects by bending the head and upper part of her body in their direction and even occasionally extending her arms toward them. Her excellent memory was revealed in the memory tests. When a box with a bell in it was given to her, she removed the bell, played with it, and then replaced it in the box before returning it to the examiner. Later when the same box was given to her without the bell, she looked about for it. When the examiner produced the bell Lorna placed it back in the box, but before returning the box to the examiner she removed the bell. Thus, she reproduced the experiment step by step. The filled box was returned filled, and the empty box was returned empty.

The psychologist was of the opinion that the advanced development of Lorna's memory plus poor tolerance of tactile stimulation since infancy might help to explain her exaggerated crying reaction to the medical examination. The psychologist also felt that the heightened "recall of danger" accounted for Lorna's preference for immobility despite her mastery of walking. By walking, one "gets nearer" to people or to things, bringing to mind conflict between pleasurable and unpleasurable memories. Thus, every object or person represents both a temptation and a danger, and the best thing is to curb the impulse to confront those possibilities.

The psychologist speculated that the negative prognosis of Lorna's first months was based, first, on the fact that she was a hypersensitive child who reacted negatively to most situations in which other children reacted positively; and secondly, that her mother was ambiguous in the behavioral clues she gave to Lorna and slow to understand Lorna's clues to her. The negative prognosis, however, did not materialize because Lorna was a child "who developed adaptive and compensatory mechanisms against difficulties." She adapted herself to the world "by keeping it at a distance and by prematurely developing a system of communicative signs. . . . This positive mastery of her defects was recognized sooner in the tests than in the clinical picture." Lorna was among the most advanced children in the study population.

At the next home visit the impression of the interviewer was that

Mrs. Bjornson assumed the role of "a pleasant and charming hostess who flitted from one topic to another in a desultory way." She mentioned that the high-school girl was no longer coming because it was too cold to take Lorna out for morning walks, and that Lorna was quite active around the house. She had learned to get down properly from places to which she climbed, and she entertained herself nicely with toys. In eating, Lorna was taking less fruit than before and as a result her stools were slightly harder. There was satisfaction that Lorna asked for the toidy in which to urinate, but bowel movements were still unpredictable. Lorna had also started drinking well from a special cup which Mrs. Bjornson had ordered. The removable lid had a spout, from which there was a free flow of fluid, and the entire mouth could surround the spout as with a nipple. It could, therefore, be considered a prelude to drinking directly from a cup.

Mrs. Bjornson had reached the decision not to buy the Childcraft materials until the new edition came out, which would include articles by several of the study staff members. She had recently read a popular pamphlet entitled "Mother-Child Relationship" but was disappointed because it did not really help her to understand child development. She said that she felt confused because she did not know what Lorna was expected to do at each age level. She was happy that her parents would soon be near her, and "in case of illness" they would be able to help each other. She felt in complete harmony with her mother, and they shared similar points of view.

The interviewer was struck by the frequency with which Mrs. Bjornson attempted to maintain the rather perfect prettiness of Lorna's attire. She constantly pulled down her blouse, straightened her hair, and made various adjustments. She also was quite concerned about Lorna becoming messy and tried to keep her away from the chocolate-covered doughnuts. When Lorna did eat a piece and became somewhat smeary, Mrs. Bjornson verbalized her distress and wiped Lorna's face and hands several times. She was far more concerned by messiness on the baby than about a cup of water which Lorna accidentally spilled on the rug. Warm physical contact and embraces were observed between mother and daughter, to which Lorna responded with joy and laughter, a striking contrast to her usual reserved and sober expression. There was also diminished anxiety towards the interviewer and some spontaneous contact. It was the first time that "the baby elicited any feeling of closeness or tenderness."

At the next well-baby clinic visit the pediatrician made special effort to explain fully the testing procedures to allay the apprehensions which Mrs. Bjornson had expressed to the interviewer. It was explained that part of the testing procedure was to determine the maximum response, and that there would always be items given which Lorna would be unable to do. Although Mrs. Bjornson seemed to understand, a few minutes later, when Lorna was tested, she could not resist pushing her to perform and she was unable to stop exerting pressure even when the pediatrician tried to get her to stop. Upon physical examination Lorna appeared to be a well-nourished and well-developed little girl, and her body had rounded feminine contours.

On the Gesell test at the chronological age of 16 months and 11 days Lorna had a general maturity level of 19½ months and a developmental quotient of 120. On the Viennese test she was also high, with a developmental quotient of 146.

At seventeen months Lorna had an intestinal upset, with some vomiting and diarrhea. Although the parents also had a similar intestinal disturbance Mrs. Bjornson worried that Lorna might possibly have appendicitis. Mrs. Bjornson's mother was quite helpful during the brief illness, and her proximity seemed quite reassuring to her. The interviewer described Mrs. Bjornson's mother as a pleasant-looking grey-haired woman with glasses who bore a resemblance to Edna. Her manner was relaxed and friendly although she said very little.

Mrs. Bjornson said that Lorna was now more able to separate from her and could tolerate being in another room. She enjoyed television and especially liked musical programs. It delighted her that Lorna showed an interest in music at this early age, and she expressed regret that during her own childhood she had had no access to a musical instrument. However, she felt that it was wrong to force a child to take up an instrument unless the desire was strong in the child. Mr. Bjornson had been forced to take lessons and consequently lost all interest in music. Mrs. Bjornson thought that Lorna would be ready for a phonograph and children's records by Christmas.

In the next well-baby clinic visit at the onset of the eighteenth month Lorna remained glued to her chair almost from the moment of arrival. There was no doubt that visits to the clinic were associated with the physical examination, which invariably produced anxiety and crying. However she was approachable with toys and took them willingly from the safety of her chair.

Her language was very impressive. According to her parents she had at least fifty words, also used combinations such as "baby-cookie," "bye-bye-car," etc. Lorna had also begun to take an interest in helping to undress herself and could pull off her socks and slip. She was finicky about spilling or soiling, would say "dirty," and insist upon immediately being washed or cleaned off. In free play Lorna was observed to play with clay but after scooping up a small bit she held it up and said "dirty." However she continued to play with it for several minutes longer. She seemed to enjoy the doll more than anything and played with it considerably.

The pediatrician talked with Mrs. Bjornson for several minutes about how well Lorna was doing, and they reminisced about the great difficulties during the early months. Mrs. Bjornson asked a question about discipline and setting limits. She wanted to establish the living and dining rooms as out of bounds for Lorna but would compensate with a great deal of freedom in her own room and some other parts of the house. Mrs. Bjornson was particularly relaxed during this visit and was scarcely recognizable as the anxious, uncertain woman of those early months. Her increased enjoyment of Lorna and greater confidence in herself were quite evident.

The interviewer was unavoidably late for the next visit and was quite surprised at Mrs. Bjornson's rather strong reaction. Mrs. Bjornson said that she had worried about the possibility of a car accident and was also afraid that she had misunderstood the appointment date. She stressed that it was terribly important for her to know with certainty about such things, in order to plan her day and to know just how she and Lorna should dress. As a matter of fact, she soon excused herself and changed Lorna from the sturdy overalls to pretty "company clothes." Mrs. Bjornson told the interviewer that a sure way to befriend Lorna was to admire her clothes. "Like any woman, Lorna is pleased by this."

Lorna was quite active during the visit, climbed up and down the sofa, bumped into the tea table, and accidentally caused the tea to spill. Mrs. Bjornson showed some exasperation and commented that the child "is always on the go."

She reported that Lorna had enjoyed the Christmas tree lights and was remarkably good about not touching the ornaments. The Bjornsons had spent the holidays with Carl's parents, and Lorna had withstood the trip excellently. Upon their return home they learned that a long-standing friend and colleague of Carl's had suddenly died of a heart attack. He was only in his forties and it was quite upsetting to the Bjornsons.

Lorna led the visitor to her toy chest, in which there were several toys that closely resembled the testing material used at the clinic. It seemed likely that Mrs. Bjornson had carefully selected such toys for their "educational value." Mrs. Bjornson showed the interviewer a 5 x 7 inch card file which she used as a record of people who sent them Christmas cards and to whom they sent cards. It was an impressive demonstration of the structured organization with which the Bjornsons surrounded themselves and upon which they relied, including authoritative consumer guides and periodicals covering all aspects of living and family life.

Lorna was not quite so fearful at the next clinic visit and walked around the toy cabinet a bit before being seated. Mrs. Bjornson expressed some vague concerns about sleeping, eating, and toileting. Upon discussion it seemed that there was an episode one evening just before bedtime when Lorna had gone down to the cellar with her father and refused to come to bed. When Mrs. Bjornson had insisted, Lorna cried bitterly and clung to her father. It was apparent from the discussion that this had aroused considerable feeling on her mother's part. Apart from this incident there was no other real trouble in regard to sleeping.

No definite problem was related to eating except that Lorna occasionally refused something. As for toileting, Lorna had begun to object to being placed on the potty and would say "can't." Then she would soil when taken off. The pediatrician felt that this was a particularly difficult area for Mrs. Bjornson, who had given evidence of distaste for "dirtiness" and had expressed concern about bowel movements. Her inclination probably was to be insistent about training but she was not able to do so without support.

The discussion led into the area of Mrs. Bjornson's tendency to put considerable pressure on Lorna to perform in terms of achievement and to be a "good girl." Yet she had conflicts about this because she was not without sympathy and understanding for the child. She also realized that she expected more mature behavior than was reasonable. There was no doubt that she found this age period a difficult one, and was eager to have Lorna more grown up.

Mrs. Bjornson spoke about having another child the following spring, when Lorna would be close to three years old. She remarked that she hoped the new baby would be easier to take care of than Lorna, otherwise she would have to spend all her time with the new baby and then "what would happen to Lorna?" She planned the baby for spring "because babies get a much better start at that time." The pediatrician was impressed with the completeness of Mrs. Bjornson's planning and felt that everything would be precisely scheduled in advance.

The mother's interviewer, who observed during the clinic visit, emphasized "Mrs. Bjornson's almost constant close physical contact with the child." She frequently touched Lorna, straightened her dress or hair, and hovered anxiously over her. Her response during testing was intense and anxious involvement to expedite the child's performance. She frequently demonstrated a solution to a problem or urged, "Yes, you can do it, dear." Her direct participation included holding the child's hand to guide the crayon, cheering successes, and urging her on. She also felt the need to justify any failure to perform with explanations such as "she's slow getting started."

At the age of 19 months and 17 days Lorna had a general maturity level of 22 months and a developmental quotient of 113 on the Gesell test.

The psychological observer again characterized Lorna as "an inactive, uninteresting-looking little girl who functions above her age." While she expected the adult to provide directions and to judge the success or failure of her contact with the environment, at the same time she perceived an element of possible danger from the adult. Hence her approach was one of caution and reserve.

Lorna's awareness of social clues from the adult gave her the capacity to carry out orders. She also had an insight for the objective structure of her immediate surroundings, which was revealed in her excellent performance. In contrast to her high capacity for perceptual and structural tasks was her striking lack of investment in motor performance. She was sedentary most of the time and left her chair only at rare episodes. During the whole observation there were but four unequivocal smiles by Lorna.

The moment the pediatrician moved towards the medical equipment Lorna's negative emotions were mobilized. She wrinkled her face, whimpered, made her body limp and passive; and finally fought directly against the danger by crying, grimacing, and pushing away the stethoscope. However, as soon as the examination was over, Lorna quickly recovered and moved about energetically and rhythmically.

The psychological examiner's concluding comment was, "Nothing in Lorna's picture indicates atypical development, either as far as her motor performance or her other performances are concerned. Nevertheless, we cannot quite rid ourselves of the impression that Lorna's difference from other children could not adequately be described by her personality alone."

Because Mrs. Bjornson was conscious of civic duty and community responsibility, she was drawn into work for a charitable organization in a leading capacity. It included considerable planning and organization, to which both the Bjornsons applied themselves diligently. Mr. Bjornson was also considering enrollment in a personality and public speaking course being given by Dale Carnegie. Despite the high fee, Mrs. Bjornson felt that it would be extremely valuable for her husband in his dealings with people. She stressed the executive level of his position and the responsibility it involved. She was proud of his status but was quick to modify this pride with the comment that "the effort is not really worth it if it ruins your health."

Mrs. Bjornson radiated pleasure as Lorna pulled toys into the room, and she joined Lorna in play with them even as she talked to the visitor. The interviewer had the impression that it was more like two children enjoying a toy together than mother and child. Customarily Mrs. Bjornson dressed herself and her daughter in similar dresses, which seemed to represent the close association between them.

Mrs. Bjornson said that Lorna was usually left in her father's care on Thursday evenings when she went to market. "They have a wonderful time playing together, and the place is always a shambles when I come home." Spontaneously she remarked that Lorna was really a pleasure now and that "she's easy-going like her father." The interviewer felt that Mrs. Bjornson and Lorna not only enjoyed each other but had similar concern for good taste, appearance, and manner. Both of them literally glowed in response to any kind of compliment or admiration. It was evident that prettiness, nice manners, and being a lady were of great importance to this mother and that conversely she was quite distressed about dirt or messiness.

One thing that continued to go badly was toilet training. It seemed that Lorna understood what the toilet was for but said "no want" and then proceeded to wet or soil herself. Mrs. Bjornson then asked about the appropriate age for children to start nursery school and whether lack of toilet training would keep a child from being accepted. She also reported that Lorna's behavior had become extremely demanding at times. When Mrs. Bjornson was on the telephone with her community work Lorna interrupted by screaming loudly in order to get her mother's attention. At meal time she sometimes deliberately pushed her dish to the floor as an "attention-getter." Because Lorna wanted undivided attention, it interfered with Mrs. Bjornson's housework, and Mrs. Bjornson felt "very uncomfortable if the house was not in order."

At 22 months and 11 days Lorna was far more tractable during the physical examination at the clinic. Although she protested with "no like" and "Lorna no want," she did not cry and permitted the examination without struggle. After the examination was completed, she was much more free and easy, lively and animated. She went to the pediatrician, leaned against her, and played a game of handing a cookie back and forth.

In her final summary the psychological examiner concluded that while Lorna gave evidence that the world might not be to her liking, she had adapted to it rather proficiently. The intrusion of outside stimulation had stopped being so painful to her, and even the dreaded medical examination had lost its terror. She had learned that avoidance and diversion served to modify the outside world and to make its impact more tolerable. Within these confines, Lorna's defenses had been marshalled to make her organized, adaptive, and capable of effective functioning. Her developmental quotient on the Viennese test was 117.

In the final home visit in the twenty-third month the interviewer found that the Bjornsons had repapered the living room to a lighter and brighter color, and had bought several new items of living room furniture. Plans were also afoot to redecorate Lorna's room and to make some changes on the exterior of the house. For Lorna's second birthday they planned to buy a sandbox and a tricycle.

There was discussion about plans to enroll Lorna in the nursery school. Mrs. Bjornson hoped that she would be continued in the study program because she would feel "absolutely lost" without its help. She said that without it she might have raised Lorna as she herself had been raised. She reviewed the deprivations of her own extremely unhappy childhood, where even a single cheap toy at Christmas was a luxury, and she pointed out that Mr. Bjornson's childhood was equally miserable and difficult. She felt that it was no wonder both of them were self-conscious about money and aspired to the better things of life.

For her the measure of the "better things" was in the tasteful comfort of her home and the status which made it possible to surround Lorna with attention, a plethora of worldly goods, and the most current concepts of child-rearing. She could only marvel, as did her parents, at the striking contrast between Old World cultural standards and the American dream come true. But the fabric of dreams is fragile, and only time will prove its real substance for Lorna and her parents.

SUMMARY

A. EXPECTATIONS

1. Maternal Expectations. Although Mrs. Bjornson looked forward with considerable pleasure to having a child, this was diffused by extreme anxiety concerning her own adequacy as a mother and fears for the welfare of the child. She read copiously about normal and abnormal infancy and wondered how she could manage the problems of child care. She dared not trust her own judgment but relied on specific instructions or advice every step of the way. Under a veneer of intellectualism Old World superstitions lingered that "something might go wrong."

There was no conflict regarding career or employment, and Mrs. Bjornson accepted her role as housewife and mother without reservations. However, despite her positive anticipation of a child, difficulties arose almost immediately.

2. Specificity of Expectations. The scope and minuteness of expectations were outstanding with Mrs. Bjornson. She feared for the health of the fetus because of her excessive nausea, and she wondered whether it was receiving proper sustenance during pregnancy. She also worried about possible hereditary defects. All her anxieties were repeatedly expressed and apprehensively evaluated.

In the hospital she had unlimited questions about each detail of child care and asked explicit instructions for every possible contingency. She was uncertain whether she could understand the child's needs and she dreaded ill consequences if she did the wrong thing. Her need for help and reassurance could scarcely be satisfied.

3. Motivational Orientation. Marked fluctuation between mother-centeredness and child-centeredness was clearly demonstrated with Mrs. Bjornson. During pregnancy she was self-absorbed about physical discomforts and her own abilities as a mother. In the first six months with the baby she was concerned about proper management of all child-care routines to the point where she failed to see her daughter's needs and wishes. She was so involved in the ritual of burping between ounces that she frustrated Lorna's desires to continue feeding.

In her reliance on outside advice and in catering to her own expectations, she often ignored the child's indicated preferences. But as she became more familiar with the baby and her own role, she became more child-centered in her attitudes and expectations. Finally she began to understand Lorna's clues and began to cooperate with the child.

In point of fact, Lorna was not an easy baby to care for. She was described by various staff members as "jittery, squirmy, trembly, and unresponsive." These qualities, combined with Mrs.

Bjornson's own helplessness in managing, intensified the strain. In the early months Mrs. Bjornson failed to recognize that her child was difficult to manage and felt that if only she "could do the right thing" everything would go smoothly. She also did not recognize when Lorna developed into a more comfortable and easy child around the age of five months. Finally, by the sixth month, she was able to speak guardedly of her pleasure in "little Lorna's advance." Even so there was still timidity in accepting the child's normality and gnawing fear that the progress was temporary.

In time Mrs. Bjornson was able to shift her orientation from self to child and to recognize Lorna's abilities and advances. When the child developed to the point where she was recognizably responsive to her mother and the environment, Mrs. Bjornson could admit her own adequacy as a mother and Lorna's as a child.

For the first time Mrs. Bjornson began to interpret and explain her child's behavior, rather than seeing it as a baffling problem. Although self-concern remained, Mrs. Bjornson became more receptive to the child's ways of communicating with her. With Lorna's development, her mother's expectations began to focus on the process of socialization, behavior, and relationship to others. However, she also remained aware of Lorna's needs for freedom, activity, and attention.

Thus, there were two types of expectations which provided some conflict for Mrs. Bjornson. The high value placed on social conformity demanded behavior more appropriate to an older child, and in this respect Mrs. Bjornson demonstrated mother-centered goals. At the same time, she tried to adapt daily life and management of family activities to allow certain kinds of freedom for Lorna, which was child-centered in orientation.

4. Role of Child in Fulfilling Mother's Expectations. Mrs. Bjornson's negative expectations about her adequacy as a mother were reinforced by the difficulties of management which Lorna presented. In those early months it was almost as if Lorna were determined to prove the validity of her mother's forebodings. Feeding problems, spitting up, fussiness, all gave Mrs. Bjornson further proof of maternal incompetence.

However, Lorna demonstrated a type of adaptation, characterized not by vigor of physical activity but by a capacity to respond to demands for achievement and social behavior. In this she fulfilled her mother's expectations, because her developmental achievements were outstanding. Her advanced language ability was a joy to her mother, who encouraged it in every way that she could. Because her expectations were so great, Mrs. Bjornson was tense and anxious in the testing situations for fear that Lorna would not measure up.

As she came to realize that Lorna was indeed capable of high standards in social achievement, Mrs. Bjornson was better able to respond to the child's emotional needs. Although she did not want to push Lorna too fast, she did all she could to stimulate the child intellectually. Mrs. Bjornson's unreasonably high standards for her daughter were matched by Lorna's consistent ability to meet them.

5. Paternal Expectations. During the pregnancy period and early months of Lorna's life Mr. Bjornson showed some of the same pervasive concern that was prominent in his wife. He urged his wife to enter the hospital during early pregnancy because of the excessive nausea, he chauffeured her around, and he privately discussed her condition at various times with the obstetrician.

Mr. Bjornson was fairly permissive in attitude toward the child during the two years, showing consideration for her limitations to conform and to go at her own pace. He had tolerance for, and interest in, the child's activities. In the early weeks there was some annoyance that evening leisure was so taken up with the baby, but he was gratified that Lorna quieted more easily for him than for his wife. In general, the relationship between father and child was relatively relaxed. He increasingly recognized Lorna's individuality and was proud of her development, but he was moderate in his praise for fear it would spoil her. When Lorna "really got to be somebody" at about six months of age, Mr. Bjornson and his daughter interacted spontaneously and often.

B. BEHAVIOR

1. Communication. Few specifics were produced in the study concerning Mrs. Bjornson's modes of verbal and physical communication with the child. It was obscured in the beginning months by the mother's concern about her ability to care adequately for the baby, and the fact that Lorna was difficult to manage. The entire process of communication was difficult and uncertain. Mrs. Bjornson could not understand Lorna's clues. Thus, she typically did not anticipate her need for food but waited until the baby cried loudly before feeding her. Under the strain of "doing it properly" she held Lorna stiffly, without any pleasure in the feeding process. The messiness of the baby's spitting up aggravated her further.

However, as better rapport was achieved, Mrs. Bjornson became more comfortable with Lorna and more adept at handling her. At first she was inclined to substitute talking and crib-rocking for holding, and throughout she reported that there was little need to hold Lorna. It was also true that Lorna was not a cuddly baby at the beginning and was not responsive to tactile stimulation. So Mrs. Bjornson talked to the child to quiet and distract her. In the second six months more physical contact was initiated. Stronger physical interchange developed as the child matured and the mother relaxed. Information about Mrs. Bjornson's response to the baby's clues was too sparse and indefinite to permit analysis.

2. Regularity and Flexibility of Scheduling. This did not appear to be a matter of major concern, although regularity was not always achieved. Between the prolonged feeding sessions and putting her baby to sleep, Edna Bjornson was occupied for large parts of each day. Her all-pervasive anxieties about child care took precedence over efforts to establish regularity in routine.

By the time Lorna was six months old a schedule of three meals a day had been achieved, to Mrs. Bjornson's delight. Although going to sleep was a problem in the early months, by the second half of the first year Mrs. Bjornson reported that Lorna's twelve-hour night sleep was "wonderful." Mrs. Bjornson accommodated herself to Lorna's nap preferences and changed daily routines according to the child's changing needs. She structured her daily life to suit the child's schedule.

3. Techniques of Management. Mrs. Bjornson used various techniques to facilitate the course of child care. She used techniques of diversion to get Lorna to eat, and pre-arrangement of objects in various areas of the home to minimize restrictions and avoid difficulties.

A particularly small proportion of non-permissive behavior was noted in the first year. In the second year reports of the mother's permissiveness decreased, consistent with changes in the mother's experiences with the child and growing emphasis on social control. In this period Mrs. Bjornson was more concerned with matters of discipline and proper behavior.

4. Relation of Expectations to Behavior. The most frequently reported behavioral areas of interaction with the infant were those in which Mrs. Bjornson had always expressed specific concerns and expectations. The major one was for the baby's well-being. Thus, activities were largely directed towards the baby's comfort and security. Feeding problems were predominant in the early months. The mother anticipated such difficulties even before the baby was born, and she developed an elaborate feeding ritual to meet the difficulties she anticipated. Even during pregnancy she was concerned about the effect of her own nausea and vomiting on the baby. Thus she was highly agitated by Lorna's spitting up. Feeding remained an anxious area for Mrs. Bjornson during most of the first year until it finally proved to be no problem.

"Normal" development of the child was also an area of great concern, and Mrs. Bjornson worked zealously to help her child's "intellectual" development. Because of intense general anxieties about her own adequacy as a mother, Mrs. Bjornson's behavior in managing Lorna was most uneasy and fearful in the first few months.

5. Paternal Behavior. Mr. Bjornson was reported to participate in caring for the child during the evening feeding and on special evenings when he relieved his wife for shopping expeditions. His care of the child was more relaxed than his wife's, and Lorna responded more easily to his ministrations. Because of his relative success in managing the child he spent as much time with her as he could. After supper there was a period of "rough-housing" between them which was enjoyable to both.

Throughout the second year, relations between father and daughter remained pleasurable to both. There was some evidence that Mr. Bjornson was a more easy-going parent than his wife because he seemed to have less investment in his daughter's superior performance than did his wife. He declared that it was more important for Lorna to be happy than to be bright.

C. SOCIO-CULTURAL INFLUENCES

1. Socio-economic Status and Values. This was a family for whom upward-mobility aspirations were quite important. Their success was measured against the financial struggle of their parents and a departure from the Old World cultural patterns of their families. Stress was placed on proper behavior, decorum, and achievement. Being a "good child" and reaching more than age-adequate developmental levels were highly important expectations held for the child.

The value of their new home was a significant material symbol of elevation from economic deprivations. Their devotion to improving its value and comfort was consistent with their goal of material betterment.

Mr. Bjornson's position as a junior executive on his way up was important to both the Bjornsons. He went on a number of business trips, often brought home work to do in the evening, and took a Dale Carnegie self-improvement course. Although Mrs. Bjornson said "that it doesn't pay to ruin your health over work," her husband's advancement was of significance to both of them.

By surrounding Lorna with space for activity, many toys, pretty clothes, and a "cultural" environment, they hoped to establish the child's role in an upwardly mobile family. When Lorna was born, an insurance policy was started for her college education. To a considerable extent Lorna conformed to her parents' expectations of social achievement.

The social activities of the Bjornsons were limited during much of the first year because of their unwillingness to trust Lorna to a baby-sitter. As she became older, however, their community contacts were renewed and both Bjornsons participated actively in community organizations. Considerable importance was also attached to social activities with friends, business associates, and family. The Bjornsons represented the process of sharply moving away from the low income and social status of their immigrant families of origin.

2. Extended Family. There was no appreciable parent-grandparent conflict, and there was consistent contact with both families of origin. Mrs. Bjornson felt more comfortable with her own mother, but she was also fond of her mother-in-law, with whom visits were periodically exchanged. In a sense the Bjornsons were remarkable for the success with which they maintained warm and active contacts with their parents, while at the same time departing widely from their social and cultural patterns.

Family relationships seemed to be compartmentalized so that the grandparents were not involved in the upwardly mobile social life of the couple. Both grandmothers played a supportive role at the time of Lorna's birth by visiting at different times and contributing actively in the household. All four grandparents also provided a wider environment of companionship and social interaction for the child. In this respect Mrs. Bjornson's family was more active than her husband's.

Mrs. Bjornson shared many similar points of view with her mother but often expressed the contrast between her values and way of life and those of her mother. While the Bjornsons were definitely moving away from their origins, they made a practical accommodation between the old and the new so that interpersonal relations did not appear to be conflictual.

3. Spatial Arrangements and Values. Mrs. Bjornson seemed to manage household affairs efficiently and conscientiously. She was careful of her possessions and intolerant of messiness. In order to maintain her well-kept home it was necessary to compromise between allowing Lorna freedom to use space but at the same time to guard the attractive appearance of the home. Lorna was allowed complete freedom in certain rooms and on the spacious lawn but certain prohibitions were established for other areas such as the living room.

Before engaging in any major venture the Bjornsons planned carefully and methodically. Mrs. Bjornson looked to household magazines and consumer guides for ideas about living arrangements and the best allocation of space. This methodical planning worked well for carpentry and household arrangements but did not always work so well for little Lorna.

The Bjornsons, more than other families in the study, made extensive use of the out-of-doors for the child's activity and exploration. Although the home contained ample space for play, Mrs. Bjornson used the spacious garden to good purpose. In terms of family management, there seemed to be mutual planning between the parents. In operational terms, they followed the customary pattern of the father being responsible for the outside of the house, carpentry, and repairs, while the mother maintained responsibility for the inside of the house, decorating, and furnishing.

D. FAMILY RELATIONSHIPS

1. Marital. This was a predominantly compatible marital relationship. Mrs. Bjornson brought dependency needs and emotional problems to her marriage, wherein emotional uncertainty and indecision became expressed in tendencies toward self-devaluation. On the surface she presented to the world a well-groomed, calm, and efficient young woman who was properly observant of social customs and manners. Beneath this, however, were deep feelings of inadequacy and self-denial.

In Mr. Bjornson she found a man whose protectiveness constituted a balance for her own dependency and feelings of inadequacy. Both were in agreement on the upper middle-class life goals and values associated with his profession. Both came from poverty-stricken Nordic immigrant families, from whom they had acquired habits of thrift and reluctance for financial extravagance in any form. Both felt that expenditures for the home were more important than those for their respective individual requirements. This was consistent with Mrs. Bjornson's psychological pattern of self-denial.

Mr. Bjornson was reserved and sometimes gave the impression of cold aloofness, but he was not without understanding and sympathy for his wife. At the same time he tended to relate to the world and to life as to a mathematical formula. Notwithstanding, these two personalities merged into a compatible marital relationship for different psychodynamic reasons. This does not mean that there was an absence of emotional tension and anxiety, but that whatever tension existed was not basically due to the marital relationship.

2. Mother-Child. The infant was one, but not the only, source of satisfaction. Mrs. Bjornson's early contact with her baby did not bring her the pleasure for which she had hoped. Her own anxieties and real difficulties in caring for Lorna acted as a barrier. When this situation changed by the end of the first year, she was able to find real gratification in her relationship with her daughter as well as satisfaction in teaching her to value the social amenities. And as the rapport between them grew the child responded more positively.

Two outstanding features of the mother-child relationship during the two-year period were the development of warmth between them, and the child's ability to conform. Mrs. Bjornson's satisfaction was reinforced by Lorna's highly adaptable behavior in meeting expectations of achievement. The child became a source of emotional satisfaction, along with at least one other interpersonal relationship.

Mrs. Bjornson continued to turn to her husband for companionship and also addressed herself to social activities, which provided satisfaction. Further she had a deep interest in beautifying her home. The increasing mutual pleasure of mother and daughter was not the only source of satisfaction to either.

3. Father-Child. From the beginning Mr. Bjornson participated in some child-care routines and spent some time with the child. He was more relaxed in his demands for achievement than his wife, and consequently was more accepting. He took pride in Lorna's developmental achievement but he made clear that he valued her happiness more than her brains. He was less inclined than his wife to be overly anxious. Father and child enjoyed each other's company, and their relationship was a source of considerable satisfaction to each of them.

E. PERSONALITY CHARACTERISTICS

1. Handling of Anxiety and Hostility. Mrs. Bjornson's problems demanded a well-developed defense against anxiety. She needed to appeal to various kinds of authorities, the written word, the study staff or others, for assurance that she was behaving properly and acting wisely. She never felt secure when, as in social situations, she was left to her own devices.

Each change in child care required the approval of some kind of authority, just as many other life decisions needed the reinforcement of those who were important to her. She was fearful and uncertain of her ability in the mothering role, and felt the necessity of converting her problems into concrete questions through which she could get authoritative direction and approval for her behavior with Lorna.

Mrs. Bjornson actually functioned better when her diffuse anxiety was directed to specific material circumstances or events, such as illness. Then she proved able to deal with them more forthrightly and adequately. Learning from staff members, books, classes, and conversation was a way Mrs. Bjornson handled anxiety through intellectualization. Consequently, at times there was a tendency to deal with her own and others' feelings in a somewhat impersonal way.

2. *Dependency and the Sense of Security*. Mrs. Bjornson had much ambivalence about her own dependency needs, but handled them in such a way as to contribute toward family integration. The deprivations of her lonely childhood led to constant need for reassurance from other adult and authority figures. In her husband she found an authority to whom she could turn. Even her interest in natural childbirth stemmed from the fact that he had learned about it in college and thought it was "good." Frequently he was sympathetic and companionable, which provided her with dependency satisfactions. But pregnancy and the anticipation of motherhood produced support needs so great that not even her husband could fulfill them.

In Mrs. Bjornson's younger years she had difficulty in making and keeping friends. In fact, both the Bjornsons tended to be shy and uncomfortable in social relations. Hence in the initial marriage relationship they concentrated on their togetherness, allowing even habitual associations such as the church to become inactive. In married life they attempted to achieve independence from their family's cultural and psychological backgrounds.

The baby's arrival posed a fairly acute problem to Mrs. Bjornson during the first six months of Lorna's life in terms of her own need "to be given to" and the need "to be a giving mother." As Lorna became more easy to satisfy, the emotional relationship improved. The issue occasionally became exacerbated when Lorna would make clinging demands upon her mother.

3. Feelings of Adequacy or Inadequacy. Mrs. Bjornson was the only one of the unitary-family mothers who was characterized by marked feelings of inadequacy. In a number of ways she expressed guilt over her possible failure to meet the family and social obligations made upon her. Each new social situation was looked upon as a possible threat to her concept of self. Her pregnancy was one such new social experience and the course of Lorna's development presented continuing new demands. Fears were aroused that Lorna's difficulties might be interpreted as failures on her part to meet the obligations placed upon her.

The sense of inadequacy made Mrs. Bjornson strive for the "perfect" in all respects. Any imperfections in the baby or her management became a source of self-derogation. Mrs. Bjornson said that she expected too much of herself, as well as of others, and that she never seemed to be satisfied with her own achievements. In many ways she was always conscious of a lack of fulfillment, both past and present. Her life was rigorously devoted to attaining her aspirations, but she had difficulty in accepting success.

4. Planning and Impulsiveness. This family seemed to have more planning compulsion than the other families. Mrs. Bjornson carried her need to plan almost to extremes. She needed specific guidelines and had a tremendous need for scheduling most life events. Her needs for predictability resulted in excessive concern when Lorna vomited, burped, or later messed with her foods. Her demands for orderliness were shown in her meticulous housekeeping and her well-groomed personal appearance. Such demands, however, were at odds with requirements for flexibility in the care of the child. Although planning was sometimes a problem, it was not sufficiently threatening to be disruptive of family organization. Mr. Bjornson, too, was a firm planner in his work, household remodeling, and scheduling of activity. Because both parents were similar in this respect, it did not operate divisively.

5. *Self-Assertion.* Mrs. Bjornson found it extremely difficult to take the initiative in interpersonal relationships. It was evident even in her initial contacts with Lorna. It was hard to assert herself in breast feeding or in the introduction of solid foods, but when Lorna became more responsive and helpfully participating, the importance of this difficulty diminished.

The difficulty of self-assertion with others was also seen in Mrs. Bjornson's trying relationship with an old family friend, whose gratuitous advice and instructions were often painfully irritating. Mrs. Bjornson found it difficult to assert herself directly face-to-face but sought refuge in complaints to her husband and staff members about this woman's intrusions.

6. *Recapitulation of Past Experiences.* Mrs. Bjornson was strongly aware of the impact of emotional deprivation in her own childhood. Both she and her husband recalled undue restriction, rigidity, poverty, loneliness, and unhappiness from which they had suffered. Cultural and material limitations were also strongly recollected by her, including lack of toys, musical opportunity, and a college education. With this in mind, she was determined not to let Lorna be similarly deprived. She tried to introduce objective devices and to create an environment which would assure her daughter of the very things which she had missed. Much of her growing satisfaction with Lorna came about when the child showed an aptitude and appreciation for such opportunities.

F. EMERGENCE OF FAMILY INTEGRATION PATTERN

1. *Family Structure.* The family tended toward unitary organization. Mr. Bjornson's confident and protective role in the family provided a partial balance for his wife's indecision and dependency. Relatively speaking, the husband-wife relationship was an emotionally supportive one. Their relationships with extended family were close and congenial, and limits of the grandparental roles were acceptable and satisfactory to all the family.

Strong dyadic relationships emerged from the very first weeks of Lorna's life, and the sense of family togetherness also developed early. Although Lorna's thorough enjoyment of her father was occasionally a little difficult for Mrs. Bjornson to take, there was a considerable amount of interaction which included Lorna from an early age. For nine months the Bjornsons had no baby-sitter to whom they would trust Lorna, and during this time the entire emphasis was upon the nuclear family. The unitary pattern remained during the full two years of study.

2. Division of Labor and Balance of Power. This unitary family contained a balance of power best described as mutual sharing. The family felt mutual security in their home, their future, and in their relationships. There was usually joint agreement on family matters, with Mr. Bjornson having ultimate charge of finances and the home remodeling, while his wife assumed responsibility for the maintenance and appearance of the home and its daily operation.

3. Development, Achievement, and Social Behavior of Child. In this family there was somewhat advanced development of the child. Lorna's first three months of life were especially difficult, but later her development proceeded at an accelerated rate. Her main difficulty was extreme shyness and aloofness towards strangers, which was a source of concern. To people outside of the family she appeared sober and seldom smiling, but she did meet her mother's high standards of social decorum and intellectual achievement.

4. Prospect of Siblings. There was considerable mention of planning for a second, and even a third, child during the course of the study. As Lorna became more satisfactory to her mother, Mrs. Bjornson tended to forget the early difficulties and looked forward to a second pregnancy with greater equilibrium. She planned on a second child when Lorna was about three years old. It seemed to at least one staff member that she would live up to her plans. During the course of the two-year study, however, there was no second pregnancy.

5. Status of Family in Community. The Bjornsons maintained considerable social contact with their extended family, though their scheme of values was vastly different from that of their parents. Neither set of parents was regarded as a model of status in community affairs, and the Bjornsons set about to make a place of their own in community life. They were active in various organizations and in social life outside the nuclear family. There was every indication that they would continue to be so in the years to come.

6. Types of Parent-Child Adaptation. The Bjornsons were a unitary family who fluctuated between parent-centered and child-centered orientations. Unlike the other unitary families, who were all mainly child-centered, the Bjornsons were considered intermediate in their motivational orientations. They were a permissive family, in fact one of the most permissive in the study. They therefore emerged as unitary, permissive, and intermediately child-centered.

POSTSCRIPT

The subsequent years did little to mitigate Mrs. Bjornson's difficulties. Her omnipresent dissatisfactions and sense of inadequacy became expressed in varying physical symptoms, health concerns, and emotional tensions. Her need for exemplary performance as wife and mother took an exacting toll, which affected not only the relationship with Lorna but with her husband as well. The marital relationship began to suffer from quarrels, a lack of communication, and Mrs. Bjornson's feeling that her husband could not share her burdens. On his part Mr. Bjornson felt that it was impossible to allay his wife's anxieties and that whatever he did or attempted to do would fail to please her anyway.

Mrs. Bjornson's chief anxiety centered around Lorna; she expressed almost phobic fears about her behavior and development. Constantly she questioned whether something was wrong with her. Lorna, in turn, gave evidence that the exacting demands of her mother weighed heavily. She was slow and resistant to toilet training, and she continued to cling to her mother, facing new situations with fear and anxiety. Thus, Lorna had to take the initial nursery school experience very gradually before she could feel secure or at ease in the separation from her mother. After that, however, she was active, happy, and in good contact with children and adults.

Relationships with extended family were not as rewarding to

Mrs. Bjornson as surface appearances had indicated. The maternal grandmother blamed Mrs. Bjornson's unhappiness on the fact that she was "too far away from God." Because she had not produced a son, Mrs. Bjornson felt that she had disappointed her in-laws. The sense of failure and inadequacy continued to haunt her, while one event after another seemed to justify these feelings.

A second daughter was born when Lorna was almost three years old. During pregnancy Mrs. Bjornson was preoccupied with herself and resentful that Lorna "still needed her so much." Physically she had symptoms of ill health, plus fantasies that the new baby might be deformed. Lorna's negativism reached new heights during this period, a further source of dismay. However, the new infant proved to be more tractable than Lorna had been.

Because Sylvia from the beginning was an easy-going and undemanding baby, Lorna began to suffer by comparison. Sylvia was characterized as "contented, affectionate, a ray of sunshine" while Lorna was "unaffectionate, clinging, never satisfied, and negative." As her own emotional stress mounted, Mrs. Bjornson found much of Lorna's behavior intolerable. Spankings became more frequent and intense. On one traumatic occasion Mrs. Bjornson stopped the car in a desolate, uninhabited area and threatened to eject Lorna, which was exceedingly frightening to the child.

Mr. Bjornson went through a period of indigestion and severe headaches, which were of great concern to his wife. She felt that his marked self-control would some day erupt in a "big explosion." Just as she demanded perfection of herself, she expected it of others, which brought inevitable disappointments. She recognized that Lorna was much like herself, somehow never satisfied or fulfilled, discontented with what she had and always seeking something more. Like her mother, Lorna was compulsively "clean" and shut out what was considered improper or unladylike by her mother's standards. At times she was bossy, complaining, and whiney but would not release hostility for fear of losing her mother's approval.

Soon situations of strife developed between the two children. Mrs. Bjornson's interventions only seemed to perpetuate rather than prevent the struggle. Sylvia became an independent, self-contained child who was persevering in getting her own way. Lorna put up little resistance, in fear that any aggression would arouse her mother's disapproval. Thus, the younger sibling became the overt aggressor and Lorna tolerated her attacks to prove "how good she was."

Sylvia was admittedly the favored child, a situation which produced guilt feelings for Mrs. Bjornson. However, her interaction with Sylvia remained warm and positive in contrast to the negative interaction with Lorna. But as Sylvia grew older, more independent, and less tractable, Mrs. Bjornson was critical of her also, stating that she was "unmanageable and impossible." As with Lorna, toilet training with Sylvia was achieved fairly late.

Mr. Bjornson's advancement in his career demanded considerable time and effort, but it gave the Bjornsons much satisfaction. His relationship to the children was one of benign tolerance and affection, although rather distant and uninvolved. Nevertheless he was quite perceptive. Accurately he characterized Sylvia "as a fighting fury who holds her own, while Lorna has so little satisfaction in herself that she seems to demand so much."

In moments of guilt Mrs. Bjornson flagellated herself as responsible for "the way Lorna turned out." At other times she was bitter that "Lorna acts this way in the face of all we have done for her." There was no doubt that Mrs. Bjornson conscientiously struggled to do the right thing but in so doing she drove herself to a point of self-sacrifice and self-pity which only exacerbated the situation.

Lorna's performance in psychological tests was in the superior range. This was highly gratifying to the Bjornsons and a further motivation "to properly develop her potential." Actually, Sylvia was also an advanced competent child according to the tests. In school, after a characteristic period of timidity and fear of the unknown, Lorna's adjustment was excellent. Later reports proved her to be an outstanding and conscientious student. Her control and the demands she made on herself remained an impressive aspect of her functioning, but she was quite successful in leading a well-rounded social and cultural life with the promise of doing well in professional pursuits.

In the last contact, when Lorna was just past 14 years old, it was evident that both attractive girls were successful in school, deportment, social, and intellectual achievements. They had adapted well and had met the exacting standards of a respected, secure, and upwardly mobile middle-class family and way of life.

The Silver Family

A CULTURAL PARADOX

Helene Silver fled her crumbling Nazi world to come to America as the German war bride of a Jewish soldier. The fears and horror of war and its aftermath were exchanged for the uncertainties of a new land and a husband-to-be whom she had not seen for eighteen months. There was no longer a future in Germany and no escape from war memories and the loss of loved ones. But in America a brave soldier awaited her, gentle and kind, a source of strength and protection.

Helene was born to a middle-class Lutheran couple in a north-eastern German town, where her father was a government official and her mother a housewife. When she was three years old her parents were divorced upon her mother's initiative. Helene lived with her mother and they "were close and meant everything to each other." But this idyllic period was shattered by her mother's remarriage when Helene was ten years old.

Helene couldn't bear her stepfather, with whom she did not get along well. She felt that he had deprived her of her mother's love. Shortly thereafter she left to live with her maternal grandparents.

Helene "got most anything she wanted" from her grandparents and from a generous aunt, more than she had ever received from her mother. She felt that her life was different from other girls', probably because she received so many more material things than if her mother had not remarried. She shuddered as she recalled the little girl who was "really terrible, very grabby" and insatiable.

Helene's personal turmoil was matched by the upheaval of the world around her. Hitler came to power when she was eight years old, and her school years became filled with the Nazi doctrines of Aryan superiority and world conquest. Her maturing mind was permeated with the cult of the master race and the myth of Jewish inferiority. "I thought that the most awful thing that could happen to you was to be Jewish."

She had great admiration for her uncle, a proud and peremptory man, "who was high up in the Nazi party. . . . He was a great Nazi. . . . The things he used to tell! . . ." The collapse of the Third Reich came as a shattering blow to her, and the disclosure of Nazi atrocities was a condemnation of ideals and loved ones which she could neither escape nor wholly accept. But her defenses were strong, and she was reluctant to blame herself. She said she "did not know these things were wrong" as she told of "the awful things that were done to the Jewish girls at school," to whom she had been "not very nice."

Helene completed the equivalent of a high-school education. She had taken four years of English and could speak the language quite well. Following this, she went to work as a private secretary for the mayor of the village, an affluent Junker estate owner, and lived with his family in well-to-do country surroundings.

Her stepfather was taken into the German army, and her family were evacuated from their town. They returned a couple of years later after the Russian occupation. As the years went by, Helene's mother had other children by her second husband, one girl and four boys, but Helene did not seem to know much about her stepsiblings. Her stepfather became a Russian prisoner of war but was ultimately released and reunited with his family.

The real impact of war for Helene started with the Russian occupation of Germany, as the Russians broke through to meet the Allied forces. "For two weeks," she recalled, "the people were between the German and Russian armies right in the front line." She greatly feared the Russians, and described them as "wild, oversexed animals who raped whatever females they found, whether they were sixteen or sixty."

Her stock of horror stories mainly encompassed sexual bestiality. She told of a forty-eight-year-old aunt who was raped by twenty-five soldiers while her twenty-five-year-old son stood by motionless "because he feared for his life." She reported that a maid was raped because Helene had not been around. She described in detail how her employer's son was shot because he intervened to protect her from the sexual attack of a Russian lieutenant. Despite the several close calls which she recounted, miraculously Helene was never actually assaulted.

Following the Russian occupation Helene was placed in a prisoner-of-war camp for about seven months. Her sympathy for the SS men in that prison was evident. "They died like flies . . . forty a day . . . because there was no medicine." She defended the innate decency of the SS. "They weren't really bad. People have a funny idea about them. They were just drafted like the rest and were given no choice." Along with defending the SS, Helene also exonerated herself. "I am not to blame because some of the Germans killed so many people and did such awful things to the Jews. I did not do these things and I don't feel I should be blamed."

Helene dwelt at length on her terrors, not only of the Russians but also of the Americans, during the occupation. She reported hiding for four days in a hole in the wall because soldiers were looking for her. Another time a soldier "tried to get her into the woods." She refused and managed to get away. She found the Americans bold and crude.

It was not surprising that Helene became attracted to David Silver, an American officer, who was "much nicer than the other soldiers" and was "gentle, courteous, and kind from the beginning." She introduced him to her aunt and uncle, who also liked him. At the time of the courtship Helene did not know that David was Jewish. Although he was rather short and slight, his wavy blond hair and blue eyes were the epitome of Aryan standards. It was also not difficult to see why David Silver was drawn to this attractive, well-dressed, carefully groomed, expertly made up blond young woman who spoke English with only a slight accent.

After some steady dating they became engaged and decided to marry in the United States. Helene recalled that before David started back home he kept saying there was something he wanted to tell her, but he did not do so before he left. In the meantime she proceeded to get her papers ready to follow him. While she was still in Germany, David's fateful letter arrived, with the belated confession that he was Jewish and had not dared admit it before for fear of losing her.

As Helene Silver told the story, she continued to smile in a friendly but impersonal way. The smile fitted the luscious curves of her rather large, well-shaped mouth but did not fit the intensity of her eyes or the calculated reserve of her words. She recounted, "David's letter was such a surprise that I did not know what to think." She considered the fact that she had liked him before knowing, and that he certainly had not changed just because he had told her. She reasoned, "It really did not make any difference; it is the individual that counts and not what his race or religion is."

Whether the de-Nazification of Mrs. Silver was really so swift, or whether her need for new security was rather so great, we shall never know. In any event, she decided to proceed with her plans. Her preparations for departure took a long eighteen months. In the turmoil of arrangements she hadn't realized what it would actually mean to leave her family behind. The full impact hit her, and she felt very much alone as she crossed the wide ocean into she knew not what.

New York was so "confusing and terrible" that she would have gone right back if it had been possible. The first days she was afraid to say anything except "yes" and "no" for fear people would laugh at her inability to use English. Many of the customs were different, "even the way Americans use their knives and forks." She had to learn the value of money not only in monetary but in personal terms.

It was a great shock when her husband made it clear that she could not spend eighteen dollars for a pair of wedding gloves, that this was impossible on his pay as a petty career officer in the Coast Guard. He told her that if this was the way she was going to spend money, they would have nothing at all. It suddenly brought home the fact that this was not the milk-and-honey paradise of her fantasies and that David Silver was not the omnipotent, affluent American savior.

Meeting her husband's family was also something of a shock. They were immigrant Russian working-class Jews in their seventies who kept a kosher table and maintained much of their Orthodox religion and Old World culture. Their apartment was in an old run-down section of New York, a far cry from the Junker estate where Helene had lived in such great comfort. Mrs. Silver felt that she did not have very much in common with them. "Both of them are older . . . more like grandparents than like parents," and "they do not speak very good English."

David was the youngest of three children. His two sisters were married. One resided in Florida because of an asthmatic child. The second sister lived in New York. She had one child and was expecting another. We do not know the conditions which led David Silver so far from his ancestral heritage as to marry a Gentile, and an attractive ex-Nazi at that. Nor could we do more than guess why this meek and gentle man elected to assume a quasi-military career.

Although his identification with Judaism had largely crumbled, David maintained relations with his parents and he continued to fulfill his filial responsibilities to the best of his ability. He had completed high school and had some commercial training. Now, with nine years' service credit, he had become a career officer in the Coast Guard.

It was an affront to Mrs. Silver that her husband's family was opposed to his marriage on religious and political grounds. She felt that if she had been able to be objective and tolerant despite her ideological background of racial superiority, surely his parents ought to be no less so.

Their backgrounds, so vitally different, laid a heavy hand on the Silvers' matrimonial debut, and the adjustments that they had to make were hammered out to a large extent alone. Partly by natural inclination, partly because of Mrs. Silver's uneasiness with American ways, and partly because of having gone so far in breaking with their respective traditions, the Silvers chose the path of relative isolation. For Mrs. Silver at least, the path proved to be lacking in satisfaction.

It was a big relief to leave New York for nearby New Haven, where Mr. Silver had a special assignment with the Coast Guard. Even so, they were not able to find a decent home to rent and were forced to consider purchasing a house. Mrs. Silver could not understand why housing was so difficult in America. She had expected it to be quite different from Germany, where so many houses had been destroyed.

A modest home was finally located in the suburbs overlooking the Sound. Although the location seemed quite isolated, lonely, and devoid of cultural activities, Mrs. Silver liked the house. While she welcomed a home of her own, the financial obligations began to loom quite large. A further complication was a possible transfer and new assignment for Mr. Silver, which raised a host of anxieties.

The Silver Family

Before their move to the new house Mrs. Silver found herself pregnant. She felt both pleased and alarmed. "The baby was not exactly planned," she said. They had thought they would like to wait a little to get themselves established in their new home first. But it had happened.

She reported that her husband was "always very considerate about sex. He isn't like other husbands who want intercourse whether the wife wants it or not." She said that she didn't know how her husband felt, but intercourse was not important to her and had never been especially satisfactory because she was slow to come to orgasm. Mr. Silver was the one who took precautions by using condoms. Now she felt more strongly about the need for contraceptives and questioned the interviewer about their availability.

Because of expenses with the house, they felt they could no longer afford the private obstetrician and decided to use the clinic at the New Haven Hospital. When they were introduced to the study Mrs. Silver thought it an excellent idea because she was going to need some help with a new baby, "such a completely new experience." Both the Silvers eagerly agreed to participate. Mr. Silver even requested a private interview so he could learn more about it. He was the only father of the eight in the study who requested such an interview.

At the interview he expressed content with his career in the service because it would provide security and a future for them. Mr. Silver's devotion to his attractive wife was much in evidence. He expressed pride in her English, compared her favorably to others, and spoke affectionately about her. Because he did not like to leave her alone overnight when he visited his ailing father, he went to New York and returned on the same day.

Mr. Silver had no preference as to the baby's sex and said of himself that he is "just like all other men . . . want to be an ideal father . . . to know what is right and wrong." He felt basically that "how a child acts depends on the parents," and he did not want his child to become a rowdy, nor did he intend to repeat his own father's mistake of being "too easy." With great solicitude for his wife, he said, "Nothing can make up for what a woman suffers at giving birth, having to give up so much and being so uncomfortable during pregnancy."

He wondered how parents learn to take care of children if there is no one to teach them and if they do not read books. To him parenthood was the greatest boon that could come to a couple, and the most fearful responsibility as well. He did his best to console his wife in her anxieties; together they would read and learn the proper way to fulfill the parental role.

During the pregnancy a typical evening at home was one of easy relaxation, with popular magazines and the evening paper spread out before them. Mr. Silver would ask his wife if she had read about a two-month-old baby that had smothered in the crib, and they would discuss the merits of having the crib in their room or in the nursery. Or Mrs. Silver would record her astonishment at the way American doctors advised things unheard of in Germany, such as insistence on dieting.

Both worried that in their zeal to do the right thing for their child they might overlook some important "don'ts" which could be disastrous to the child or its personality. Or Mr. Silver would read aloud about natural childbirth from a current weekly and then, patting his wife's hand affectionately, would insist, "Nothing can make up for the pain and inconvenience you are having."

Mrs. Silver told the interviewer that her mother almost dropped her shortly after she was born when trying to bathe her. She was afraid that something like that could happen to her if she had no help in learning. Although the baby had not been planned, she was looking forward to it with much satisfaction and was "very happy . . . because it will be someone who will really belong to me."

Mrs. Silver thought it would be "very unfortunate" to prefer one sex over the other, and she was careful in all interviews to allude to the baby as "it" rather than "he" or "she." Occasionally she referred to the "baby." Names for either a boy or girl had already been selected, and she "would not think of using anything except American names." She had prepared two baby outfits, one pink and the other blue. Parts of the outfits had been given to her. Whatever color wasn't used she planned to give away because she didn't contemplate having another baby, "at least not for a few years."

For Mrs. Silver the physical course of pregnancy was not difficult. She had no vomiting and only some nausea at the beginning. The discomfort did not disturb her because "feeling bad in pregnancy is to be expected." She had thought about the pain at delivery, but "other women go through this and if they can, so can I." She took some comfort from the fact that her husband would be there and she would not be "with strangers only." But in a strange land she felt there were few to whom she could turn for support in the problems of motherhood.

The child began to move earlier than she expected. When it kicked actively at night, she was unable to sleep, but when it was quiet for more than a few minutes, both she and her husband were terribly anxious that it would be stillborn.

The moving and "jumping" of the child made her uncomfortable, and she was embarrassed to go out in public for fear that it was so noticeable. At night, especially, she had the feeling, "The space in the middle of my body is not long enough for the baby." She also had pains and cramps in her legs occasionally.

She was surprised that Americans made such a fuss about breast feeding because she thought it was considered old-fashioned in this country. At first she did not want to breast feed, then changed her mind. The exercise class also held some fears for her because she thought its purpose was to encourage her to have natural childbirth. She said she was "really very frightened and scared" of the delivery because she never had been able to stand pain; "even going to the dentist frightens me . . . The fact that other women go through it does not make me feel any better about it."

Mr. Silver's solicitous attitude presented some problems for his wife. While she approved of his great interest, she was annoyed by his frequent questions and gratuitous advice from his reading. "I am afraid I am going to have a hard time with my husband because he is so worried and anxious that he will not dare touch the child." She had adopted an attitude of barely listening and was becoming very impatient with him. "It is very nice if fathers are interested in their children . . . anyone has to learn how to take care of their first baby . . . but they have to use their common sense."

Mrs. Silver's great fear was that her husband would be reassigned elsewhere before the baby arrived and before they moved to the new house. In this event she would have the problem of moving and caring for the baby at the same time. The thought that she might be "alone to face everything" was almost too much to bear. If he should get a permanent assignment, she considered joining him. But Mr. Silver was opposed to relocating elsewhere at this time because it might have disadvantages for the baby.

Mrs. Silver wished she were "like other girls who take changes easier." In thinking it over, she said, "It's not the actual change that bothers me so much as the uncertainty of what I may be going to." She disclaimed any credit for bravely facing a difficult situation and said, "Don't think I haven't cried too. I'm not so courageous. I have cried gallons of tears." At this point her eyes misted, but she went on to say that she knew "crying will not help" and they would have to figure out how to "make the best of it."

Mrs. Silver often wished she were back home and kept in close touch with her mother and the rest of the family, all of whom were eagerly awaiting news of the delivery. She was also "troubled about bringing a baby into this world" and expressed her dissatisfaction and disillusionment with the way things were in the United States. "I do not feel safe here either. . . . Democracy is a fine thing, but I don't know . . . In times like these . . . someone should be running things. . . . I wouldn't want to give Truman any more power . . . but when I hear how they bicker about things . . . and the way they just let anybody into the State Department who might be a Communist . . ."

Her impression of American soldiers had also been disillusioning. It surprised her "how little they appreciate opera." She remembered that in Germany the American soldiers would sometimes go to the opera, but "it didn't mean a thing to them. . . . Even with the language problem, I would think that they could have enjoyed the music." She herself missed the opera very much, and there was little opportunity for it here in the States.

Mrs. Silver commented on the amount of prejudice she had noticed in this country. One of her German girl friends was married to an Irishman, and another to an Italian. Each was prejudiced against the other. The idea of prejudice in the United States seemed quite threatening because of her own position as an alien. She said, "People think that all Germans are bad because some did bad things. But I didn't do those things, so why blame me?"

Mrs. Silver's anxiety was diffused among many problems and continued unabated throughout the interviews. She knew a family in Germany who had a child that was born without any arms, "just little stubs." She remembered how the little stubs would move when it tried to make the motions of a normal baby. "I know that such things happen very rarely, but one cannot help but think and wonder."

Most of all, she questioned how she would be able to be a good mother. She had been "so grabby as a child," how would she be able to give? "The baby should be most important. . . . Nothing should matter more than the baby. . . . The mother should take care of the baby and give it love and affection. I want to be a very good mother but do not know if I will know how to be."

Around this time the question also arose whether to keep or sell their house. They were almost sure that Mr. Silver was to be transferred elsewhere. The thought of selling the house was extremely disturbing, especially since one of the rooms had been fixed up as a nursery and "the baby will have so little time in that lovely room."

As the time approached for her delivery, Mrs. Silver became "hungry all the time." She knew she should restrict herself, but a meal without potatoes was especially unsatisfying and she did love sweets. In Germany she had never heard about pregnant women being put on a diet. "There they are allowed to eat all they want. . . . The doctor may want the baby small, but I don't want a small baby." On the other hand, she said she knew that delivery would be easier with a smaller baby. The days began to seem interminable to Mrs. Silver and she especially longed for her mother.

In terms of help after the baby was born Mrs. Silver said that her husband planned to stay home for a while but "what help could he be when he's so afraid?" Also, a German war bride friend who had a three-year-old child said she would come in as much as she could. The final waiting period was quite hard on Mrs. Silver and produced new fears and nightmares.

"Could it be possible that I am going to have twins?" She told of feeling one night that there were "two equal protrusions" on either side of her abdomen. She had also read in one of the papers about "a woman who was told that she was going to have twins, and it turned out to be just one baby that weighed seventeen and one-half pounds!"

Mrs. Silver smilingly confessed that she had indulged herself two days before the anticipated delivery date by buying a pound of chocolate-covered cherries and eating almost all of them herself. Nothing had happened except that she was two pounds heavier!

During the day she felt well, but at night there was discomfort and difficulty in breathing because of the pressure. One night she suddenly realized that she felt no movement at all, and Mr. Silver became even more upset than she. It was a great relief when the baby started to move again after a couple of hours and they could go to sleep. She fervently hoped that labor would start while it was daylight. She hated to think of coming to the hospital in the middle of the night.

In the meantime, "nothing seems to be getting finished up. . . . The baby is delayed and even selling the house seems to be delayed. We have still not found an apartment, but on the other hand, we don't want to go ahead and rent one before we are sure that the house is sold."

At this interview Mrs. Silver was quite determined to breast feed and practically gave a lecture on the advantages of breast feeding, which she had read and learned from various persons. It was not clear whether she was really firmly convinced or was trying to convince herself.

As time went on, Mrs. Silver's questions became more specific. In addition to rooming-in, natural birth, breast or bottle feeding, she asked about "self-demand." Did it mean feeding the baby "every time it cries?" She seemed relieved when told that such frequent feeding was a misinterpretation of ad lib feeding. It was the interviewer's impression that "she now has so many questions about how to take care of the baby, that she does not even know how to begin asking them."

She began to express a great deal of apprehension about delivery and seemed more concerned with how she might act and what people might think of her than about the actual pain. There was also considerable relief at being told that she could have something for pain when needed.

The baby was born seventeen days later than Mrs. Silver had expected, and the pink outfit was required. She explained smilingly that everybody had thought it would be a boy except Mr. Silver. "My husband was right."

The delivery was not easy. Labor lasted approximately twenty-two and one-half hours and was a mid-forceps delivery with episiotomy. The interviewer said that Mrs. Silver was quite courageous throughout the ordeal. The day after the delivery Mrs. Silver remembered that the doctor had tried to turn the baby around and could not. He told her that he had to give her some gas to help a little. When she woke up her hands were strapped down and her legs were still in the stirrups. She started to cry. Then she saw the baby across the room and asked, "Is that my baby?" The doctor asked if she knew what sex it was. She answered "a boy." "No, a girl," he replied.

The baby girl had little resemblance to Mrs. Silver's image of a friend's baby, who had "bright blue eyes and long pigtails arranged around the top of her head." "Poor little Ruth has hardly any hair at all," said her mother, who nevertheless appeared very happy with her "poor little Ruth." To the staff, Ruth's lack of hair was of the least concern. They described her as badly battered up by the mid-forceps delivery, and they were deeply shaken by the sight of her.

The severe molding of her head made it seem as if an "extra head" came out of her skull, and the instrument had left bright red marks on her skin, which was deadly white with a slightly bluish tinge. Her fingernails were dark, and she looked fragile, although not really skinny. Her large mouth was mostly open, as if gasping for air. The observers commented that it was the largest mouth they had ever seen in a baby. There was a ghost-like quality about her, as if she were not fit or ready to live in this world. This impression was accentuated by the oxygen tent, which gave the impression of tragedy "hardly prevented."

Nevertheless, it was soon clear that Ruth's organism was well equipped to fight hard and that one could be sure she would win. If a baby's world centers around its mouth, Ruth found her world soon after birth. In the space of five minutes the right hand was in her mouth and vigorous sucking movements succeeded in quieting her completely.

But success was not always so complete. A later observation at twenty-seven and one-half hours showed the arms moving slowly and constantly in large circles seeking the mouth. They seemed to miss the mouth each time by a fraction of an inch. When the mouth was missed, Ruth tensed with hands fisted and legs flexed stiffly. In another observation at forty-nine and one-half hours Ruth was crying but the intensity increased or decreased depending on the hands' success in reaching the mouth. When contact was established, her crying diminished in intensity. In the mouth the hand became active and the fingers opened and closed, whereupon the hand slipped out. Then Ruth startled, which separated the hand even further from the mouth, and crying reached a peak. This record of tension and relaxation in terms of hand-mouth contact so early in a newborn was quite rare.

It was striking how Ruth's behavioral sequences started with the mouth, which changed readily to push her tongue out, suck, blow, spit, vocalize. Whenever something occurred in her mouth, her arms started to move. At fifty-two hours she was seen lying in prone sucking her right fist, at peace with herself and the world. When her blanket was removed she seemed to wake up, and her hand lost contact with the mouth through greater activity. After the interrupted hand-mouth contact was again made and the blanket restored, Ruth appeared fast asleep.

Ruth's behavior seemed gratifyingly well structured, but always on the over-intense side and accomplished with her whole being. As she matured hour by hour, the observations showed that the hand-to-mouth search proceeded under certain circumstances and not under others. The particular circumstances that prompted or ended the mouth search could not be defined. But whatever the cause, Ruth startled and restartled, occasionally trembling all over. She became red as a poppy, yelled like mad, her breathing became irregular, and she spit up. Her responses seemed almost always to involve the cardio-respiratory, the autonomic, and the sensory-motor systems. The motor response to acoustic stimuli was in all instances a startle. Whereas sound excited her, touch calmed her.

When she started fussing, her mother picked her up and she quieted down immediately. Her head rested on her mother's arm, and she seemed to look at her mother's face. Mrs. Silver commented, "She likes to be picked up and held."

Ruth's response to the blanket removal was immediate. She startled upon its removal and became more active. Upon the blanket's reappearance she calmed down. It seemed that temperature changes also had a rather consistent effect on Ruth, in combination with the sensory modalities of warmth, touch, and change of position. Her movements were well defined in an individualized way. If she was searching for her mouth, her fingers opened one at a time, starting with the index finger and progressing slowly until the little finger, the last one, was stretched out.

Despite the trauma of her birth, the staff was satisfied that Ruth's newborn equipment was not badly organized. If she was not too attractive and startling in some of her responses, she was nevertheless easier to describe and therefore less puzzling than were some newborns.

She seemed more at peace and at ease when relaxed in the prone position with her head turned to the right. In the first few days sleep patterns were poorly integrated, and it was difficult to estimate whether she was asleep or awake. But if differentiation between sleeping and waking is a sign of maturity in infants, by the third day it seemed that Ruth had successfully overcome whatever traumatic damage might have occurred at delivery. At slightly over fifty hours there was no further doubt as to whether Ruth was awake or sleeping.

Breast feeding went well, and the infant had no difficulty in finding the nipple and sucking immediately in a rhythmical and sufficiently strong fashion to be efficacious. Her large mouth permitted her to absorb the entire areola, and her body was relaxed and quiet.

Mrs. Silver cuddled Ruth gently in her right arm, with her hand curved around the baby in her blanket. Her left hand supported her breast, and her head was bent down to Ruth in a tender gesture. When the baby's hand moved from the breast to her own face and sucking became irregular, the mother delicately replaced the little hand on her breast, saying, "What did you do?" Again the baby's hand moved towards her mouth and the scene repeated itself. Mrs. Silver gave up and allowed the hand to remain close to the mouth.

Upon Ruth's dismissal from the hospital the pediatrician wrote, "This is a well-developed baby girl of six days, moderately active and not unattractive. Her cry is vigorous, respiration normal, and there is no evidence of congenital defect or cerebral injury."

The pediatrician's opinion was shared by the interviewers, who felt that there was something decidedly attractive about Ruth despite the large mouth and ghost-like appearance. An "intensity" or "liveliness" appeared in the small organism, and there was positive response to the human contact of touch, warmth, and being held. For Mrs. Silver, who wanted a baby all for herself, it augured well that her wish would be fulfilled.

The house to which Ruth was taken by her mother was immaculately clean, new looking, and tastefully furnished with contemporary furniture. There were a number of books on the shelves, including that of Spock, several recent novels, a couple of encyclopedias, and a copy of *Mein Kampf*. But her stay there was of short duration.

Approximately two and one-half months later the house was sold and the Silvers moved into the third floor of a large, freshly painted white frame-house, with a spacious and inviting back yard. The kitchen was large and sunny and held Ruth's playpen. The living room was not as light as the kitchen but had the same tasteful furniture. The Silvers' bedroom had everything except their bed, which had been placed in Ruth's room. Mr. Silver insisted that they sleep in Ruth's room lest "something happen," and he made even more trips to the crib during the night than did his wife. Mrs. Silver worried if Ruth slept too long because she was fearful of smothering and Ruth "had a habit of pulling the blanket over her head."

She also worried about Ruth's color changes. "Could Ruth have inherited the heart condition of Mrs. Silver's mother and aunt? Why do her feet turn blue in the bath? Ruthie breathes heavily and excitedly when we pick her up. Is this the beginning of seizures and convulsions?"

She compared Ruth with a girl friend's baby boy, who had rolls of fat, while "my poor little Ruth is so much smaller." The pediatrician assured her that Ruth was doing very nicely, but Mrs. Silver was still unconvinced. However, nothing of this anxiety was visible in Mrs. Silver's contacts with Ruth, whom she handled with the utmost ease, competence, and warmth.

Mrs. Silver found it quite hard to take care of a young baby and also get her housework done. The baby kept her busy until nine o'clock in the evening. Mr. Silver helped with the house cleaning, but he was not of great help with Ruth, as he was afraid to handle her.

Mrs. Silver soon recovered her good looks, and at her first appointment with the interviewer she appeared quite glamorous in a red flaring overcoat and snugly fitting clothes. As she waited for the bus, a man offered her a ride in his car, which she refused but was pleased that it had been offered. She told the interviewer flatly that she did not want any more children, and "I mean it."

Her aversion to having more children stemmed from the many anxieties about Ruth and the fear that her husband would be called away, leaving her alone to cope with life. Mrs. Silver dreaded being alone at any time and laughingly recounted that when she and a girl friend were alone in the apartment they heard noises and barricaded the door. She had not been nearly so scared in Germany, but "horrible things happen in this country." She read of them constantly in the newspapers.

The urge to see her mother remained strong. She said that as soon as she had her citizenship papers, she wanted to visit Germany, whether or not her husband could join her. She had sent Ruth's photo to her mother, but "would like to show her the real Ruth."

Mrs. Silver was quite the proud mother and found her daughter cute, "even if other people might think her homely." She said Ruth was homely only when she cried, and she could not stand Ruth to cry. "It is unfair that such little babies should feel uncomfortable." At Ruth's slightest cry, her mother picked her up and comforted her in a soft musical voice. If this did not help, Mrs. Silver herself started to cry.

Her solicitude for the child knew no bounds. In the Silver household, by mutual consent, life revolved about Ruth's needs. Her mother was willing to abjure all opportunities for contact with the outside world in order to care for her. And her father proved himself a surpassingly anxious parent who could scarcely take his eyes from his "beautiful little daughter."

When Ruth was one month and nine days old Mrs. Silver went for her first obstetrical checkup to the hospital. It was the first separation from Ruth, who had been left with her father. Mrs. Silver called home several times to be assured that all was well. After the interview, but before the obstetrical checkup, she again telephoned. Suddenly she looked as if she would faint and rushed away without having the checkup.

Later it was learned that the nervous father had tried to give Ruth a bottle, which she took quite well at first but then suddenly turned pale. Her father believed she would die. In alarm he called a neighbor, who burped Ruth and thought that she was all right. When Mrs. Silver arrived home in an agony of fear, Ruth was rosily and peacefully asleep.

Breast feeding had gone well in the hospital, but at home Ruth seemed to suck slowly and to interrupt herself for periods of five minutes or longer. Mrs. Silver complained that she did not seem satisfied with her morning feeding. The pediatrician advised substituting a bottle for the morning feeding. It was not surprising that breast feeding decreased to one a day and finally was completely abandoned when Ruth was three months old. "There is not enough milk to be worth continuing," her mother said.

The switch to the bottle was made because of her anxiety that Ruth did not get enough milk. Throughout, Mrs. Silver's expectation was that a healthy baby should be plump, and because Ruth seemed to be a small child, she attempted in every way to make her eat more. At first Ruth did not like the bottle, but she then began to take her formula well and weaning apparently did not present any great problem. In addition to the formula Ruth also took her solids well. From two months on, she flushed rather than paled during feeding.

Ruth was not the kind of child who was difficult to put to sleep. She slept well at night and awakened only for her feeding. By three months of age she mostly slept through the night and rarely asked for a meal. At four months she could be counted on to sleep from 6 or 7 P.M. in the evening until 6 A.M. in the morning. Her favored sleep position during the first weeks was in prone, but at two months she preferred to go to sleep on her back or side. A month later she definitely refused to be put down in prone and slept in supine. At four months her left arm always lay over her eyes in sleep.

From two and one-half months on, she was reported to have "found her thumb." At three months Mr. Silver called to ask whether it was "all right for Ruth to sleep alone in her room." Apparently the reassurance was insufficient, for at a later interview it was found that the parents' bed was still in Ruth's bedroom.

At first Ruth did not like to be undressed or have a bath, but by four months she was happier without clothes and enjoyed her bath very much. She was quite sensitive to touch, and showed frequent color changes of her skin. Noises did not disturb her except when she was just falling asleep and then she startled. She lifted her head well when in prone and was exceedingly well developed for her age.

She was most responsive to visual stimulation. When she saw people she cooed and chuckled, grunted and squealed at toys or objects in the room, was excited in anticipation of being picked up, and smiled at her mirror image. At 3 months (13 weeks) the Gesell tests placed her between the 16- to 20-week levels. On the whole, she was a docile, placid child who developed well and gave her parents no particular difficulties in management. She was not given to excessive crying, but her parents were intolerant of any wails. It was their feeling that "babies should not have to cry if their parents properly fulfill their responsibilities."

The observation of Ruth at the well-baby clinic during the fourth month bore out that Ruth was basically a happy baby. The "poor little Ruth" impression was entirely gone. She was not only healthy but robust looking, with a round and full body, and a smooth, white and rosy skin. Her hair was silky, thin and blond, and her definitely blue eyes were quite striking. They were wide-set and large and concentrated intently on people and the environment.

At four months of age it appeared that Ruth had begun to discriminate strangers, and she displayed a somewhat cautious reaction to the pediatrician. While she was not acutely frightened, she evidenced some restraint and could be comforted only by her mother. No matter how deeply upset, she could always be comforted by her mother.

The tie between mother and child was so strong that as long as her mother was near, Ruth was not even interested in toys. Her mother's presence was sufficient to absorb all of Ruth's interest, and the world to Ruth was only one object, her mother. She provided the impulse to move, to act, to live. Everything was judged by its likeness to this one object and could be enjoyed only if the mother also liked or did not object to this enjoyment.

When Ruth was on her mother's lap, her left hand was used predominantly. When she was separated from her mother's lap, the right hand was more consistently used and became the center of activity. Play objects did not yet provide any real diversion. Although she mouthed the objects, they had no meaning in themselves, just happening to be in the hand as it journeyed to the mouth to be sucked.

All in all, there was a general feeling of health and happiness about Ruth. A happy child is gratifying to a mother, and in spite of her expressed worries we saw that Mrs. Silver enjoyed Ruth and therefore created conditions under which Ruth might develop well.

From the sixth month on, although Ruth's parents continued to worry about every developmental change as possibly abnormal or pathological, their worries seemed to have calmed down somewhat. Mrs. Silver was frightened of the injections and preferred that her husband be the one present when they were given. She was concerned that Ruth should not handle anything which might have fallen on the floor, and she warned her husband about the dangers to come when Ruth started to crawl. He concurred anxiously that "little children need watching" and referred to "freak accidents like falling into the washing machine," of which he had read. For this reason the pediatrician believed that Mrs. Silver did not encourage Ruth to move a great deal.

Otherwise Mrs. Silver was delighted with Ruth and proud of her accomplishments. "We think that Ruth is doing just fine, and we're pretty lucky to have such a good baby." In general Mrs. Silver had greater peace of mind, partly due to Ruth's smooth development and partly because her husband refused to take a post elsewhere, even with a promotion, rather than separate from his family. She was both relieved and reassured that there would be no drastic change in their life.

Ruth had never been a big eater and still was not. It took her considerable time to finish a meal, and she had neither great appetite nor enthusiasm. "She simply does not feel about food the same way as the neighbor's baby does," Mrs. Silver said. However she appeared philosophical about it.

During this period Ruth learned a number of things and was able to amuse herself in her crib with toys or with a string from the bumper. Sometimes she was interested in her feet as a toy substitute, and if toys were out of reach she pushed them nearer with her feet. At the sight of her mother, Ruth's face would light up joyously and she began to imitate the mother's hand gestures and her head-shaking "no." She did not yet crawl but otherwise was well developed, had good grasping patterns, rich and varied vocalization, and a great faculty for imitating. "She looks wonderfully well," the pediatrician commented, "and she never seems to cry at home."

In the well-baby clinic at six months Ruth's stranger reaction was more marked. She screamed at first, and her mother had to pick her up to comfort her. After ten minutes she became less anxious but was still perturbed. It was clear that she could sharply differentiate between people. However the stranger anxiety was still mild and Ruth was tested easily. She even smiled at the pediatrician fairly early in the examination.

The need for constant visual contact with her mother had diminished somewhat, and Ruth's responses to the test material and the toys were more immediate and of longer duration. Her right hand was still the more active in contacting objects, but both hands were used equally for mouthing. She seemed to derive the same comfort from mouthing objects as she formerly had from her thumb. Mrs. Silver occasionally interfered with her mouthing.

While Ruth's development had progressed satisfactorily, a perceptible change was seen in her mother, who for the first time showed some irritation and was not quite so gentle as before. To the staff it appeared that Mrs. Silver was reacting to Ruth's growing independence.

The Silvers' apartment remained in a rather unfinished state, as Mrs. Silver had no time to sew curtains nor was she inclined to fix up the bedrooms. Ruth and her mother spent afternoons in the park, where they were accustomed to meet Mrs. Silver's girl friend and baby, with whom they socialized.

When Ruth was seven months old the interviewer reported that she found the apartment immaculately clean. Even the rubber toys were so scrubbed that all the paint was gone from them. Although Mrs. Silver looked attractive, well groomed, and friendly, she seemed somehow ill at ease and apologized that the house did not look as it should because every waking moment was so consumed with Ruth.

Mr. Silver so objected to leaving Ruth alone at any time that he strung up a laundry line in the living room so that his wife needn't leave the house. He also did not agree to a high chair because Ruth might fall out of it, and he was against taking Ruth to other people's houses where she might catch a disease. Thus, social life was limited to a bare minimum, and Mrs. Silver complained that he thought of nobody but Ruth and that she "was nothing but Ruth's mother" to him.

This was not to say that Mrs. Silver was less attached to her daughter. She lovingly anticipated Ruth's every wish, she spent much time with her in gentle play, and she exercised zealous care that Ruth should touch nothing dirty. The usually immaculate housekeeping was augmented by daily scrubbings of the floor as the child began to creep.

The suggestion of difficulties in the Silver home became a reality with Mrs. Silver's case of the flu a month and a half later. Both parents panicked that Ruth might catch it. The pediatrician advised Mr. Silver to take over the baby's care, since he remained at home during his wife's illness. But this was easier said than done. He was unsuccessful in feeding Ruth, who sensed his anxiety and twisted her head from side to side so that "he just could not manage it." Finally her mother had to feed her after all.

He also couldn't manage her bath, and Mrs. Silver had to take over and give Ruth a daily sponge bath. About all he could do, according to his wife, "was to put some clothes on her," but even then he needed assistance with the sweater. He was unsatisfactory in changing diapers and Ruth developed a rash. Moreover, he proved to be a poor housekeeper, and Mrs. Silver worried about the accumulation of dirt in her home. When he took Ruth out for the daily walk he pushed the carriage along the gutter, afraid to tilt it in getting up and down curbs. Mrs. Silver said, "The neighbors must have thought he is out of his mind."

It was hard for Mrs. Silver to lie there and watch the zealous but ineffectual efforts of her husband. "He did what he could, but after all, he is only a man." Mrs. Silver was left tired and exhausted after her illness. Soon other problems developed: a vaginal discharge that did not disappear after medication, and some fluid discharge from her breast. The only two explanations that came to her mind were "pregnancy" or "cancer." It seemed that both carried equal dread for her.

As Christmas approached Mrs. Silver was nostalgic for the family celebrations of other years in Germany, with a large tree, gaiety, and singing around the table. Mr. Silver also looked forward to having a tree because as a Jewish child he had felt cheated out of

Christmas. Both hoped that Ruth would enjoy the tree and not be scared of it. As for singing, Mrs. Silver commented that "it would be silly with just us two around the table."

Ruth had a slight respiratory illness in her seventh month, but it did not seem to excite her parents particularly. Later Mrs. Silver became concerned about poor eating and a possible weight loss. However, the pediatrician found her weight the same, and she looked rosy and healthy.

Mrs. Silver's concern about Ruth's eating nevertheless persisted. She thought that solids were terribly important for a child of this age, and she tried to distract Ruth in many ways in order to get additional spoons of food into her mouth. To reassure Mrs. Silver the pediatrician prescribed vitamins, and two weeks later Mrs. Silver reported that "they worked wonders" as Ruth's appetite had increased.

At 7 months and 17 days (33 weeks) Ruth's developmental quotient on the Viennese test was 128. Her general maturity level on the Gesell tests was on the 39-week level, with a developmental quotient of 118.

Night sleeping and naps continued to be problem-free. Up to eight and one-half months Ruth napped for half an hour in the morning and early afternoon. Then she stopped sleeping during these periods but vocalized and played in her crib. There was never a problem in putting her to bed, and she never woke up crying in the morning. Her elimination was always regular, and Mrs. Silver never expressed any worries in this connection. It appeared to the pediatrician that Mrs. Silver was hesitant to start toilet training. She said that she did not mind diaper washing and that it was too early and might be hard on Ruth.

Baby Ruth knew how to keep herself busy without relying on toys. She interested herself in banging coasters, tearing up old magazines, playing with her father's old gloves. As might be expected, both Mr. and Mrs. Silver took great pleasure in Ruth's developing abilities and devised many little games to keep their daughter amused. Throughout the entire period of study, her level of development was above average.

In all her waking moments Ruth Silver enjoyed the attention of one or both of her parents, but she rarely saw outsiders. This, plus acute visual perception of her surroundings, might have been partly responsible for her marked anxiety with strangers and new situations. Thus, at the next well-baby clinic she screamed with fear and never once lost sight of her mother's face. The pediatrician commented that this was "the most marked stranger anxiety she had ever seen."

When Ruth was nine months old she screamed with fright not only at rearrangements of the furniture in her house but at changes in her mother's clothing or hairdo. Mrs. Silver said that Ruth would not let anybody touch or take care of her, and she worried "about how badly Ruth will behave" at the next clinic visit. However, it did not turn out badly because Ruth was tested on her mother's lap, and as long as her mother was around, she did not object to being in the playpen. She still did not crawl around a lot but otherwise was active and vigorous. Her mother called her a "happy little girl who enjoys life tremendously." The pediatrician found her attractive and responsive.

Between the ninth and tenth months Mrs. Silver reported proudly that Ruth "must be a German girl because she likes potatoes so well." She ate well, but only if distracted and amused, and she had not yet started to hold the bottle herself. At mealtimes she held a toy in her hand and passively permitted her mother to coax her into eating. Once her parents gave her a bit of meat, but she choked, frightening them out of their wits.

Some changes in her behavior began to be seen. If she was prohibited, Ruth became quite furious and red in the face, doubled her hands into fists, stiffened, and shook. If something was out of her reach, she would determinedly take her mother's hand and move it to the desired object. If her mother didn't join her in play, she would "just sit around and moan." Her anxiety towards the stranger was diminishing, but she seemed to have developed definite fear reactions to certain toys, particularly a little black furry dog which she dared not touch.

While she did not yet creep on hands and knees, she got around well in a kind of rolling and hitching motion. Her fine motor development was more advanced for her age than the gross motor development. She was beyond her age in adaptive behavior, language production, and language comprehension. She started to show an interest in picture books and television.

Mr. Silver had long wanted to buy a television set, but his wife did not believe in going into debt for such luxuries. At last they bought one. For several nights they looked at it until the wee hours and Ruth awoke to join them in viewing. Mrs. Silver commented that "the stuff was not worth looking at" and that she "preferred to read a good book anytime." However, the television served a good purpose in motivating them to rearrange the living room furniture, which now looked more attractive.

Mrs. Silver would have liked to purchase some original paintings by young artists for the wall, but she realized that it took time to select pictures and she did not dare to leave Ruth for more than half an hour. She would not entrust her to a baby-sitter, as she had read that "terrible things can happen, like the strangling of a nineteen-month-old baby by a baby-sitter." It was hard not to have a relative available so she could get out more, and Mrs. Silver complained that social life was very limited.

At the interviewer's next visit she broke into tears because she was so lonely and had nobody to talk to. The people she knew here were hardly the ones she would choose. In Germany she was happy-go-lucky and did interesting work. "But Ruth needs me and Ruth's happiness is all I want."

In speaking of her loneliness, she said that her family all now lived in West Germany and were very badly off. Her stepfather was without a job and her stepsister, a bright girl of seventeen, had to interrupt schooling to accept domestic placement. The uncle who had been a high Nazi official was waiting for his de-Nazification. He was in a camp where "Negro soldiers deliberately threw things on the floor and made the German officers pick them up." Mrs. Silver said that her uncle hated the Americans, and she could partly understand his resentment "because some GI's behaved very badly."

A month after this discussion Mrs. Silver's worries again shifted to her health. She had lost weight and was fearful of having contracted tuberculosis. "What would happen to Ruth if I had to go to a sanatorium?" She did not take her temperature, however, and no X-rays were made. No illnesses were reported for Ruth.

Ruth's interest in food was still limited, and she had acquired some definite likes and dislikes. She favored eggs so much that the parents gave up their eggs at breakfast for fear Ruth might insist on eating them and they might be too much for her. She also developed the habit of gagging on lumpy foods, so Mrs. Silver avoided anything the slightest bit lumpy. Usually Ruth refused chopped or junior foods, but she liked mashed home foods prepared by her mother. Generally she was wary of new foods.

At 10 months and 9 days (44 weeks) Ruth's developmental quotient on the Viennese test was 128. On the Gesell test her general maturity level was 53 weeks and her developmental quotient 120.

In the eleventh month a toilet seat was purchased and training began. It seemed a huge success. Mrs. Silver would place Ruth on the toilet after the morning bottle, and this seemed to be an appropriate time for Ruth to respond. In the afternoons Ruth announced her need for toileting by grunting and saying "aach."

During the second year of her life Ruth continued to be a rather advanced child, somewhat small but very attractive to those who saw her. The general pattern of her environment did not change markedly, and her parents continued to sleep in her bedroom despite several abortive attempts to move into their own quarters. Feeding continued to be discouraging to Mrs. Silver, but unproblematic from the point of view of the study staff. In order to overcome Ruth's "lack of interest" in eating, the Silvers devised all sorts of distractions. In this and other ways her parents tried to keep her always happy. It was the opinion of the study staff that "if it would help, her father would have been glad to stand on his head for her." The same could be said for her mother.

Surrounded by such solicitude, Ruth expected always to get what she wanted. Deprived to a large degree of outside contacts, she demanded the constant presence of mother and/or father. As she became mobile and exploratory, this insistence on adult attention increased. Any illness accentuated the child's demandingness. As with all children, it became increasingly necessary to discipline her during the second year.

Mrs. Silver utilized a whole hierarchy of management devices, ranging from substitution and prearrangement to verbal prohibitions and an occasional slight spank. Games were frequently used to elicit Ruth's cooperation. But if the child remained obdurate or sulked at a scolding or a light slap, her parents typically capitulated and gave her what she wanted. As for Mr. Silver, he refused to discipline his daughter at all: "I have too little time with her to spoil it with that!"

In the twelfth month some sleeping problems started. When Ruth was put to bed at 5:30 she could not fall asleep and cried. She also showed resistance to her afternoon nap. Her mother coped with these problems by allowing Ruth to remain up during the parents' supper time, after which she readily went to sleep. Also, her naps were postponed until times when Ruth was more receptive. All in all, her mother was able to recognize clearly whether or not Ruth was sleepy and accommodated herself to it.

At the beginning of Ruth's second year the sleeping problems became somewhat more acute. She woke up at 5 A.M. and insisted on being entertained. Although she was dead tired during the day, she resisted morning and afternoon naps but succumbed to an hour and a half sleep around 5:30 or 6:00 P.M. Then she would wake again. Mrs. Silver found herself completely exhausted by the end of the day.

Her parents considered changing the sleeping arrangements but without confidence that it would work. Two attempts were made during Ruth's fourteenth month. Once she was moved into their bedless bedroom, but she objected. Then they tried to sleep in their own room, leaving Ruth in hers. Ruth slept very well but Mrs. Silver hardly closed an eye. After three days the Silvers' bed was again placed in Ruth's room. In contrast to her early months, Ruth's sleep was now very light.

During this period Ruth seemed to have a greater need for motion. She fussed to leave her mother's lap and did not want to stay in the playpen anymore. She was able to pull herself to standing and cruise around an object, and she crawled from room to room through the whole apartment, even venturing into the unfamiliar bedroom of her parents.

The outstanding feature at this time was her wish and capacity for communication. She imitated sounds so that they sounded like words and conversation. She vocalized almost constantly at home, said "bye-bye" and played pat-a-cake spontaneously. She became most interested in household objects, pots and pans, spoons and bric-a-brac, from which her mother tried to distract her. But Ruth had a mind of her own and constantly returned to the object of her original interest. Her mother needed to interfere quite forcibly before Ruth desisted.

New situations and experiences continued to produce stranger anxiety in Ruth. Under such circumstances she started to use a very artificial smile, which looked like a "switched-on" grimace of the mouth while the eyes remained serious, frightened, and even sad. This smile appeared on her face whenever she felt ill at ease or uncomfortable. At her first party with other children Ruth clung to her mother and yelled at the top of her lungs when a child approached her.

At 1 year, 1 month, and 12 days (13½ months) on the Viennese tests Ruth's developmental age was 1 year, 4 months, and 19 days. Her development quotient was 124. On the Gesell tests her general maturity level was 15 months and 12 days, with a development quotient of 114.

Mrs. Silver's preoccupation with her own health continued during the early part of Ruth's second year. The X-rays proved negative in regard to tuberculosis but soon Mrs. Silver began to report "terrific headaches." Recognizing her need for distraction, she occasionally went to the theater or movies with a girl friend while her husband cared for Ruth. As long as it did not involve any extensive physical handling, he now seemed able to cope with her.

The staff saw Mrs. Silver's various physical symptoms as reactions to events which were disturbing to her. One was Ruth's development toward greater independence and less tractability. Another troublesome concern was the financial situation, because her husband had to provide substantial support for his aging parents. His ailing father could no longer work. Once Mr. Silver had suggested that it would be cheaper if his parents lived with them, and this prospect was most alarming to Mrs. Silver. She said that her parents-in-law were strangers to her, their kosher food was not her food, and she couldn't see why the daughter in Florida could not provide them with a home.

When she was fourteen months old Ruth had a small uneventful bout with diarrhea, which was well handled by her mother. After a few days of somewhat restricted diet she returned to normal. In general, she became more interested in food than before and took a sudden liking for Coke. Mrs. Silver was relieved to hear that this would not harm her. She continued to be a light sleeper, and her mother had to be absolutely quiet or Ruth would be disturbed.

Ruth was now a charming mixture of coyness and friendliness. She approached strangers in a flirtatious way and seemed perfectly at ease with them. She was very tender and affectionate towards a toy bunny, but continued to neglect most of her toys. The telephone had captured her attention and she tried to dial.

With the increase of mobility it was not surprising that Mrs. Silver had to resort to more "no's." Ruth talked all day long and loved to play peek-a-boo with her parents for hours. When she fell, she did not wait to be picked up by her mother, but said "up" and went on with her activity. Only if she was really hurt did she walk over to her mother for consolation.

The well-baby clinic evaluation disclosed that Ruth still had some difficulty in separating from her mother. She whimpered when put down on the floor unless her mother stayed close to her, and she did not touch any toys unless they were first offered by her mother. One could see the result of her mother's efforts to prohibit mouthing. Ruth did little mouth experimenting with toys or material. Before reaching for something, she seemed deliberately to postpone herself, as if awaiting possible prohibitions.

She walked surprisingly well, with coordination and security, and had also developed both a sidewards and backwards walk, which helped to maintain visual contact with her mother in whatever direction she went. She was deft in picking something up from the standing position and showed good body mastery. The artificial smile was still there, but now it seemed to have acquired the specific communicative function of seeking permission or warding off interference. Ruth had acquired a number of new words and could imitate whatever word she was asked to imitate. She moved easily, vocalized considerably, and played more vigorously. However, Mrs. Silver appeared to be inhibited and rather tense during the observation.

Between Ruth's fourteenth and seventeenth months Mrs. Silver became even more bothered and worried about her health. The unbearable headaches reminded her of the migraines she suffered as an adolescent. She could not take the pills prescribed by the doctor because they made her drowsy and interfered with her care of Ruth. Fortunately the headaches began to disappear even without medication, but then she developed an irritating throat-ache, which she differentiated from a sore throat. The threat of cancer arose. "What would happen to Ruth if I died? It would be hard for a child to be without her mother and life would not be the same anymore." She recalled her own feelings when her mother had remarried.

Mrs. Silver asked her interviewer to arrange for a thorough checkup and complained that "doctors were always in such a hurry." After the checkup her symptoms still remained. One and a half months later she was again in the middle of a thorough checkup. In the course of wandering from one doctor to another, she saw an internist, an obstetrician, an orthopedist, and others. None of them found anything, but her troubles persisted and were even augmented. In addition to the headaches and throat-aches, she had pains in her shoulder and back, constantly saw a speck before her eyes, and felt very, very tired. Every practitioner whom she consulted told her that the problems were functional and many suggested psychiatric help.

It made her feel even worse because she could not stop worrying. At night she woke up feeling "there is no one to turn to, no one with whom to share the responsibility. . . . I am so alone and my family so far away." She made no reference to her husband as a possible source of moral support and only commented that he would be completely unable to care for Ruth if something serious should happen to her.

The relationship between Mr. and Mrs. Silver seemed, superficially at least, to be compatible. Mrs. Silver constantly reported how "good" her husband was to her and compared him favorably with the spouses of acquaintances. Mr. Silver was, in fact, as anxious and solicitous of her welfare as he was of Ruth's. Although he stood a good chance of winning a promotion, he failed to pursue it because it involved periods of sea duty and he could not bear to frighten Mrs. Silver by leaving her alone.

When she complained of not feeling well, he was not only sympathetic but concerned to leave no stone unturned in tracking down the cause of her maladies. Yet although he was gentle and solicitous, he could not help transmitting his own anxieties. Unable to cope decisively with domestic situations, he proved to be a poor leaning post and gave Mrs. Silver little real psychological support.

Characterizing herself as "a very dependent kind of person," Mrs. Silver expressed the hope that Ruth would not grow up to be like that. She felt that responsibility for a home and a baby was a difficult experience for her, very different from what it had been with her first marriage. This was mentioned very casually as though it had been frequently discussed.

Thus, for the first time in the study it was inadvertently learned that Mrs. Silver had not been totally innocent or sexually untouched during the war years. Actually she had been married to a German soldier and had had a spontaneous abortion in the third month of pregnancy. This fact may not have been mentioned earlier by Mrs. Silver because of her understanding that the study was for mothers having their first pregnancy. Conceivably she may have concealed the earlier pregnancy lest she be excluded from the study.

Mrs. Silver recounted that while she was working for the wealthy estate owner she met the man who became her first husband. He was a "tall, blond, and handsome twenty-six-year-old officer in the Luftwaffe and a law school graduate." After six months' courtship she was married at the age of eighteen against her mother's wish. But her bliss ended all too soon. Her husband was transferred to France, from where he sent her many beautiful clothes. "I have never since been dressed so well."

Later he returned to Germany as a paratrooper but subsequently was drowned in the Rhine while trying to save one of his friends. At that time Mrs. Silver was already pregnant but soon lost the baby. She felt that she aborted "due to the strain of putting on and taking off her heavy boots." At first she mourned deeply for the loss of this baby, but then felt it might be better not to have a baby under the circumstances.

Mrs. Silver now reported that her family in Germany was better off and had a five-room apartment. She hoped to visit them in two years, when "Ruth would be old enough to remember the trip." She said, "Maybe I should never have left Germany!" There she had had no responsibilities or symptoms of ill health.

Her social life remained as sparse and unsatisfactory as ever. Because they refused to leave Ruth with a baby-sitter, the Silvers went nowhere together. Even a visit to a girl friend in Boston had to be abandoned because her husband couldn't lose that much time from work. Mrs. Silver wanted to go alone with Ruth, but her husband felt it might be too much for the baby. In her eagerness for some change of scene Mrs. Silver even looked forward to a visit with her in-laws in New York!

Her only diversion was the daily excursions to the beach with Ruth. She said, "Maybe the sun will bake all the troubles out of me." Ruth was self-sufficient at the beach and quite adventurous in the water. Her mother said she had to watch her closely. Ruth was also inclined to do the opposite of what she was asked. This was hard for Mrs. Silver, who became impatient and over-disciplinarian at times. On occasion she slapped Ruth's hand and spanked her on the behind. It seemed to the interviewer that "a real battle of will" had developed between mother and daughter.

Mrs. Silver was also irritated that Ruth trailed her wherever she went and kept her from accomplishing the housework. She was also resentful of the mess Ruth made in water play. Another thing that bothered her was that Ruth did not defend herself against other children. Ruth's newly acquired habit of grinding her teeth was particularly objectionable. When she did it, her mother pinched the sides of her mouth, saying sharply, "Stop that!" But Ruth resumed the offensive trait as soon as the mother's hands were removed.

During this period Ruth ran a high fever and developed roseola. Both parents were solicitous to the point of permitting her to become an absolute tyrant. In order to get Ruth to take aspirin they resorted to every conceivable device. Ruth sensed their apprehension and refused the pill every time. The pediatrician visited often during this illness, and Mrs. Silver was genuinely grateful for her help and attention. At this time Mrs. Silver spoke more warmly about her husband than ever before, especially to say that she did not know how she would have managed during Ruth's illness without his help.

Finally Mrs. Silver stopped worrying about Ruth's eating and was convinced that the food intake was adequate. Ruth still disliked junior foods but had developed a taste for meat and chicken. She did not like to feed herself, except that she would finger-feed from her mother's plate, and all milk was still taken from the bottle. At nineteen months she first started to use the spoon. Her mealtime still remained quite a production. While watching a television program, and occupied with a toy in her hand as well as a picture book in front of her, Ruth hardly noticed that she was being fed.

During the next five weeks sleeping became a real problem. Ruth would not go to sleep in her crib so she was put on the couch or her parents' bed, or would fall asleep cuddled in their arms. She would awaken several times during the night and had to be taken into the parents' bed until she again fell asleep. It was quite disruptive to their rest. The sleep difficulty ran its course, and then Ruth's regular patterns were restored.

At about nineteen months Ruth had all her bowel movements on the potty and was very proud of it. If she had an accident, she was ashamed and insisted on being changed immediately. She had become especially attached to a yellow blanket with satin binding that she called "mom." She rubbed the satin and woolly parts alternately against her face and sucked her right thumb.

Her disposition during this period was not regarded as sunny. She was described several times as "smiling less" than before and being "in a cross mood, half whining, half crying." The staff was not certain whether this was due to a real change of temperament or to the tense maternal atmosphere. Ruth would not take "no" for an answer and responded to the threat of spanking by withdrawal and a reproachful look. She went on with forbidden activities despite her mother's prohibitions, then substituted another activity equally annoying to her mother.

Despite the apparent antagonism between them, Ruth wanted her mother's presence and full attention. If Mrs. Silver closed the bathroom door for privacy, Ruth ordered "open up." But Ruth no longer wanted her mother's cuddling. With an unmistakable gesture she indicated to the mother that she should sit in a chair across the room. Only if Ruth fell and really hurt herself did she want to be picked up.

Ruth enjoyed being admired by people but kept them at a distance with a display of friendliness but reserve. She liked older children who were nice to her but left her alone. Her interest in toys was still limited except for a doll which she hugged and carried around. Most of all she loved water play, with which she busied herself for hours. It was hard to get her out of the water at the beach, and she adored the big bathtub at home.

Ruth liked to run around naked but began also to be very fond of being dressed up. She would go to the mirror and admiringly say "pretty." She did not help with her own dressing except for attempting to lace her shoes. Although she had a large vocabulary, she preferred to make up names for certain objects and activities which she consistenty used, and she became quite angry if one did not understand her.

The furniture had again been rearranged in the Silvers' living room, which looked very clean but cheerless. The reason for this rearrangement was that Ruth had taken to opening the door leading to the fire-escape porch. Therefore the sofa was placed against the door. Now Mrs. Silver had to move the sofa each time she wanted to use the clothesline — quite an inconvenience.

During this time Mr. Silver's father was hospitalized with a "ruptured stomach," and Mrs. Silver was again concerned about the possibility of additional financial obligations. When she first heard about it, she got one of her unbearable spells of headache. Otherwise, the headaches were better now, but the throat still ached, and she was bothered by lymph nodes behind her ears. The doctor advised her "to stop running to doctors" and said her husband should help her to relax.

Mr. Silver suggested inviting his wife's stepsister from Germany to visit but this proved to be impossible and was a further source of unhappiness. Minor irritations nagged at her: discomfort with the American language; the feeling that her table manners were wrong in this country. "In Germany it was not important to shave one's legs or have perfect makeup." Trifles grew out of proportion. The noise of the dry cleaning establishment in the next building "was driving her crazy." But she was fearful and refused to sign a petition to regulate the hours when the machine could operate.

Ruth's thumb-sucking was increasingly hard for Mrs. Silver to tolerate, and she wondered "whether Dr. Spock was correct in saying that thumb-sucking was a sign of not enough stimulation and affection. . . . Surely this is not true for Ruth." The result of these difficulties made her more impatient and disciplinary with Ruth.

The earlier toilet training success broke down almost completely. Ruth cried when put on the seat and refused to sit on it. She reported her bowel movement only after it happened. Mrs. Silver told the interviewer laconically, "It's too late for us to do anything about this now."

There was no doubt that Ruth had become adventurous. She would not stay on her mother's lap, climbed on tables and chairs, ran away, and wanted to be chased. She was also noisy and banged whatever she could lay her hands on. Prohibitions were still without success, and if the parents tried to slap her, she slapped back, saying "smack." It became a hilarious game with her.

At the well-baby clinic evaluation in Ruth's twentieth month both mother and child seemed out of kilter. Both of them looked fatigued and Ruth's hair was not well combed or shiny. Mrs. Silver exerted more direct control over Ruth and tried to force her to remain in the testing chair. With the testing material Ruth seemed sure of herself only when she received adult assurance and approval, otherwise she was inhibited.

During interviews in the following two months it was noticed that the Silvers' apartment had once more been completely rearranged. Now the former living room was Ruth's room so as to give her more space, and the Silvers' old bedroom had become the living room. It was a chilly, fairly unattractive place, much cluttered with Ruth's toys.

The Silvers finally visited their friends in Boston and seemed to have enjoyed the trip. Mrs. Silver got along very well with her friends, and Ruth had fun with their little boy. However, an unpleasant episode occurred on the return train trip, when a Negro soldier persisted in speaking to Mrs. Silver. She said, "He was quite drunk and offered to show her New York." Then he became very hostile upon learning that she came from Germany, and "he mentioned that his brother was killed by the Germans."

Although Mrs. Silver's health was fortunately much better, she was hardly in a rosy mood during this period. Christmas was again disappointing. Their futile efforts to trim a crooked little tree reminded her once more of the beautiful tree in her grandfather's house, which he so carefully decorated with the assistance of the whole family. Mrs. Silver believed that all the presents they had chosen for Ruth were mistakes and that the celebration excited her to the extent that she grew pale.

Also, Mrs. Silver suspected that her parents-in-law lacked affection for Ruth, and she became resentful towards them. There was also impatience with her girl friends and their limited interests. Further, she was sick and tired of Dr. Spock's new child-rearing dogma, "Avoid frustration!" She said, "That's just what I am — frustrated." She said, "A child should learn that it cannot have whatever it wants, or do entirely as it wants." And she commented that it was utterly "unfair that I am always the one to discipline Ruth because my husband fails to do so."

Ruth had been exposed to mumps and came down with it. Mrs. Silver herself diagnosed the illness and was more amused than perturbed by Ruth's appearance. She became concerned only when Ruth refused liquids and her temperature rose. Then she called the pediatrician in some alarm. Mr. Silver, who had never had mumps, was only slightly concerned that he might catch them. But he declined to separate from his family, "as he probably could not catch anything bad from a little girl as cute and sweet as Ruth." The pediatrician was more realistic with her warning that "mumps is mumps."

Ruth ate a variety of foods at this time but was very positive about her likes and dislikes. Sleeping was also well in hand, and Ruth slept through the night as long as her "mom" blanket was in the crib. She napped after lunch regularly. Mrs. Silver had given up toilet training for the moment and planned to wait until summer, when she could put Ruth in training pants.

Ruth talked "a mile-a-minute." Her vocabulary and syntax still seemed quite spectacular. She was reported to be capable of reading her own name and the names of products in advertising posters. She wanted to be admired and would cooperate to any extent if one told her that "she will look pretty." Dressing and undressing seemed to be quite a game, and Ruth imaginatively contributed by fetching her father's gloves from the drawer and insisting that the mother, interviewer, or even the doll wear them.

At the twenty-second month well-baby clinic observation Ruth again looked well groomed, neatly combed, light and dainty. She had an air of "charming assurance" and her play progressed smoothly. In water play with a pan and spoon she was careful not to spill any of the water. When a few drops spilled despite her precautions, she sought for something to wipe it up and carefully did so. She showed no disgust in playing with the clay nor undue excitement. Her habit of discarding toys was exceedingly neat. She never threw a toy on the floor but put it back in its place on the toy shelf, even making room for it. After a while Ruth started to lift and pull at her skirt as an invitation to be undressed for the expected medical examination. The implication was, "I know I'm here for a medical examination so let's get on with it."

At the next home visit three reproductions of French watercolors were noticed on the living room walls, which made the room less dreary looking. But Mrs. Silver's physical symptoms had again reached a new height, concurrent with her husband's notice of an imminent transfer and possible overseas duty. She had hit her elbow, which gave acute pain; she had spells of morning coughing that nothing would relieve; and she was so nauseated and dizzy that she could hardly eat anything.

When the interviewer questioned her about the possibility of being pregnant, Mrs. Silver said that it had been ruled out but "it would be the last straw." In the course of this new accumulation of symptoms Mrs. Silver had again changed doctors, but the new one also failed to find anything specifically wrong. She rejected the idea of seeing a psychiatrist, not from misconceptions of the psychiatrist's function, but because she was convinced that she had some specific physical ailment.

Mr. Silver's gentle patience for his wife's complaints began to run thin as he worried over the threat of overseas duty. It was very hard to plan for his family, as he did not want to drag his wife to New York and then leave her there if he had to leave. Mrs. Silver dreaded moving to a new city and having to meet new people. Suddenly her present situation seemed very desirable and filled with friendly sympathetic people whom she was about to lose. She was consumed with sadness and anxiety about the future.

About this time Ruth entered the nursery school of the Child Study Center as part of the on-going study. She attended approximately two hours in the afternoon twice a week. Her adjustment was better than anyone would have anticipated. She separated from her mother with comparative ease and used the nursery school equipment with little hesitation. She held her own with even the most aggressive of her age-mates and kept them at a distance by the glance of her eyes. Ruth's first painting in the nursery school was an experience of sheer enchantment for her. She was oblivious to the world, entranced by the appearance of the blue strokes on the paper in front of the easel.

Shortly after her second birthday Ruth was "christened." Her mother reported that throughout the ceremony she loudly said, "I want to go home," and screamed when the water was sprinkled on her. Mrs. Silver had been very embarrassed but said it was her fault because she had waited so long for what she called the "christening." Nothing was said about Mr. Silver's reaction to the religious rite, whether he was a party to it, or whether he was present for it.

At slightly over two years Ruth was described as a little girl "who is dressed like a doll, has blue eyes, and a big and mobile mouth. She is not pretty, but very attractive." In her development she was almost solidly on a thirty month level, and in language and the personal-social area she reached the three year level on a number of items.

At the final well-baby clinic evaluation at the age of twenty-six months there was a dual impression of Ruth. She looked small despite her average weight and height, but she also looked adult. The contradiction in appearance was not so much from individual features, which still retained their young child look, or from her build, which was sturdy without any roundness or plumpness, but from her expression, gestures, and movements. These seemed superimposed on her, as if borrowed from somebody else. One did not have to seek far to see the source of the borrowed elements. Ruth was a replica of her mother.

Ruth's former elf-like, delicate, shiny appearance had dovetailed with her mother's former glamorous self. But as Mrs. Silver shed her glamour, Ruth suffered the same transformation that had overcome her mother. Mrs. Silver now appeared heavy and pedestrian, as if she no longer cared how she looked. And this same quality was duplicated in Ruth. Mrs. Silver's tensely set look in the moments when she forgot to smile was emulated in Ruth's hard, set, and unsmiling expression. When Ruth did smile, it suggested irony rather than pleasure or relaxation.

At this visit Ruth was somewhat inhibited in her movements, not from lack of agility or body mastery, but from the need to relate every movement to a "one-ness" with her mother. Her attitude towards the adults in the room was not entirely friendly, and she exhibited an element of provocativeness in small actions, such as rolling the truck just a little too far so that it fell from the table, or ignoring the helping words and gestures offered by her father. When a task was unfamiliar, or if for some reason she felt the threat of failure, she brushed her hand over her forehead as if wiping sweat from it.

Rather than rebel overtly against adult jurisdiction, Ruth's way was indirect, seeming to comply but actually limiting compliance to a self-chosen minimum. In contrast to her positive activity with material, she was passive when being dressed or undressed. She permitted her arms and legs to be moved without the slightest effort on her part to facilitate the procedure, not even to the extent of removing her fist from her mouth. Ruth simply allowed the necessary manipulations to take place.

She similarly tolerated the examination, including inspection of her throat, without protest and with surprising cooperation for a child only twenty-six months old. Nevertheless, there were a number of signs that the examination was provocative of anxiety. She intensely followed each move of the pediatrician with her eyes and held her body tense, as if the posture helped provide emotional tolerance.

Her expressional defense pattern was a miniature version of her mother's, heroically bearing life's assaults while at the same time dramatizing and belittling them. However, Ruth gave promise that her own experiences would be permitted to determine her own independent world, because the intense mother identification was born of love rather than of fear.

There was no doubt that Ruth was the focus of life for both her parents, and it was probably true that the validity of their marriage lay in the ability to be good parents. Within the limitations of their apparently neurotic constitutions the Silvers were attached to each other and together attempted to create a good home for their daughter. There was no reason to believe that either felt that they had failed in this aspiration.

Yet it cannot be ignored that the Silvers came from strangely diverse backgrounds and acculturations, each with the trauma of past experiences that cast a pall of guilt even in the fulfillment of their most cherished desires. Ruth's future will not only tell the story of their success in family integration but will be a measure of her parents' emotional accommodation to each other's respective heritages.

SUMMARY

A. EXPECTATIONS

1. Maternal Expectations. Mrs. Silver experienced concern and diffuse anxiety about her adequacy as a mother, but she anticipated the child with considerable pleasure. She was very happy at the prospect of having someone who would "really belong" to her but at the same time she wondered if she would know how to be a good mother and fulfill the responsibilities of caring for her baby. She felt she would need much help in learning and would have to overcome traits in herself which might prevent her from being a "giving mother." She felt that parents were obligated to provide the baby with love, care, and attention. There was no interest in assuming the role of wage earner or engaging in work outside the home.

2. Specificity of Expectations. Mrs. Silver demonstrated a growing number of specific expectations during pregnancy related to the care, well-being, development, and management of the child. She was outstanding in the scope and minuteness of her expectations in these areas. Would the child be healthy, would it be "normal," would "something happen"? These considerations were repeatedly expressed and accompanied by intense anxiety.

During the first six months of Ruth's life, Mrs. Silver repeatedly asked questions about how routines should be carried out, about dangers that might occur or develop, whether she would be able to understand and respond to the child's needs, and the possible consequences if she did the wrong thing.

3. Motivational Orientation. Mrs. Silver was predominantly child-centered throughout the study despite her considerable anxieties. Her expectations continued always to be directed toward the child's needs and well-being. In the second year there was some shift towards self-centeredness related to feelings about herself as an individual. At that time she began to focus on fears about her own health, isolation, and feelings of dependency. However, this was not a departure or a diminution of child-oriented expectations but a redirection of some of her feelings toward herself.

4. Role of Child in Fulfilling Mother's Expectations. A number of Mrs. Silver's original anticipations were hardly fulfilled at the beginning. Instead of a plump, fair-skinned baby, Ruth was fragile and her skin mottled easily. She was not a big eater and not too "pretty." But all of this vanished in Mrs. Silver's loving acceptance and pride in her child. Demands for achievement and conformity were rather lenient in comparison with other mothers, and Mrs. Silver greatly appreciated Ruth's qualities. In the second year there was some concern that Ruth "did not hold her own" against other children, and some exasperation with her willfulness, but on the whole she thoroughly fulfilled her mother's expectations.

5. Paternal Expectations. Mr. Silver was quite concerned with the question of his ability to fulfill the paternal role, to be an "ideal father." During his wife's pregnancy he demonstrated great anxiety about his adequacy as a father. When he did talk about his anticipations, he spoke of school and relations with other children. His image of the coming infant appeared to be of a school-age child rather than an infant. A pervasive anxiety continued after the birth of the child and was expressed in relation to his own functioning and to the well-being of the child. The anxiety was so strong that little else was learned beyond this point.

B. BEHAVIOR

1. Communication. Mrs. Silver talked to convey love and express her feelings for Ruth rather than for direction or control. It was accompanied by much physical contact, holding, love, and comforting for the entire two year period. By the end of the first year she was more able to diminish her need to be physically close to her baby.

Mrs. Silver was always quick to respond to the slightest clue of the child relating to mood or affect, and she exerted herself to interpret and comply with Ruth's desires. Games were improvised to entertain, enticements were provided to make eating time pleasant, food likes and dislikes were catered to, no effort was spared to make the baby happy and contented. The communication between child and mother was so close and strong that it could be said that each was the other's world.

2. *Regularity and Flexibility of Scheduling.* Management of routines fell into fairly regular patterns, but Mrs. Silver was prepared to adapt herself to the child's preferences. When Ruth had difficulty with sleep or naps, the mother's schedule was adjusted to fit the baby's desires rather than her own plans. The same applied to eating, play, visits to the park, or any other activity. But from the beginning Ruth herself was a remarkably "regular" child. From three months on, she slept mostly through the night. She was rather uninterested in eating, but her mother paced feeding to Ruth's desires on the whole. Consequently the "demand" schedule assumed a regularity which was derived by mutual consent, not imposed by the mother.

3. *Techniques of Management.* Mrs. Silver used various devices to avoid difficult situations and provide contentment for Ruth. She made a game of a task, provided diversions to get the child to behave willingly, and used prearrangement to set the stage for feeding, sleep, and play situations. To encourage Ruth's eating, her mother provided toys, books, television, and any other distraction. When Ruth took to nibbling from her parents' plates, they deprived themselves of eggs for breakfast lest she eat too much egg.

As Ruth grew older, more control became necessary, and Ruth learned to test her mother to extremes. Mrs. Silver was preponderantly permissive in both the first and second years, although slightly less so in the second. Occasionally during the second year, and especially during her period of self-concern, she resorted to some prohibitions, but mainly her management was accommodative to the child. Mrs. Silver wanted her husband to be more of a disciplinarian, and she resented his reluctance to be involved in disciplining Ruth. Consequently, both parents avoided difficulties with, or pressures on, Ruth.

4. Relation of Expectations to Behavior. Mrs. Silver felt that a baby should come first in the mother's life. She suited all of her behavior with the child to this premise. Although she had misgivings about her own ability to be a "giving" mother, her behavior strongly verified her expectations that "the baby should be most important and get love and affection."

The most frequently reported behavioral interactions were in areas where Mrs. Silver had expressed most of her specific concerns and expectations, namely for the baby's comfort and security. In the first months Mrs. Silver spent much time holding, watching, and comforting Ruth, suiting all activity to what she saw as the child's needs.

Despite intense and diffuse anxieties Mrs. Silver handled her baby with a certainty that was in direct contrast to her convictions that she never could be a competent mother. Even when Ruth was ill, her mother's behavior was sure and effective. Her anxieties did not get in the way of her caring for Ruth nor were they communicated to the child.

5. Paternal Behavior. Mr. Silver endeavored to be the "ideal father" and did not want to be "too easy" like his father, but he refused to discipline Ruth, as she could do no wrong in his eyes. He was anxious even during his wife's pregnancy but so much so after the baby's birth that Mrs. Silver was convinced her husband could do no more than baby-sit (although he was even fearful about that). It was mainly because of his fears that Ruth's parents slept in her room during most of the first two years, in dread that something might happen to her during the night.

Mr. Silver's main role was to read, study, and pass on information about child care and protection to his wife. He played with Ruth and was concerned with all aspects of her care, but the fear that he might do something wrong practically immobilized him. He mistrusted his own adequacy to the point where he was in mortal fear of being alone with her. Mr. Silver's career took second place to the welfare of his wife and child, with every move predicated on what would be best for Ruth. On the whole, he was a fond, indulgent, protective, and extremely anxious father. His behavior was predominantly permissive throughout the study.

C. SOCIO-CULTURAL INFLUENCES

1. Socio-economic Status and Values. The Silvers were characterized by equivocal strivings toward achievement. Like many other career servicemen, Mr. Silver aspired to promotion, but he did not put it ahead of the interests of his family nor did he seem to find it difficult to adjust to peacetime status after having been a wartime officer. Throughout the study there was frequent ambivalence about promotional aspirations, but they were compromised by his own personal needs and his unrealistic wish to undertake no new venture which would result in separation from his wife and baby.

With no close friends or family ties, the Silvers had few informal sources of pediatric advice and no real models for their own approach to child-rearing. Neither of them regarded friends among other foreign war bride couples as outstanding examples of parenthood or child education. And aside from an occasional exchange with her sister-in-law, Mrs. Silver was alienated from her husband's family. The Silvers, therefore, with their habit of reading, came to rely on written and professional advice. In this reliance they came to accept standards of child-rearing which may have been significantly more "middle-class" in orientation than those by which they had been raised.

Mrs. Silver's social values were generally of a higher level than those of her husband. She identified herself with the upper middle-class life that she had experienced in Germany, and which was also represented by the important official rank of her uncle in the Nazi hierarchy. Consequently she felt a sharp change in status and a shock to her middle-class values upon exposure to the working-class background of her husband and his family. However, she tried to re-orient herself towards more "democratic and unprejudiced" viewpoints.

The social implications of this Jewish-Lutheran marriage between an American war veteran and an ex-Nazi are not entirely clear. The ambivalence of Mr. Silver, who maintained a filial relationship with his Orthodox parents, may have stemmed from the loss of an important source of emotional support. His great anxiety, sense of inadequacy, and desire to please his wife and baby to the exclusion of all else may have been a concomitant of the untraditional marriage. As for Mrs. Silver it was undoubtedly true that both her socio-economic status and social values were inexorably changed and that she had had to make and accept adjustments beyond any of her expectations.

2. Extended Family. The Silvers were an exceptionally isolated family, in a category almost by themselves in this study. There were virtually no contacts with either set of grandparents, few friendships, and limited social activity. The German war bride had little social contact with the tradition-oriented Jewish paternal grandparents, whose ways she little understood or liked. Mrs. Silver's great fear was the possibility that her husband's mother might have to live with them in the event of his father's death.

Mr. Silver's sense of allegiance to the Jewish faith did not appear to be great, though he fulfilled his parental obligations by means of visits and financial help when necessary. Although these visits indicated a sense of responsibility and concern for his elderly parents, there was no evidence of a wish to share his family life with them.

On her part, Mrs. Silver was isolated from her family by the separation of an ocean and half a continent. While she maintained written contact throughout the study, it was most unsatisfactory, and often she spoke longingly about going back to visit. In reality she had few close ties left with her family, apart from her mother. There had been only the most meager past association with her step-siblings and certainly no affection for the stepfather, with whom she never got along. But in her loneliness and isolation, Mrs. Silver spoke nostalgically about her family and the many traditional things now lost to her.

3. Spatial Arrangements and Values. In the Silver household, where everything was geared to the baby, there was no question about limitation of space with regard to Ruth. Every room in the apartment held Ruth's paraphernalia and toys. In fear that something might happen during the night, the Silvers gave up the privacy of their own bedroom and shared Ruth's. Several times during the study the bedrooms and living room were changed functionally and in decoration for the greater convenience of Ruth.

Immaculate housekeeping was augmented by daily floor scrubbings so the child would touch nothing dirty. The Silvers relinquished both television and their easy chairs for weeks at a time, remaining in the kitchen, so that their whispered conversation would not distrub Ruth, who was a light sleeper. In this home all spatial arrangements and values were totally sublimated to the child, and in this respect there was always complete unanimity between the parents.

D. FAMILY RELATIONSHIPS

1. Marital. Mrs. Silver had many emotional difficulties, which affected the relationship with her husband and her satisfactions in marriage. Her feelings of loss upon her parents' divorce and her mother's remarriage fostered a need to have someone exclusively her own. This may account for the closeness that immediately developed between her and her baby. The wartime hazards reinforced her feelings of insecurity and intensified her dependency needs. In the face of such strong emotional needs it was doubtful that gentle and irresolute David Silver could appear as a pillar of strength.

On his part, Mr. Silver also appeared unsure, anxious, and uncertain. Certainly he found the adult responsibilities associated with marital and paternal roles difficult to cope with. Possibly he turned to the maritime setting for satisfaction of his own dependency needs. There were many questions brought to mind about the meaning of this union between the daughter of a militaristic German family and the son of immigrant Russian Jewish parents. These questions were not answerable in this study. All we can say is that such a marriage must surmount formidable cultural barriers.

There was a considerable amount of unresolved tension, but the marital relationship seemed to be generally satisfying to the Silvers, despite the evident sexual disinterest of Mrs. Silver. The couple shared the anxieties brought to their marriage by their own individual feelings of doubt and insecurity. With trepidation they together faced the unknowns that lay in store for them and their very precious child. Mrs. Silver's chronic worry that her husband's assignments might separate them was no more severe than his anxiety that he might be separated from his family. Similarly, Mrs. Silver's every worry about her daughter's health or development was matched by her husband's.

Mr. Silver always spoke with high regard and praise for his wife. Mrs. Silver was always guarded and poised in referring to her husband, blandly asserting, "Naturally I will see only good in him, for he is my husband." Hence, there was every reason to believe that the marriage functioned as smoothly as possible within the limits set by their respective and somewhat neurotic personalities.

There were occasional points of friction, although these did not loom large. Such differences arose mainly from Mr. Silver's refusal to discipline Ruth or after one of his visits to his parents. Sometimes Mrs. Silver was intolerant of her husband's lack of confidence with Ruth; sometimes Mr. Silver was impatient with his wife's chronic complaints of illness. A characteristic limitation in their relationship was Mr. Silver's apparent lack of sensitivity to his wife's moods and wishes. He would try to be helpful and understanding but appeared to miss his cues frequently. To what extent he experienced a similar lack of response from his wife was not indicated in the records.

2. *Mother-Child.* For Helene Silver the infant was her chief source of emotional satisfaction. Her psychological, cultural, and familial isolation, her great need to have someone all her own, and her difficulty in sharing loved ones led her to invest much of her emotion in the child. This channeling of her feelings was reinforced by her husband's tendency to intensify rather than lighten her anxieties about herself, the child, and their life together. It was inevitable that the mother-child relationship would become the all-absorbing focus of Mrs. Silver's life.

Mrs. Silver took some months to realize that she could enjoy her child and that her fears about the baby were unrealistic. But as she experienced a diminution of these doubts and fears, she turned her anxieties inward and developed hypochondriacal feelings. At the point when she became reasonably reassured that Ruth was healthy, her own well-being and physical symptoms began to engage her.

Remembering the loneliness of her own childhood, Mrs. Silver brooded about her possible ill health and how disastrous it would be for Ruth without a mother. Under no circumstances could she visualize her husband filling the breach. Her focus was on love and affection for Ruth rather than on material things, although she saw to it that Ruth wanted for nothing. As if partly in response to this feeling of love and devotion, Ruth's development was normal and uncomplicated by undue stress. In this family, Ruth seemed to meet the very important psychological and emotional needs of her mother.

3. Father-Child. Mr. Silver's devotion to Ruth was unquestionable. He spent considerable time in play with her and left no stone unturned to provide every care and protection. His joy in Ruth was tempered in good part by chronic fears for her well-being, which immobilized him when he was required to undertake practical management of the child.

Mrs. Silver was aware of the extent to which her husband's life revolved about his beloved Ruth, and she made laughing reference to the fact that she was "only Ruth's mother to him." Along with Mr. Silver's complete emotional involvement with his daughter there was an expressed feeling of inadequacy in the paternal role, which was demonstrated by his reluctance to have any part in discipline and his refusal to deny Ruth anything. It appeared to observers that Ruth served some very important emotional needs for her father, which were only hinted at during the period under study.

E. PERSONALITY CHARACTERISTICS

1. Handling of Anxiety and Hostility. While Mrs. Silver experienced a great deal of anxiety flowing from one person to another and from one event to the next, she nevertheless managed to handle all phases of child care adequately and without undue problems. Because of the emotional deprivations of her own childhood, and the tremendous sense of mother-loss, which had not been assuaged by the material things provided by her grandparents, Mrs. Silver held the value of emotional satisfaction to be above that of material goods. Hence, she expressed her ideology of love as the most important element in child care.

Mrs. Silver's prime psychological mechanism for handling hostility was the use of displacement rather than direct expression. For example, she camouflaged her own feelings of prejudice by observations about existing prejudice and intolerance in the United States. Ambivalence about her Nazi past was evident in implied criticism of American democratic values and the "carelessness" with which the American government tolerated "Communists." A self-concept of cultural superiority was overt in her evaluation that Americans were disinterested in and lacked appreciation for opera.

Criticism and negative feelings toward her husband or baby were rarely expressed. Any criticism of her husband was implied in a laughing, humorous, anecdotal way and then hastily masked. Thus, when irritated with her husband's fears about the prospective baby, she would say contemptuously, "What use will he be, he's so afraid." But then she would quickly add, "Everyone is like that with a first child, but he will be a good father." Mrs. Silver mostly praised and admired her daughter, finding little to criticize. Even during the later period when Ruth was somewhat willful, provocative, and negative, Mrs. Silver was never wholly critical or derogatory.

This did not mean that Mrs. Silver lacked ego strength. On the contrary, she gave evidence of a very considerable amount. One example was her extraordinary persistence in coping with eighteen months of red tape before she could come to America. Although authoritarian figures were significant in her past, these same authorities were deemed inappropriate to her life in America, and she did not hesitate to be critical or annoyed with them when necessary.

The acceptance of appropriate authority, such as the study staff and child-care books, was difficult for her. She had tremendous need for reassurance and yet could only ambivalently use such sources of assurance as were available. She could and did express disagreement with many American customs concerning child care, and on occasion she decided against incorporating them into her own way of thinking. One example concerned restriction of diet during pregnancy. Mrs. Silver never accepted this and only grudgingly accepted dietary restrictions.

Mrs. Silver was indeed a lonely woman, having few friends and no relatives with whom to share tension and from whom to gain support. Her husband was only partly satisfactory in this respect. Nevertheless, there was some comfort in each other, and little Ruth was not called upon to carry the burden of parental anxiety.

2. Dependency and the Sense of Security. Mrs. Silver's great need for emotional reassurance was partly an outgrowth of her lonely childhood. She needed to have the assurance of affection from others and also to have someone who would look to her for the emotional "giving" that she so strongly wanted to express. Lacking friends and intimate family relationships, she felt separated from the idealized "family life" that she had experienced when working on the estate in Germany. Though sympathetic, Mr. Silver was not very effective in meeting her needs for reassurance and support. We know little about his own dependency needs except that he gave evidence of their existence. Thus Helene Silver's problem of dependency was only partially solved.

The Silvers were unlike the other nuclear families, who had opportunities for resolving their dependency needs in the day-to-day interaction and functioning with other family members. Mrs. Silver demonstrated her dependency needs not only in her intense interdependent relationship with her husband but also by redirecting her concerns to her own health — visiting many physicians in her attempts to assuage her fears. Dependency was a problem to Mrs. Silver, but the handling of these feelings did not significantly intrude upon the achievement of family unity and a sense of identity between father, mother, and child.

3. Feelings of Adequacy or Inadequacy. The management of feelings of inadequacy was not a major problem. Mrs. Silver had a marked tendency toward self-devaluation and indeed had many inadequacy feelings, although these were protected by a glamorous smile and a well-groomed appearance. She looked upon herself as just an ordinary person with no special talents or abilities. Although her inadequacy feelings were at times severe, her handling of them did not interfere with family unity.

4. Planning and Impulsiveness. Planning did not seem to be significant. Mrs. Silver found Ruth to be a remarkably regular child who did not require a high degree of flexibility in her care. The data are insufficient to show whether Mrs. Silver was either impulsive or markedly future-oriented in her management of Ruth. Mrs. Silver did have many concerns about coping with the future if her husband were reassigned, but these fears were more tied to dependency and insecurity than to the need for future-oriented planning. We have already described the large amount of psychic energy which Mrs. Silver put into her daily life. It is likely that an undemanding husband and Ruth's regularity combined to make planning less important than it might otherwise have been.

5. *Self-Assertion.* Self-assertion did involve some problems for Mrs. Silver. In many instances her favorable comparisons of life and customs in Germany as contrasted to the United States reflected the need for self-assertion, as did emphasis on her own cultural interests. However, this need did not significantly reflect in her relationship to Ruth or impinge on the family in any decisive way.

6. *Recapitulation of Past Experiences.* There was strong reaction by Mrs. Silver against perceived childhood deprivations and strong motivations that Ruth should not suffer similarly. The determination that Ruth should have full and undivided mother-love influenced her daily life and practices with the child. The gnawing worry about her own health revolved about what might happen to Ruth without a mother. She relived her own childhood traumas, and was intensely determined that life would be otherwise for her daughter. These past experiences also influenced Mrs. Silver strongly to want someone completely her own. She found in Ruth the answer to such a "oneness" and "belonging," which she had lacked in her early life.

F. EMERGENCE OF FAMILY INTEGRATION PATTERNS

1. *Family Structure.* In the absence of intimate extended family members and friends, the Silver family early established themselves as a tightly knit threesome. Despite their emotional uncertainties and anxieties, there was a kind of emotional nexus between the two parents which tended to be more ego-supporting than threat-

ening. Hence, the Silvers were regarded as a unitary family, although they varied from the overall pattern to an appreciable extent.

In their individual relationships with Ruth, both parents were anxious and fearful. Ruth created few problems herself and the focus of anxiety shifted to other concerns, such as job uncertainty and hypochondria. It was psychologically difficult for Mrs. Silver to share Ruth with her husband because of tremendous needs to have someone all her own. Yet she managed to do so, and a mutual relationship of mother, father, and child developed. There were many common family activities and emotional satisfactions in this relatively isolated unitary triad.

2. Division of Labor and Balance of Power. The Silvers had a mutual, but anxious, sharing enterprise, in which the husband showed slightly more initiative than his wife. Mrs. Silver managed the home and child care almost exclusively, except for the few occasions when Mr. Silver unsuccessfully took over. Mr. Silver seemed to be influential in decisions on family, household, and job matters. It appeared that Mrs. Silver accepted his decisions concerning financial matters, trips, and general conduct.

3. Development, Achievement, and Social Behavior of Child. Ruth was somewhat advanced in age adequacy and physical and social development throughout the two years of the study. While she had some outstanding sensitivities at various times (excessive fear of strangers, of toy animals, etc.) she was an appealing and attractive child. Her language development was especially advanced during the period under observation.

4. Prospect of Siblings. There was no evidence of any real desire or prospect for future pregnancies. In fact, from the beginning of her first pregnancy, Mrs. Silver insisted that she did not want another child, "at least for a few years," and she was greatly interested in learning about the use of contraceptives. Mr. Silver did not express any desire for a larger family.

5. Status of Family in Community. There was no pronounced extended family conflict, although there was a minimum of social contact. The relationship with Mr. Silver's family was mainly conducted by himself, with only very occasional visits by his wife and daughter. Mrs. Silver was continually alarmed that should her husband's father die, his mother might live with them.

The Silvers also tended to be relatively isolated from community influences and pressures. Attachments to their few friends were not based on very strong ties. The new world and its customs were enigmas to Helene Silver, and even frightening in some respects. The differences between the German Christian and the Jewish cultures, the difficulties of life in a new community, and their retiring personalities worked to make the Silvers the most socially isolated nuclear family in the study.

6. Types of Parent-Child Adaptation. The Silvers were decidedly child-centered in motivational orientation. Their entire lives revolved almost exclusively about the child. They were among the most permissive of the unitary families. Thus, the family was seen as unitary in structure, child-centered in orientation, and permissive in management.

POSTSCRIPT

The family departed from the area some six months after the two year study had ended, because Mr. Silver was transferred elsewhere. However, Ruth did have an opportunity to attend the nursery school for approximately four months. Despite the fact that she missed fully half of the nursery school sessions because of slight colds or other reasons, her time there was pleasurable and rewarding.

Mrs. Silver, who had hitherto never relinquished Ruth's care to anyone, had ambivalent feelings in the beginning about the separation. The overly-sheltered and protected child, however, took the separation surprisingly well. At first, her approach to other children and play objects was careful, methodical, and gradual. But as she became familiar with the surroundings, she was at ease, purposeful, poised, and mature in activity and interaction.

The staff had been particularly careful to ward off any precipitous experiences, but their efforts were hardly necessary. Ruth conducted herself with authority and independence. In fact, she even took it upon herself to lend a helping hand to other children in an offhand and slightly domineering manner. She overcame her fear of outdoor equipment and developed greater freedom of movement and increased body gracefulness. Shyness and timidity with other children decreased considerably.

A letter from the Silvers several months after they had moved warmly thanked the staff and described Ruth's superb adjustment to her new surroundings. From the first night she slept alone in her own bedroom and played outside with other children with no evidence of timidity or fear. All told, the family seemed contented with the move, secure in their tightly bound threesome. As ever, Ruth was the focal point of the family and brought deep joy and gratification. With no clear indication of future offspring, it appeared that her sovereignty would remain undisputed.

The Grasso Family

COMING TO TERMS WITH REALITY

Real life is far removed from childish make-believe, and Eleanor Grasso had to come to terms with this fact as she faced maturity and motherhood. "My girl friend and I used to play and plan that some day we would be married and bring our babies to see each other. She had her baby, and now I'll have mine, and it will be just like we planned."

She had realized her romantic, girlish fantasy by capturing a handsome, happy-go-lucky husband who had been the "heart throb" of many of her friends. There were some who warned against marriage with an "irresponsible guy" who drifted along, seeking the aimless pleasures of the street-corner gang. But "boy-crazy" and impetuous at sixteen, Eleanor paid little heed to seasoned advice. She fell madly in love with Salvatore, ten years her senior, and within a year and a half they were man and wife.

Though she had known that he was hospitalized in the Armed Forces, she did not learn until the time of her honeymoon that her husband had had tuberculosis. Early in the marriage, active disease was rediscovered, and for the first year of marriage Sal was confined to a sanatorium. When he was discharged, he faced a long period of convalescence, but Eleanor was so happy to have her husband with her again that it was of little consequence.

And now her dream of having a baby was about to come true. All things considered, Eleanor Grasso felt that she was very lucky. It was hard to bring herself down to earth, or to consider the real problems which had to be faced by a married couple.

It was just as hard to speak of herself or her past. "I wouldn't know what to say to you," she told a staff member. "I won't know the answers. I mean . . . I don't know what I mean myself." Mrs. Grasso was a little over five feet tall, slender, attractive, and neatly dressed. She wore lipstick and nail polish, and her dark brown hair curled in bangs toward the middle of her forehead. Shyly the twenty-year-old woman looked at the floor when she wasn't talking, and hesitated about joining the study group.

Mrs. Grasso had been trying to have a baby since her marriage almost two years ago. Once she had had a spontaneous abortion after a two-month pregnancy. Then she underwent a suspension operation and had a cyst removed. One month later she became pregnant and was delighted with the quick result. She felt a little nauseated but had no vomiting. Her only discomfort was being very sleepy. She still worked at her factory job and put her earnings "in with the rest." The "rest" came from a pension which Mr. Grasso received from the government as a result of the tuberculosis which he had contracted in the Army. Mrs. Grasso banked his pension each month and used it "as if it were a regular salary."

Mr. Grasso was overjoyed about the coming baby. He wanted a little "Sal" to carry on his name, but he would be satisfied no matter what it was. Both of Mr. Grasso's parents were deceased. His three sisters had children, but it was still up to Sal to carry on the family name. When talking about the baby Mrs. Grasso's face lit up enthusiastically and she seemed quite self-assured. She looked forward to buying baby clothes the next week and mentioned names they had prepared for either a boy or a girl. She hoped the baby would have black hair and blue eyes. When asked if she might want to go back to work after the baby was born, she said, "I may want to work, but I want to stay home for two years and have time to enjoy my baby."

The Grassos lived in a four-room apartment next door to Eleanor's mother and father. Nothing was said of her father, and he remained almost totally unknown and hardly mentioned throughout the study. With obvious satisfaction she reported that she and her mother "get along good" and "it's great to be by my mother." When it was suggested that the mother could be of help with a new baby, she said, "I don't think I'll need any help."

Mrs. Grasso lit up a cigarette and discussed the question of whether she would raise her baby as her mother had raised her. She replied that she would be stricter. In her opinion, her mother had been too good to her and had gone without many things because she sacrificed so much for her children. As to the ways in which she would be stricter, Mrs. Grasso said, "I don't know what I mean, but I won't let her go out so soon. That is, if it's a girl." As for herself, "I was sixteen when I started going steady with my husband. That is too young."

When asked if she planned to nurse the baby, Mrs. Grasso said she would like to try, at least in the hospital, but planned to give a bottle once in a while because "when you go out you want to take a bottle along for the baby." Spontaneously she reported that she had bought a number of pretty suits and received many clothes from her sister, all for boys. "I don't know what I'll do if it's a girl." She had also bought a book about rabbits for the baby and her husband had said, "Are you going to teach him to read already?"

Mrs. Grasso didn't plan to stop working until after Christmas because there was "no point losing the bonus." But the work was too strenuous to continue beyond that. She said, "My mother is so good to me. She makes little kimonos for the baby and helps me with the house because I work." Mrs. Grasso spoke about a friend who already had six children. "That's too many," she said. For herself she wanted "as many as we can afford and have room for, but six or seven are too many."

When the interviewer closed her notebook at the end of the meeting, Mrs. Grasso became more at ease. She told of a wart on her knee which had been removed but had grown back. She was a little concerned because someone had said it might be cancer. Even though the doctor who had removed the wart said it wasn't cancerous, Mrs. Grasso said, "Yes, but things are done so quickly that you can't believe them." She added, "You know, I still can't believe everything is all right, and that I'm pregnant. I asked the doctor and he said I was pregnant but it's so hard to believe."

The interviewer pointed out that she was getting larger. Mrs. Grasso replied, "I'm two inches larger in the breasts and three in the waist, so it is happening, I suppose." She said she would be so glad "to finally feel it move." Concerning her weight, she said, "I only gained a pound or two, but I eat like a horse, everything I feel like." When asked if she wanted special things to eat, she laughed as if it were an old wives' tale, but said, "It's so funny. I want turnips and crabs. I tried to get my husband to bring some home. But he forgot every night for a week so finally I sent him out to get some."

In her sixth month Mrs. Grasso still appeared quite slender. She wore a green sport sweater, which was a good camouflage for her pregnancy. She said she felt fine and had gained six pounds in the past six months. Her appetite had increased with her pregnancy, and she put no limit on her diet. She believed that long walks helped to keep her weight down. Spontaneously she confided that they wanted a boy but wouldn't really care if it were a girl, "because a girl is always closer to the mother." "No matter how you bring up a boy, he's bound to leave you."

Throughout the interview Mrs. Grasso tended to look away and seemed quite embarrassed. Then suddenly she blurted out, "I don't see why you interview me. I haven't anything to tell. It embarrasses me to talk to you this way." The interviewer explained the purpose of the study, but Mrs. Grasso was not particularly reassured and said again, "I really don't see the point of all this."

The Rorschach test the next month evaluated Mrs. Grasso as "a person of average or limited intelligence and interests." "Her concepts were child-like and immature, and self-identification probably rather infantile. There appeared to be little or minimal emotional contact with people although no actual withdrawal."

As time passed, Mrs. Grasso became more interested in the study, but still there was hesitancy to talk about herself. She looked more pregnant than before and was always dressed in some shade of green. She seemed extremely happy in her pregnant state and had a rather soft, dreamy look when she talked about the baby. Now she was somewhat worried about her weight gain because "they don't want you to suddenly start gaining."

Mrs. Grasso said that her husband could not yet return to work, and she found it important to put his pension in the bank or she was "likely to spend it all at once." "Living on a pension sometimes means that you must pinch pennies." There was plenty for everyday needs, but they were not able to save anything for the future.

Concerning breast feeding, she said at first she had thought she wouldn't, but then had changed her mind and thought it was most likely a good idea. Her breasts enlarged considerably and there was some caking. "It won't hurt to try it for a while to see how things go, and after all you can always stop." She said her mother had nursed her, and "the family thinks it's the natural thing to do." The interviewer felt that she was rather cool towards breast feeding and would not be upset if she could not nurse.

When asked about the onset of menstruation, she said that it had started when she was sixteen years old and that she had been jealous of other girls who had begun to menstruate early. However, her mother also hadn't started to menstruate until quite late. Mrs. Grasso said she "learned all the facts of life" from her mother when she was eight or nine years old, that her mother was modern, and that they were good friends. The other day her mother commented, "The way my belly button is popping out, she guessed it would be a boy."

In the interviewing room there was a small bottle with a fetus in it. Mrs. Grasso walked over to look at it and remembered that a nurse had once said it might be upsetting for her to see it. She commented, "Things like that never upset me," and proceeded to examine the fetus very carefully, stating her amazement that a three-month fetus was developed so far.

At the pediatric interview Mrs. Grasso was neatly dressed, and the pediatrician found it hard to believe that she would be delivering in less than a month. Mrs. Grasso outlined her previous history, including the spontaneous abortion, the laparotomy, and removal of the cyst. She smiled and said, "I got caught the month after. The doctor said I should wait at least a month." She talked a little about her husband's tuberculosis when that question was raised, and responded to the question about his occupation by saying he was "a disabled veteran." She said that she hadn't wanted to breast feed at first, but her husband wanted her to "because it is better." Now she was increasingly desirous of breast feeding, she said.

At the next interview Mrs. Grasso learned about the results of her psychology tests. It was explained that she had done well on the Bellevue-Wechsler test except for remembering numbers. Mrs. Grasso corroborated that she simply couldn't remember numbers and had had trouble with that part of it. She added, "Well, then if I did pretty well, I'll have an average baby." She was assured that as far as her tests were concerned, there was every expectation of a normal and average youngster. As for the "ink blot" test, Mrs. Grasso said that she couldn't see anything in the ink blot cards and "they all looked like splotches of dirt and nothing much else."

Mrs. Grasso said that "although she wasn't as big as some women, she felt terribly large." She no longer felt like making up her face because it had broken out, and when she awoke in the morning her nose and lips were swollen. Also her ankles swelled a bit. She felt, "It's not worth the trouble to fix my hair." Her attitude was that in this condition she wouldn't be very attractive anyhow so there was no use doing anything about it. Mrs. Grasso hardly looked as unattractive as her words might indicate. She wore her lipstick nicely applied, and was neat in a maternity skirt and one of Sal's shirts.

The name "Vince" had been definitely picked for a boy, and "Lillian" had been chosen for a girl's name. Mrs. Grasso was still undecided which sex she would really prefer. "I always wanted an older brother, so it would be nice to have a boy first, but then I see baby girls and realize how adorable they are, how much fun it is to dress them up, and then I want a girl."

She had seen the delivery room and commented that it had frightened her and looked "pretty scarey." She hated the idea of "having her legs way up there," but her girl friend said that "you didn't think about anything like that when you were having a baby and didn't mind all the funny things they do to you because you're so busy having a baby." Mrs. Grasso imagined she would feel the same way and not be embarrassed. But she said that she definitely wouldn't want her husband to be in the delivery room and "see the head come out." Although she knew that babies could be two weeks late or two weeks early, she'd like it very much to be on the two weeks early side.

Mrs. Grasso's attitude at this meeting was most cooperative, and the interviewer finally felt sure that she would remain a member of the study group and that she was genuinely interested in the services which were offered. The interviewer's impression was that the psychological tests had been the turning point that proved to Mrs. Grasso that the staff was interested in her development as a person and as a mother-to-be.

Six days later Mrs. Grasso came to the hospital. For several hours prior to admission she had had irregular contractions. In the hospital the contractions became regular and lasted almost nine hours. The nurses noted that "the patient was cooperative," and during delivery she pushed with the contractions as told. There was spontaneous delivery of an apparently normal male with no anesthesia except for two percent Novocain for the episiotomy repair. After delivery Mrs. Grasso was described as being radiantly happy and enchanted with her little boy, who was called Vincent Rudolpho Grasso.

"My husband thinks he has too long a nose, but I think he's beautiful," Mrs. Grasso commented. The staff tended to agree with Mr. Grasso. Vince's nose was indeed long, with a cherry-red spot on it. His complexion was yellowish and there was nothing round or cuddly about him. There was no doubt to observers that he was a boy even though he had on a diaper. His movements precluded any impression of femininity, and his "masculinity" conveyed a sense of independence as if he would "go his own way" regardless of whether it achieved happiness or contentment.

Vince was far removed from contentment. He cried incessantly during eight of the ten times he was observed during his hospital stay. The observers found his ear-splitting cries nerve-wracking and could hardly imagine so small a lung with so much strength. He seemed impossible to comfort. The crying did not seem to be despair, but rather irritation and a vast fury.

His leg positions were quite awkward. The observers wondered how he could hold such an "impossible" leg position, in which the feet were turned inward to a point where it seemed the ligaments did not exist at all. The continuous rhythmical bicycling movement of his legs and the circling movement of his arms made Vince look like a robot machine. Usually movements in newborns are expressive of states of peace or of restlessness, of peaks of distress and then of relief. But Vince's continuous movements and crying were always at a maximal pitch. In general, his stiff movements were accompanied by a trembling or jerking of the whole body.

His reactions were not to outside stimulus but seemed to come from a stimulus inside himself. Noise, light, sound, or touch rarely elicited response from him. He was reachable only when his equilibrium was involved, such as when he was picked up or his position changed. He could also be quieted from his state of fury if one put a finger in his mouth. Then he calmed down and sucked vigorously. Two different people independently found this means of comforting him.

His own hand-to-mouth contact was precarious. No dominant hand pattern emerged, and he sought mouth contact with both hands, equally unsuccessfully. This seemed due to head movements which were poorly timed with the arm movements. When the mouth-searching activity was carried on by the right hand, the head was turned to the left side if Vince was in supine. When he was in prone his head seemed to get stuck in the middle position. Another factor that seemed to interfere drastically with the hand-mouth contact was the movement of his legs. As he tried to get the hand into his mouth, such a violent movement of the lower extremities began that the hand seemed to be pulled away from the lips.

Vince obviously preferred the prone position, in which he cried less, was not so stiff, and trembled less frequently. Also the prone position limited his leg movements, thus making hand-mouth contact more successful. It seemed that Vince was obsessed by some continuous discomfort, but whether this was hunger or an inner disquieting milieu remained to be seen. After being fed, Vince usually succeeded in sucking his hand and falling asleep. In sleep he seemed to liberate himself from the discomforting forces. The yellowishness of his skin tended to disappear, he became quite rosy, and his expression was described as blissful. If one disturbed this state of bliss, he awoke and resumed his maximal "fury."

Mrs. Grasso's experience in nursing Vince was not rewarding. Her good cheer of the first few days gave way to discomfort and depression as she began to have difficulty nursing him. "He just eats and eats and is still hungry. I have enough milk but it doesn't seem to satisfy him. I don't know whether to feed him or not. He goes to sleep after a few minutes at the breast, then when I put him down he spits up a mouthful and is hungry again in thirty minutes." She was near tears, her gown soaked with breast milk, her hair uncombed, and her face not made up. She could hardly talk to her husband for weeping.

The pediatrician assured her that she could breast feed or not, as she wished. The doctor also felt that reality was catching up with Mrs. Grasso and that she was not prepared for the vicissitudes of caring for a baby. It surprised her that babies spit up from time to time, or cry, or are not hungry at strictly regular intervals. It seemed as if she had fantasied only sweetness and light and now she was faced by crying, regurgitation, and her own discomfort with breast feeding. She remained undecided about nursing and thought she might try it for a day or two after she got home. Then if things were no better, she would put the baby on formula. She seemed glad, and even relieved, to be going home, where she could do as she pleased with the baby. Before leaving the hospital Mrs. Grasso had Vince circumcised.

The Grassos lived in an ugly old house, but their apartment was strikingly attractive and immaculately clean. The kitchen had a modern new-looking stove, which Mrs. Grasso had secured second-hand. In combination with the kitchen was a baby's room, which held a new bassinet, diaper can, stacks of fresh diapers, and all of the paraphernalia for baby care. Off the kitchen was a small living room, which was clean and nicely furnished. It had rather ornate lace curtains at the window and was chock-full of knick-knacks and various novelty decorations. They did not look particularly junky.

Mrs. Grasso reported that the baby was "fussy" because of excessive gassiness. This was usually relieved by picking him up. She was a little concerned about spoiling him if she picked him up so frequently. Also, she was worried about a "knot" in the left groin, which proved to be a lymph gland. After a couple of weeks of breast feeding Mrs. Grasso had stopped because it was "too messy" and the baby needed both breast and formula. She said she wished she had never started nursing in the first place.

Mrs. Grasso's mother was introduced to the interviewer. She was a very slender, trim-looking woman, with smartly arranged gray hair. The relationship between mother and daughter was almost sisterly. When Mrs. Grasso was out of the room, her mother expounded on her daughter's home-making talents and her great devotion to her husband. She contrasted her with Eleanor's older sister, who was "devilish and wild" and had never cared for children.

Mrs. Grasso commented to the interviewer that Vince was "every bit as handsome as his father." The interviewer, however, described Mr. Grasso as "a sheik-like, frail-looking man, with carefully arranged dark hair, thumb-nails close to an inch long, and bad teeth." In conversation with the interviewer, he told of his poker-winning exploits and his fascination with horse-racing. He had traveled around a great deal, done odd jobs, and resisted his father's attempts to get him steady work. After the tuberculosis attack, which now appeared arrested, he had calmed down and was resigned to the fact that his days of adventure were over.

Mrs. Grasso reported that the baby ate very well and also slept through the night. To cope with his gassiness she removed various fruits or cereal from his diet with little effect, so she decided "that's just the way he is." While she held the baby on her lap, he obviously started to have a bowel movement, which went on for a few minutes. Mrs. Grasso smiled at him throughout, and from time to time she would say fondly, "You stink." The interviewer felt that Mrs. Grasso was perceptive to the baby's needs and able to satisfy them to his complete pleasure.

At the first well-baby clinic Mrs. Grasso was pleasant but seemed shy and rather uncomfortable. She knew about the observers in the booth and avoided looking at the screen throughout most of the session. She seemed very proud of her baby and reported his accomplishments. At seven weeks the baby was taking solids well and "can't wait a minute when he's hungry." Mrs. Grasso had a number of questions about additional solids and seemed eager to add them to his diet. She said that Vince was still moderately gassy but had less discomfort than before. He "works hard" at having his stools, and in the crib he "hollers and grunts." Bath time was enjoyable, and he smiled and babbled in his bath. He usually slept soundly.

The pediatrician reported Vince as a well-nourished, active, slightly hypertonic infant. He had a social smile and an alert expression, with interest and attention toward people. Postural adjustments and development were advanced, hands were still mostly fisted and feet inverted. Mrs. Grasso was told how to massage the feet to make them more flexible. At 7 weeks Vince's general maturity level was 10 weeks, and on the Viennese developmental quotient he attained the score of 147.

At the next well-baby visit at twelve weeks Vince had his first immunization. Mrs. Grasso was anxious. "You going to give him the needle? Someone told me that they don't give babies needles in the summer because it's the polio season." The pediatrician explained that this might be true for older children but did not pertain to infants. Mrs. Grasso held Vince in sitting position and talked to him and the examiner. "You're going to get the needle. . . . When he got circumcised I almost had a fit when they gave him the needle." The doctor laughed and said, "It won't hurt him."

During developmental testing Mr. and Mrs. Grasso looked on with much interest and smiling. They did not seem at all concerned with how the baby performed the various test items and looked with good humor on his attempt to sit in the little chair and his grimaces as he tried to reach objects.

The interviewer spoke with Mr. Grasso when his wife and Vince left the room to go for the physical examination. He told her how much his wife loved to go swimming. "She likes swimming more than a baby. . . . She's really more of a baby than the baby is." He said he had considered renting a cabin at the beach, but he "wouldn't pay that much money." He spoke of playing poker "with the boys" on weekends and sometimes winning from 300 to 500 dollars, which "comes in handy." During his Army training period he "cleaned up and would go to bed covered with money belts, sometimes 4000 to 5000 dollars." But "when the boys didn't have any money to go home on leave, I gave it back so they could get home before going overseas." He went on to say, "Before you're married, it's all right to fool around and do anything you want to do but after you're married you have to settle down and not have as much fun."

The pediatrician examined Vince's feet, which were kept inverted a good deal of the time. Mrs. Grasso showed some apprehension and asked if his feet were all right. The pediatrician had not even suspected that she was aware of the inverted foot position. It was her impression that Mrs. Grasso pretended to be rather offhand and matter-of-fact about the baby as a cover-up for much anxiety, which she found difficult to express. The doctor also was mindful that Mrs. Grasso never at any point thus far had mentioned her husband's tuberculosis in relation to the baby.

About three weeks later Mrs. Grasso called the pediatrician on a Sunday because Vince had a cold and was running a bit of fever. She was apologetic but genuinely worried, and uncertain of his illness. The pediatrician found a mild upper respiratory infection, for which she prescribed, and urged Mrs. Grasso not to hesitate about calling if she was upset. On this day the doctor raised the question of Mr. Grasso's tuberculosis and the need to check the baby at regular intervals to be on the safe side. Mrs. Grasso said that she herself had to go for regular checkups and that her husband had "to take air for several more years — pneumothorax." She seemed quite willing to discuss the situation in a matter-of-fact way.

At the clinic visit when Vince was slightly over four months old, Mrs. Grasso enthusiastically reported all the things he could do. He played with his hands and feet and was able to get his toes into his mouth. Since he bit everything reaching his mouth, she wondered if he was teething. She said he squealed, grunted, growled, and laughed aloud. When a record was playing, he "sang like a little dog howling." Also, he had begun to pull at her hair and slap at her face to some extent when he was held.

The pediatrician reported Vince to be a well-developed, husky boy, who was much better looking than in the newborn period. He was alert, well nourished, and socially responsive and entered into the testing situation and handling of material with considerable interest. The psychological examiner, however, felt that Vince's response to the human partner, including his mother, was mainly through movement which the adult produced in him. She felt that he did not seek the human partner by eye or ear but experienced the adult only in terms of movement, which stimulated his own movements. She speculated on the quality of human relationship which he might develop.

A few days later the pediatrician was again called because of a cold, fussiness, and a fever. Mrs. Grasso had become quite anxious because Vince also was reported to have a dry hacking cough. She seemed relieved that nothing was seriously wrong. Both Mr. and Mrs. Grasso had also wondered why Vince's head perspired so much and if this was normal. Undoubtedly there was a connection between the fear of the cough, the concern about sweating, and Mr. Grasso's tuberculosis.

Mrs. Grasso also took this occasion to tell the pediatrician that she had really been frightened this month because her period was eight days late and she thought she was pregnant. She had immediately started to make mental plans for rearranging the house to accommodate the two babies. Her husband had said that she ought to wait a few days before making all those plans, but she replied, "I'd rather think I'm pregnant and find out that I'm not, than to think that I'm not and find out that I am." Mrs. Grasso added that though she wouldn't want another baby right now, she could manage all right if she did have one.

A few days later at the regular clinic visit Mrs. Grasso seemed tired and looked as if she had lost some weight. She said she didn't get to bed very early and that Vince's night-time waking had "gotten to be a habit." He wanted to play an hour or so when he woke up, and as a result she was always terribly sleepy.

The tuberculin test was given to Vince as planned. Mrs. Grasso asked what would happen if it were found to be positive: "Would he have to go to a hospital somewhere?" For the first time the magnitude of her anxiety about this became evident, and she was able to talk about it. The occurrence of Vince's cough, her own weight loss, and the tuberculin test all served as coincidental happenings to intensify her anxiety.

The interviewer visited the Grasso home during Vince's fifth month. The outside of the house looked more dilapidated and run down than ever in sharp contrast to the clean neatness of the apartment. All types of furniture and play equipment had been bought for Vince. The baby was in a swing hanging from the doorway between the kitchen and living room. He seemed rather placid and unresponsive to the interviewer's smile. Mrs. Grasso said that lately, when a stranger approached, he "cried and howled miserably."

Mrs. Grasso looked very thin and haggard. She reported that the doctor had found her to be anemic and to have low blood pressure. There were also small tears in the cervix, which accounted for her long periods of menstruation, and the doctor had prescribed medication. While on his mother's lap, Vince was in almost constant movement, standing on her and grabbing at her. He gave the feeling of a very strong, active, almost overpowering boy constantly trampling on his mother. She took it in good grace but seemed slightly irritated.

The conversation turned to Mrs. Grasso's sister in Nevada, from whom she had recently heard. Mrs. Grasso said her sister was an impulsive person with whom she had never gotten along well. As a child she had hated her sister but was too young to understand her problems. Mrs. Grasso recalled that in girlhood they had come across papers disclosing that the sister was the offspring of a prior marriage by their mother and had been legally adopted by Mrs. Grasso's father. It was a great shock to her sister, and she became constantly jealous of Eleanor. Mrs. Grasso did not know anything about her mother's first husband or how her mother had remarried. She said, "It's her business and I think you ought to let people alone if they don't want to tell you things." Mrs. Grasso's sister had been divorced and was currently dating a married man who had children.

A month later Mrs. Grasso looked and felt better. She told the pediatrician that things were going well. The fact that her chest X-ray and the baby's tuberculin test were negative may have contributed to her state of well-being. Also, the fact that the baby had gained a pound and a half since the last visit pleased her very much. Vince looked very compact and well built. While he was not a handsome little boy by any standards, his great responsiveness and general alertness made him a very attractive infant, especially when he smiled.

Vince was taking whole milk, which he did not like quite as much as the formula. He refused anything at all from a cup, but Mrs. Grasso was not concerned over this. He ate well and she had no feeding problems. Also his night waking had ceased and he slept through the night. Mrs. Grasso had been placing him on the potty for several weeks and "was satisfied with the results." She planned to buy Vince special shoes which the doctor had suggested, and preferred a more expensive shoe shop, "where they have good fitters."

At 6½ months the baby could sit briefly alone, was able to support a large fraction of his weight at the standing position, and bounced actively. He seemed greatly interested in motor activity for its own sake. Although he was not actually creeping or even crawling, he was able to pivot in prone and move from back to side. He was quite interested in exploiting the testing material and had even more interest in the adult. His general maturity level was at the 7½-month level, with a developmental quotient of 116. He was highest in body and social areas, the social level being at 8 months. His lowest sector was learning, which nevertheless was at the 7-month level. Physical examination was normal except for a slight rhinitis.

To the interviewer Mrs. Grasso elaborated on Vince's success with bowel training. He usually performed in a high chair with a potty in it, either before or after his lunch. On a visit to her sister-in-law's home he needed the potty, according to Mrs. Grasso, but retained the movement until they could get home to use his own potty. In her various descriptions it sounded as if Mrs. Grasso did not scold Vince for lapses but only praised him for success. The interviewer was struck by the loving way Mrs. Grasso handled the baby and the amount of endearing phrases she used with him.

At home Vince "grabbed everything in sight," and Mrs. Grasso said, "Last week I turned my back for a minute and he pulled a scarf to break one of my lovely vases." She described Vince as a happy baby, "but he also gets terribly mad." When he was angry he would clench his fists and hold his breath. The first time he held his breath she laughed at him; "now he thinks that it's something funny."

With great enthusiasm Mrs. Grasso reported that she had a job selling cosmetics from door to door at friends' homes. She did not try to sell to strangers but was trying to work up a business among friends. The money "would come in handy for Christmas." During the conversation, Vince's expression was sober, and he smiled very little. When he did smile his face looked much more attractive. Most of the time he climbed on his mother, chewed on her blouse, and bit her arm.

In a home visit at eight months Vince was in a playpen that took up almost all available space in the kitchen. The playpen was filled with toys and a large teddy bear. When the interviewer arrived, Mrs. Grasso excused herself for a hurried trip to the grocery. Vince did not seem at all concerned to be left alone with a stranger. He stared at her and was unresponsive but not fearful. He did not look like a particularly attractive child until at last he smiled.

Mrs. Grasso looked somewhat healthier and said that douching had helped the cervical area and she felt better. Her report of Vince's schedule was rather sketchy, and it appeared to vary from day to day depending on Vince's desires. She said that if she scolded him for touching something, "he hangs his head to one side and looks shy." When Mrs. Grasso held Vince, he bit her hard on the shoulder and she winced. At one point he was so active kicking at her, climbing on her, and pulling her hair that she said quite sharply, "Stop it," whereupon he quieted for a bit.

To the inquiry about her husband's health Mrs. Grasso replied that it was fine and that after the first of the year he hoped to get a job, "something like the work of a janitor or custodian in an institution."

About a month later Mrs. Grasso called the pediatrician in great alarm because Vince had a temperature of 104. She had left him in her husband's care while she went for a physical checkup. Her husband had called about the high fever just when she was about to see the doctor so she immediately rushed home by cab. The pediatrician came at once and found that Vince had an otitis media, for which she gave him an injection of penicillin. After this Mrs. Grasso relaxed and talked of herself and the fact that she had again not felt well.

Vince was waking up quite early in the morning and wanted his complete breakfast as well as the bottle, so she had to get up to feed him. The visiting nurse had suggested that the baby be put in a separate room for sleeping. Mrs. Grasso reacted with considerable anger. "I think it would be nice if he had a room for himself, but where would I put him in this house? I don't have any room."

She also said she wished her husband were able to work now. His being at home so much and getting up at 10 or 11 meant that she had to prepare breakfast three times and she did not get her housework done until afternoon. It seemed to her that she was "cooking and cleaning all day."

At the next clinic visit when Vince was just past nine months his mother still looked somewhat thin, worried, and harassed. She asked several questions about the nursery school and expressed her approval of its activities for young children. Vince was reported to be taking some table food and enjoying it, particularly Italian bread. He loved fruit so much that all she had to do to get him to open his mouth was to say the word "fruit." She said that he was not particularly interested in playing with toys.

Mrs. Grasso mentioned that Vince had been having trouble with hard stools and that her sister-in-law recommended suppositories instead of enemas. This was the pediatrician's first inkling that Mrs. Grasso had been giving enemas to Vince at least once every week or two for several months. Both she and her husband had become quite adept at it. Lately she had used the Neocultol, which the pediatrician had prescribed during Vince's last illness, and this had kept his stools soft. Mrs. Grasso also reported in an unconcerned way that when Vince was placed on the potty he frequently manipulated his genitals.

The pediatrician described Vince as "a cute-looking, socially responsive, attractive little boy who at present gives the impression of considerable preoccupation with mastering standing and walking." He appeared well nourished, in about the 50th percentile in weight and slightly above this in length. The slight varus attitude of his feet seemed to be correcting itself with his well-fitted shoes.

At the chronological age of 9 months his social responses were at the 10-month level, and intellectual performance was at the 11-month level. He was low in learning, remaining at the 7-month level, the same as at the last examination. This was because of lack of interest in the testing material, and insufficient drive to uncover or pursue an object.

The psychological examiner at this same clinic was somewhat nonplussed at Vince. "He appears well built and well covered but in no way plump or cuddly. . . . His lack of expression makes Vince especially hard to understand. . . . Despite his advanced motor coordination, his perfectly age-adequate manipulation of toys, and his developed physique, he looks less a person than children of his age usually do." The main reason for this impression was lack of a developed relationship to a human being, especially no detectable warmth in relation to his mother. His face was mostly turned away from her, and he looked at her only twice, the same as at the pediatrician. Despite his many body movements Vince appeared to lack "the animation or soul of a loving relationship," which would give pleasure and meaning to his movements.

The interviewer was invited to share dinner with the Grassos one evening. Mr. Grasso's skin appeared blotchy and he looked rather haggard. He took the occasion to voice his dissatisfaction with Army "red tape," the inadequacy of his pension, the poor food he had received in the hospital, and the fact "that almost anything you have to do with the government doesn't work out." His usually soft voice became very loud, harsh, strident, and explosive.

He felt that the course of his disease had been poorly handled by the government doctors and that they had let it go until his condition had become extreme. In a plaintive way he added that he must keep himself well to protect others. "I won't do things to my wife and son against their good health." Mrs. Grasso interjected, "Oh, that's silly, it doesn't matter." In terms of going back to work, Mr. Grasso mentioned that he was considering a sandwich stand or some such small-business operation.

Mr. and Mrs. Grasso had a rather heated discussion over the fact that child-rearing today was more complicated and difficult than in former years. Mr. Grasso took the position that "women are softer now and complain more." His wife felt that "things were simpler years ago when women just took care of the baby and let the house go." The discussion just missed developing into an argument.

At this point Mrs. Grasso's mother came over and played with Vince. She picked him up and threw him around rather roughly. Both grandmother and baby laughed aloud. She said that her husband had wanted to visit too but she had discouraged him from coming. Then she made some disparaging remarks about him. Mrs. Grasso quickly replied, "Don't talk about my father that way."

Some five weeks later at the well-baby clinic Mrs. Grasso looked rather tired and somewhat depressed. She was considering taking a factory job if her mother would quit work and take care of Vince. She was not particularly eager to work, she said, but she would try it for a while and if it proved too exhausting she would stop because she didn't want to let herself get run down again. Then she went on to say how difficult it was to manage on their income, and "I'm awfully tired of having to scrimp and save and worry whether it is all right to buy this or that." She looked at Vince tenderly and said she really hated to leave him but she had to try and earn some extra money.

At ten months Vince was reported to eat fairly well and was interested in finger-feeding himself. The sleeping situation, however, continued to have its ups and downs. Occasionally Vince had periods of night waking and fretfulness when he needed to be rocked or fed, or both, to get back to sleep.

Mrs. Grasso also reported that recently Vince had begun to fuss over being placed on the potty. She said that she didn't pressure him and that she did not punish him if he soiled his diaper. However, one of her reservations about going back to work was that she felt he was almost toilet-trained and she didn't want him to "slip back."

With respect to language ability, Mrs. Grasso thought that Vince imitated a great many words and was quite advanced in this respect. His interest in toys continued to be minimal, but he was greatly preoccupied with moving about the house very quickly "and constantly getting into things." He was also doing a great deal of throwing and trying to push things over. What seemed to concern her most was Vince's behavior. She said that when she told him to do something or prohibited him, he hit her in the face or pulled her hair. She then spanked his hands but "he doesn't care, he just goes on hitting me." She recalled her distaste for a young nephew who was unmanageable and had hoped during pregnancy that her baby would not be like that. "But now Vince is getting just that way."

The examination by the pediatrician showed an infant of almost eleven months whose body contour had already lost a great deal of the baby look. His legs and arms were like that of a much older boy, and he already looked quite muscular. He handled his body quite well and moved about very rapidly. Language development was appropriate for his age, and some of his social responses were similarly advanced. However, his behavior with the testing materials was somewhat disturbing, since he showed only very brief interest. He used all the items except the mirror for banging, some mouthing, and then casting. He had a very strong left hand preference and threw like a fifteen-month-old child. He was not at all interested in situations demanding problem-solving or combining things. His imitation of tapping the drum was a qualitatively poor performance. He became easily distracted and was not inclined to use the materials for the purpose for which they were intended. More interest was shown toward the inanimate objects which supported his locomotion, such as chairs, tables, etc.

Three weeks later in a home visit Mrs. Grasso was still debating whether or not to go back to work. It was now "more yes than no" and depended on whether her husband would go back to work. The doctors were very pleased with his progress and said he was well enough to work at least four hours a day, "but it is hard to get such part-time jobs." She discussed their difficult financial situation and said, "You need more money to raise children right." "When I see those poor children playing in alleys and streets, I feel sick, because no one has the right to have children unless they know they can give them the best."

The interviewer asked how she felt about limiting her family and whether birth control ran counter to her religious beliefs. Mrs. Grasso said it disturbed her to practice birth control because "it means we can't go to communion," but her husband had said he found nothing wrong with birth control.

Although the apartment looked immaculate and in good condition, Mrs. Grasso complained that her house was getting to be a mess because Vince "is just into everything, and scratching and nicking my furniture." She said she knew she would have to get over being so worried about what he was doing to her things, and she thought she was better about it than she had been a month ago.

When Vince awoke from his nap he smiled brightly and looked very attractive. He hugged his mother hard and kissed her cheeks and chin. She remarked, "You could kiss and love me all day." Vince walked about with excellent balance on the slippery waxed floors and then he went after the cookies in a closet. Mrs. Grasso said "no" in a very harsh voice, quite different from her speaking voice. Finally she threatened to get "the big spoon," a large wooden salad spoon, with which she gestured at him. She said it was the only thing that really frightened him. He did look frightened and stopped what he was doing.

Mrs. Grasso said that Vince often visited a downstairs neighbor, "who adores him and lets him get away with everything." When he came back from there he got into mischief and had to be scolded and spanked. She wondered "why he always hits back after you've hit him." She said that when her husband spanked Vince, the baby would start hitting her, "and that isn't fair."

Shortly thereafter Vince had another siege of illness, an acute upper respiratory infection, moderate fever, and an otitis media. During the illness he was moderately fretful, woke up frequently at night, and required considerable rocking. Mrs. Grasso felt, "He gets by with murder when he is sick."

At the next examination the pediatrician described Vince as "a well-nourished, cute but not handsome infant." On this visit he was tested at the beginning of the session because it was felt that his performance regressed when he became fatigued or fretful. He accepted the testing materials rapidly and with good humor and exploited them in a satisfactory manner.

On the Gesell examination at 1 year and 9 days his gross motor development was close to 15 months. He could stand, walk quite well by himself, creep up a few stairs. His fine motor ability was slightly awkward but effective, and he was able to accomplish what he wished. Reflexes were brisk but not hyperactive, and there were no pathological reflexes. His language was approximately at the 14½-month level. He had four to six words, including names and incipient jargon, and understood a few objects by name. In personal-social adaptation he was at the 14-month level, quite responsive to people and very discriminating, although not anxious about strangers. He was very socially aware and able to anticipate danger situations. Upon seeing the doctor's stethoscope he immediately went to his mother and began to cry, even though he had been friendly and playful with the pediatrician before. In general maturity he was rated at a level of 13 months and 3 weeks, with a developmental quotient of 111, which was somewhat advanced development for his age.

On the Viennese test he also did much better than on the previous visit and showed real interest in the testing materials. Except for imitation, which was poor and brought down his score in learning, he was above his age level in other areas, with body mastery at 17 months, social response at 15 months, and learning at 11 months. His developmental age was 1 year, 2 months, and 1 day, with a developmental quotient of 114. The psychological examiner commented, "Vince looks more like a little man than a baby. His facial expression is sober but occasionally lights up with a rather endearing smile, which is directed both toward people and inanimate objects."

The psychological examiner noted Vince's frequent biting-like mouthing and his tendency to throw objects even while in the process of working with them. His mother tolerated these activities until all at once she would lose her composure and temper. In spite of this, or because of it, Vince frequently engaged in these pursuits. In one instance of throwing, she suddenly yelled, "Stop it" and slapped his hand rather hard. He did not really cry after the punishment, but his body coordination deteriorated and his interest in inanimate objects became absolutely limited to throwing and mouthing. This lasted for about five minutes. Thus, a vicious circle was created, wherein the punishment produced more of the undesirable behavior, which in turn received more punishment, ad infinitum.

It was speculated that the child emulated his mother's disintegration of composure by regressing his own behavior to more infantile levels. He was unsure of when to expect the danger of his mother's violent reaction, since she ranged from tolerance, warmth, and tenderness to strong irritation and need to punish within the space of a very few seconds. There was no doubt that there were times when this very active, demanding youngster was capable of exasperating his mother to the utmost. But it was also true that many of the limits she set for him were inconsistent ones, and he was permitted to get by with things at one time which she limited very strongly at other times.

The psychological examiner speculated that this unpredictable environment must produce some negative effect on the child's faculty to imitate or to memorize. His approach in problem solution had no consistency and gave the impression of a divided energy between alternatives based on whatever attracted his momentary attention. She also pointed out that Vince recognized danger if it came from an adult via a "prop" such as the stethoscope, but that he was not perceptually aware of danger from the physical environment. He ran into a corner of a desk while trying to grasp a toy and would have walked off the bed if he had not been restrained. From an extremely active child with little perceptual awareness, "who acts before he thinks," such behavior impressed the psychologist as accident proneness and the "tendency to seek accident-punishment."

About this time Mr. Grasso began to work for a few hours each morning. He and a man for whom he had once worked arranged to sell fish in various neighborhoods. The Grassos sold their car and bought a truck for this purpose. Mrs. Grasso was glad that this work was not physically taxing and hoped it would last at least through the summer months.

A few weeks later Vince had another bout with fever, a mild otitis on the left, and tonsillitis with a cervical adenitis. Temperature subsided, and the infection cleared up within three days upon treatment. When the interviewer visited Vince in his thirteenth month, the boy looked strong and well. He had a bit more hair and was good-looking except for his ears, which stuck rather far out and made him somewhat short of handsome. Mrs. Grasso was happy that he now slept until 9 A.M., which gave her more morning rest, but her housework was delayed. She attributed this later awakening to the fact that she now kept him up until 8:30 P.M. at night.

Mrs. Grasso enjoyed going to the beach. Vince was still frightened of the water and would not go near it alone, but he would wade if she held his hand. He was fascinated with the sand and played with it at length. Mr. Grasso never went to the beach and maintained that the doctors said too much sun was not good for him. Mrs. Grasso indicated that the fish-selling enterprise was running into difficulties with the partner, and she had decided to go to work in September. Her mother planned finally to leave her job and take care of Vince.

Mrs. Grasso went into the details of a law suit in which her mother was involved as a result of a car accident. A settlement was forthcoming which might bring 8000 to 9000 dollars. With this money her mother planned to buy a two-family house, and the Grassos would move into one half of it.

Apropos of the new housing possibility Mrs. Grasso said she very much wanted to have another baby and would try at once if she had another place to live. She very much wanted a baby girl. In looking back on pregnancy, labor, and delivery it all seemed very easy to her. The most difficult part, she said, was the first six or seven months of Vince's life, when "he had so many little complaints." Now, within the last month or so, he had changed into "an almost perfect baby," was able to play by himself, and made fewer demands on her. But it still annoyed her that he was so very difficult when she took him visiting, to the point where relatives had asked what she had done to make him that way.

In the fourteenth month Mrs. Grasso spoke at length about Vince's extreme activity and her difficulty in managing him. She reversed an earlier opinion, saying that as a baby he had been really very easy and "just wonderful" but that he had now become increasingly difficult. He "wants to go all the time" and was unaccepting of the limits she tried to impose. There was no doubt that Vince received numerous spankings throughout the day and responded to them by counter-aggression. In an effort to discourage this pattern the pediatrician said that this was a difficult age to cope with, and Mrs. Grasso admitted that she couldn't control herself "because I get so out of patience when he gets this way." The pediatrician felt that in many ways the relationship between mother and child was warm and tender but that Mrs. Grasso would heave a sigh of relief when Vince became old enough to go to nursery school.

In the testing situation Vince did fairly well with the materials but after a time began to regress, becoming fretful, increasingly active, hurling himself about the room, falling frequently, and getting banged up. The pediatrician described Mrs. Grasso at this point as "a chronically harassed, tired young woman, with a husband who does not work to provide for his family and a son who is hard to manage. She loves them both, yet wishes they would be a little different."

At the next home visit Mrs. Grasso told the interviewer that she was extremely disappointed because Vince was so "fresh," and that she had made every effort to bring him up to be a "good boy." Now he had begun to hit other children and get into small fights with them. At this point Vince became somewhat fussy, and Mrs. Grasso gave him a small piece of banana. When he reached for more before finishing it, she yelled in a rather shrewish tone of voice, stating with some disgust that he only wanted to mess with it. Apparently Vince often liked to mess with his food.

This led Mrs. Grasso to a discussion of the current state of toilet training. Although Vince was now completely trained for bowel movements, he had begun "teasing." He made the characteristic sound for toileting but then declined to go. As for urinary training, she had just about given up. She felt that Vince urinated so frequently that she couldn't catch him and he "teased" her by refusing to urinate on the toilet but wetting himself the minute he was taken off.

Mrs. Grasso mentioned that she had been having very severe cramps with the last two menstrual periods and that she had been under care for some kind of gynecological infection. If her cramps continued, she planned to contact the women's clinic again. Concerning her husband, she said that he was working only erratically doing odd jobs and that she would not "push him any more," but go to work herself instead. Vince became quite distracting at this point, and Mrs. Grasso became irritated. She shouted at him, but the irritation passed quickly, and she was again warm and smiling. The interviewer felt that despite the many problems which beset this young attractive mother and despite her need for an obedient, clean child, there was a good deal of warmth and pride in her relationship with Vince.

In September, Mrs. Grasso told the interviewer that the summer had been fine, but then she went on to describe all the problems which had occurred. Her mother was in the hospital "with some kind of tumor on her side." Mrs. Grasso herself had recently been seen at the gynecology clinic, where "a growth was removed" on an out-patient basis. Since its removal she had been having less severe pain during menstrual periods, although she still felt irritable and fatigued.

In August she had noticed a couple of little lumps on Vince's arm, but the pediatrician who was substituting during the vacation period had "laughed it off" and did not feel the need to see the baby. He said that it was a post-injection occurrence. Later Vince developed an irritation of the mucous membrane in the mouth and again Mrs. Grasso called the pediatrician. She felt that he minimized her concern and regarded her as an over-anxious mother. Finally she decided to have her dentist look at Vince, and he said it was just a place in the mouth where he had bitten the buccal mucosa and there was no infection. However, she was waiting the return of the permanent pediatrician before she could be truly reassured.

Mrs. Grasso was much concerned with growths of one kind or another, her own, her mother's, or Vince's. Yet it was striking that her deep anxiety about health problems was not revealed either in her voice or the way in which she described the problems. Because of her mother's illness Mrs. Grasso could not go ahead with her plans to start work, since it would be too much for her mother to cope with Vince. She said, "I've learned not to plan definitely on anything because the plans don't work out." Although her husband was making attempts to find work, it seemed that he always arrived a little too late to apply, and the job was already filled. It was evident that Mrs. Grasso was guarding her real feelings about these events and making a considerable effort to be casual and philosophic about them.

According to Mrs. Grasso, Vince was now considerably less "fresh" and had also stopped attacking his playmates. She felt that he was so extremely friendly with everyone that he would never hesitate to go off with a stranger, which was a matter of concern to her. In interaction with the child Mrs. Grasso displayed considerable inconsistency. She verbally prohibited him several times from touching a particular piece of bric-a-brac and threatened to spank him. At first her threats discouraged him, but each time he went back on the chair to reach for it. Finally she did get out a large wooden spoon and whacked his buttocks. Vince cried for a few minutes but then appeared happy again. Right after the spanking she was as warm towards him as before. A few minutes later Vince repeated the activity for which he had been punished, and this time Mrs. Grasso ignored him, although she was quite aware of what he was doing.

When Vince was sixteen and one-half months the psychological examiner saw him as "an extremely attractive child, well built, muscular, with a golden skin and strikingly dark eyes." His blond hair was sparse and gave him a "masculine" look. His body movements were agile, and his facial expressions displayed a wide gamut of emotions: interested and intense, searching and serious. At this same visit the mother's interviewer simultaneously commented on Mrs. Grasso's "considerable variation of facial expression that reflected a range of tense and sad feeling, smiling animation, annoyance, sulkiness, and outright anger."

From time to time Vince smiled. This smile was a feature that made him most engaging. It created contact and conveyed a sense of happy self-satisfaction. His motor development was excellent, and he mastered his body without fear or hesitation. He walked without difficulty on even or uneven surfaces, climbed successfully, and stood on one leg without loss of balance. Running was distinctly and intentionally different from walking.

In his actions he always used maximal motor effort, beyond what was called for. When throwing a ball he lifted his arm almost fully extended, bent it backward in full swing, and then threw. The exaggerated movement seemed to create special pleasure for him with no special strain. But it was striking that there was no attempt at constructive activity on his part. The general impression was that he could produce chaos within a few minutes. He crumpled and tore paper into pieces instead of drawing, hit at the mirror instead of looking into it, and used one object to hit or throw at another.

Vince did not mouth as much as before, but he still mouthed each new object as if undecided when to start his destructive game with it. Also, he regularly mouthed when play material was being taken from him. In such instances his fingers closed around the object, which either touched his closed lips or was pushed into the mouth.

A second type of mouthing was distinctly different. For this he used only objects shaped like a cigarette (crayon, pencil). He held the object with only two fingers and then inhaled. It appeared as a special activity itself, an exact imitation of his mother's smoking, and gave insight into a behavior dependency on his mother. There was more evidence of this dependency. Despite Vince's constant motion and activity, he never lost sight of his mother's face and checked on its expression at regular intervals. He seemed to know and feel that she watched critically.

All of this exaggerated motor behavior seemed to serve as armament in the battle of child against parent, as a weapon against the mother. The disorder and destruction of which he was capable could be especially disturbing to Mrs. Grasso's wish for a well-organized household. The way the mother and child looked at each other revealed the nature of their battle quite clearly. She looked at him like a tamer of wild animals who both savored and feared the job, while he responded by testing the limits, knowing that she was master but venturing to become stronger after all.

The closeness of the mother-son relationship was also evidenced in positive terms. Most striking was Vince's compliance with his mother's teaching of language. He had the most elaborate vocabulary of all study children his age, pronounced each word clearly and distinctly, and chose them appropriately. He showed great capacity to repeat words in a parrot-like way but had not yet reached the stage where he used language to initiate and carry on his own communication.

When Vince was engaged in destructive activity he seemed to

synthesize the dual roles of his mother, that of critic and of model for his gestures. His facial expression was far from relaxed or happy and he frowned at himself while in the act of destroying. Similarly, when he succeeded at an approved task he applauded himself by clapping his hands.

Despite the gestures and language imitative of his mother, Vince did not imitate in any organized fashion. He performed activities fairly well on a spontaneous level but did not pay attention to any modifications demonstrated by the examiner, nor did he attempt to reproduce them in any way. It seemed that his energy was so tied up by the battle with his mother and his defenses against it that there was little left for autonomous performance. He gave the impression of being driven into a fight and inclined to act out by vehement impulsive motor behavior.

At the next meeting with the pediatrician Mrs. Grasso reported that her mother was now home from the hospital and feeling better. She had had a cyst removed from her lip and one from her neck, and had been given an injection for the low back pain. As a consequence she had less back pain than in many years. Mrs. Grasso said nothing about going back to work but discussed her desire to have another baby while Vince was young and she herself was still young. She had been trying to persuade her husband of this, but he said they couldn't afford it. Her feeling was that "one could always manage."

During this period Vince was again an early morning riser, which did not please her. He ate table foods almost exclusively but still took his milk in three daily bottles. His mother reported that he played best with older children because they "give in to him more." With children his own age, he tended to take things away from them, hit them, and become aggressive. For this reason she did not often let him play with children his own age. She was delighted that Vince would soon participate in a forthcoming Child Study Center play group. As yet he showed no particular interest in toys but preferred all kinds of motor activity, such as playing ball, climbing steps, getting up on the dining room table, crawling on chairs. She said that he didn't look where he was going and impetuously ran into many things in his hurry. He cried briefly but was easily comforted and went about his business.

Vince continued to speak very well and was beginning to use

words more and more for communication. He called many things by name and understood complicated directions. Generally he told his mother when he needed the toilet and was proud of himself when he performed. He seemed more compliant in this area than in others. In addition to having impressive language ability, Vince revealed high social response on the Viennese test. However, his behavior with most of the test materials was to take them quickly, sometimes exploit them appropriately, and then resort to banging or throwing. He had a wonderful smile, which lit up his entire face.

To the home visitor Mrs. Grasso reported that her husband was in excellent health but still worked only occasionally on part-time jobs. Although her mother had recovered, Mrs. Grasso had decided not to look for a job herself. In this decision she was supported by her husband's sister, who also felt that if she went to work before her husband settled into a full-time job, she would "be left with the responsibility." She said vehemently that she would work only on the condition that it was "fifty-fifty" with her husband. She also mentioned that Mr. Grasso took Vince out with him occasionally but only when she suggested it. Most of the time he didn't think of it himself. She guessed "that men are like that." On the other hand, she felt that he was quite competent with the baby, and when Vince was ill her husband could even give him an enema.

A month later Mrs. Grasso appeared quite thin and tired. She told the interviewer that it was extremely hard to get her housework done in the morning because her husband usually slept until noon. She had not been feeling well for over a week, suffering from nausea and severe headaches which nothing could relieve. One night she got out of bed at 4 A.M. and gave herself an enema in the hope that it would help the headache. She mentioned, "I'm only twenty-two years old, but I feel tired most of the time and I can't get things done." She didn't think she was pregnant because she recently had had a menstrual period, and "I've had nothing to do with my husband since then." Although she had very much wanted another baby, now she felt she would be completely overwhelmed if she had one, "because of all I have to do."

Mrs. Grasso complained that Vince was "so fresh" and messed with everything in the house, including the household appliances, which might be dangerous to touch. During the discussion Vince indeed was into and upon everything. The Grassos now had a stray kitten, with which Vince played tenderly at first; but then he took hold of its tail and inserted the tip into his mouth as a nipple. His mother said, "He's so cute that I have to laugh at him even when he's doing something wrong."

Mrs. Grasso's mother dropped in to visit. She looked smartly groomed and well dressed. Her voice was quite "cultured" compared with her daughter's. When Vince started touching the toaster Mrs. Grasso went for a wooden fork, with which she threatened him. She said this substituted for the wooden spoon that Vince had taken and hidden. A crisis occurred when Vince knocked over and broke one of the cocktail glasses on the sideboard. Mrs. Grasso lost her temper and gave him several very hard spanks with the wooden fork. She scolded for a minute or so, then spanked him again, saying, "At moments like this I would like to kill him."

After a few minutes Vince quieted down and Mrs. Grasso noticed that he had wet himself and made a puddle on the floor. Again she exploded in anger, spanked him, and scolded harshly. Roughly she removed his pants, told him, "You're a very bad boy" and then changed the pants. In a few moments she relented and took the initiative to interest him in a mechanical horse-and-buggy toy. Then she held him tenderly in her lap, kissing the top of his head several times. Mrs. Grasso expressed her great discouragement, saying "Sometimes I really could weep because Vince doesn't mind me."

She referred again to the desire for another baby and said, "In fact, I would like three children." Since she had never been close to her only sibling, a sister, she had felt lonely and had always envied large families with many children. She was sure that Vince's problems arose from the limited space in the house, and she despaired of ever having a home of her own because of her husband's employment difficulties. She felt that Vince's behavior was a phase "which he must go through if I can stand it while it lasts."

When Vince was nineteen months old Mrs. Grasso reported to the pediatrician that he "fusses and picks at his food." It came out that she was really concerned that he no longer cared for meat and had an increased tendency to refuse things. She "scolded him and called him a bad boy" and tried to persuade him, although without actually force-feeding. It was quite obvious that some of his refusal was from his need to struggle with her. Since he did appear rather thin and pale, the pediatrician put him on a combination of vitamins and iron as long as he was not eating so well. As for Vince's sleeping, "It's pretty good; it's off and on." He slept most of the night but wakened enough to rouse his mother so that she either had to give him a bottle or take him to bed with her. Although the sleeping situation was somewhat irregular, it did not seem to be too bothersome to the family.

Vince was still exceedingly active in getting about and had little interest in toys. The cat tolerated his approaches until it could stand no more and then ran where it could not be reached. Mrs. Grasso said that she tried to teach him to be gentle, "and he is part of the time, but then squeezes too hard." Her method of discipline was to yell at him or produce the wooden fork. When she corrected him, he "screamed for daddy" or stuck out his tongue at her.

Vince had recently submitted to his first barber-shop haircut and was surprisingly good about it, which pleased Mrs. Grasso. He had also been taken to see a department store Santa Claus, which turned out to be a real fiasco. He shrank from Santa, saying "bad boy," began to cry as they got close, and refused to go near him. Since then, whenever he saw a picture of Santa, he continued to say "bad boy."

The first week in January the pediatrician was called because of a quite high fever and paroxysms of coughing. She found numerous piping musical chest rales, a large amount of purulent post-nasal drainage, and several quite enlarged tender cervical glands. The throat was moderately red. Medication was given and the asthmatic symptoms began to decrease. After the third day the temperature remained normal and there were no further symptoms. Since this was the first episode of asthmatic breathing in Vince's respiratory infections, it frightened both the Grassos considerably. During the ten days that it ran its course, Vince was particularly hard to live with and his mother was exhausted. "I felt bad that I hollered at him but sometimes I had to. . . . One night I just sat down and cried."

In the middle of January, Vince had a cold and cough for several days without fever. Mrs. Grasso told the home visitor that

Vince had been very good about not touching the Christmas tree and was enthralled by the lights. She was happy to learn that he would soon be starting in the nursery school. Regarding her own health, she said that it was better and that the headaches had not recurred. In December she had gone to the hospital, where "two growths were cut off my private and a wart removed from my knee." She had had the wart for a long time and it tended to become irritated. Its removal was a relief because "I don't like having something that doesn't belong to my body. . . . You hear too much about cancer cases these days."

Mr. Grasso had at last found a full-time job in a bowling alley. He was supposed to start the following week, but Mrs. Grasso said, "I won't believe it until he begins." She felt that the chronic unemployment had been extremely bad for him, as he slept late and didn't get anything done during the day. The one saving grace was that he had more time for Vince. "Now daddy is everything to Vince."

Mrs. Grasso had started to attend an evening adult education sewing class and displayed the clothes she was making. She wished she could own her own console machine some day "but it's impossible now." Later on, she planned to go to one of the wood-working classes and hoped Mr. Grasso might also be interested. During the conversation Vince started to pick up a miniature salt and pepper set from the sideboard. Mrs. Grasso put it out of his reach, saying, "It's better to avoid trouble before it begins." This was the first time she had been observed to remove prohibited objects from temptation.

Later Vince climbed on a chair, which toppled over, and he was left hanging from the edge of the sideboard by his hands and chin, yelling urgently for "mommy." She quickly responded. Then he said a word that sounded like "vermouth," a bottle of which was on the sideboard. Mrs. Grasso poured some into a small glass and gave it to him, saying "Vermouth is a good tonic for a child." He drank some, set down the glass, and disappeared.

There was complete silence for a while and then Mrs. Grasso said she had better find out "what he's up to." The next sounds were shrill scolding and spanking. She returned to the dinette, followed by Vince holding his buttocks and crying vigorously for "daddy." In a gentle tone of voice his mother explained that "daddy will be home soon." She told the interviewer, "Every time he gets in trouble with me he wants his daddy." Vince pleaded, "Rockie, Mommy," whereupon Mrs. Grasso took him in her arms, sat in the rocking chair, held him close, and rocked with a tender expression on her face.

When Vince was seen at the age of twenty months and twenty-six days the pediatrician felt that he looked quite slender but was not surprised in view of his recent illness. He weighed no more than he had a month before. He climbed into the crib and the physical examination proceeded. He seemed to accept the reassurance of "no needle" from the pediatrician and only objected to the removal of his training pants, obviously remembering the penicillin injection in his buttocks less than two weeks before. The pediatrician was surprised to find him so cooperative, since she had given him injections on the many occasions of respiratory illnesses.

Mrs. Grasso reported that toileting was proceeding smoothly and Vince usually told her of his needs. He seemed quite proud of his ability to use the toilet. He now had so many words "that it's difficult to count." He also said his prayers, but Mrs. Grasso remarked, "He's stubborn and when he's supposed to say Father, Son, and Holy Ghost, he will only say Son and Holy Ghost but not Father." His refusal to say Father seemed to her just perversity because he clamped his lips and adamantly refused to say it. He also had picked up a number of words which were not to her liking, such as "Oh, Christ," "damn," etc.

The psychological examiner noted "the manliness of Vince's build, the serious intensity of his face, and the smile, which is as engaging as ever." While Vince was easy to describe physically he was hard to evaluate. An outstanding characteristic of behavior was the "speed" which cloaked his movements. They appeared "like a continuous acting with no beginning and no end." It was impossible to predict the level of motor functioning, which was agile and advanced in some areas, clumsy in others. He was an incredible climber, yet he looked awkward and dejected when he was sitting. Although he moved along smoothly, suddenly he could fall down without any warning.

The examiner believed this was due to a discrepancy between the continuous impulse to move and the staccato-type movement produced. Vince also behaved as if he did not perceive the realities of environment. Light things were lifted as if they were heavy, small things as if they were large. He reached for near things as if they were far away, he moved on any surface as if it were slippery. He seemed not to notice changes in environment or to cope with them at different levels.

One of the most confusing features was the impression Vince gave that he always wanted to do more than one thing at a time. Not only his mind but also his body seemed simultaneously to aim at two different goals. The left hand held an object ready to put down, the right hand held another object ready to throw. Even the legs seemed to participate in the division. The left leg was still and controlled, the right leg dangled in a relaxed fashion. He also appeared to move simultaneously in two directions at once. While his right arm tended forward, his left tended backward. If his left arm climbed upward, his right drew down. He seemed not to have realized that one can move only in one direction at a time.

It was also difficult to predict his behavior in terms of social response. Although he responded well to prohibitions and even accepted suggestions occasionally, he worked without zest if he was not particularly interested. At other times he became genuinely interested in the task. But he clearly showed determination for independent goals against the will of the adult. His refusals were stated verbally, accompanied by facial expressions of annoyance and followed by a motor action which made it final. It was hard to determine under which circumstances he cooperated and under which he became negative. It rather looked as if Vince genuinely wanted to obey but as if some rising tension in him prevented it. For Vince, social compliance had the impact of physical restraint, which he could tolerate for only a short while but then had to rebel.

The mother's observer on this visit felt that Mrs. Grasso appeared quite tense despite the attractiveness of her appearance. She leaned rigidly forward, with her legs tightly entwined around the chair, and when she left the chair her motions were very darting and rapid. This same intense quality appeared throughout Vince's testing. Although she appeared to be amused with some of his errors and found one reason or another to excuse his failures to perform, there was no question but that she was concerned about how he performed.

Her relationship to the child was consistent with that observed in home visits. When he was in any physical difficulty she immediately went to his rescue. When he was in emotional distress she comforted him with verbal soft conversation and tender holding, but in such a way as not to interfere with the necessary procedures. The only difference at the clinic was that she did not directly prohibit Vince or fly into a shrill rage as she did at home.

A month later Mrs. Grasso told the interviewer that it was wonderful to be able to get her housework done early since her husband was up and out of the house in the morning. She also believed that Vince was doing quite well in the nursery school and was pleased to have him there, although there were transportation problems. She doubted that she would want to continue with nursery school the following year because it took three mornings each week and "I'm not able to get the housework done." She was rather vague as to whether afternoon sessions would solve the problem.

She then mentioned that it still gave her "a funny feeling" to talk to various people about herself. "I can't help wondering what they all think of me." She said that it was perfectly all right, however, and she didn't mind because "they have to know the mothers, too." But the interviewer felt that there was more to it, which Mrs. Grasso was unable or unwilling to verbalize further.

Mrs. Grasso had become discouraged with sewing after she had run into difficulties with a satin blouse. She said, "I know I get disgusted and give up too quickly." She guessed that "Vince inherited those traits from me." Recently toilet training had not been going too well because Vince "would play with himself" or with the toilet paper and not produce any result. During the conversation Vince started to play with his mother's cigarette case, throwing the two separate pieces repeatedly to the floor. When he did not respond to her prohibitions, she finally flared up in anger and went to get the wooden spoon. He then quieted down.

In retrospect the interviewer felt that Vince's adjustment to the nursery school had been hard on Mrs. Grasso and also that she was still uncomfortable about her own relationship to the study. The interviewer was also struck by the impulsive nature of Mrs. Grasso's responses to many areas of her life, the tendency to become quickly angered or discouraged and to withdraw from an activity or situation. One felt that "her reaction was often disproportionate to the provocation."

In Vince's twenty-third month Mrs. Grasso told the home visitor that she had decided to have another baby. A couple of months back she had thought she was pregnant because her period was late and she had asked her husband whether there had been any "accidents." "There's always the possibility that a condom could have a slow leak." She was disappointed not to be pregnant, but now her husband had finally agreed to a second baby even though he was out of work again.

His job in the bowling alley had petered out and he was seeking a night-shift job, which he preferred to day work. Nothing had yet been found, and Mrs. Grasso felt very discouraged, especially since his government pension was going to be cut back in August. This had prompted her to take a selling job. However, the night before her job was to begin, Mr. Grasso had agreed that she could become pregnant again. As a consequence, she worked only one day, and that only "because I promised them." Her thinking was that if they did have a second child, her husband "would really have to settle down to a full-time job."

At 23 months and 20 days, in spite of his over-activity, Vince scored a developmental age of 27 months on the Viennese test, with a developmental quotient of 114.

As the second year drew to a close, the quality of interaction in the Grasso household remained inconsistent and ambivalent although the relationship remained basically warm. The economic jeopardy of the household seemed inclined to continue as an important undercurrent which would affect the family's adjustment throughout its history. Under the circumstances the goal of a second child would seem likely to complicate further the tenuous financial realities.

But this is a value judgment far removed from the nonstriving, low-income, blue-collar values of the Grassos' world, where impulse rather than planning and restraint is the fundamental level of actual behavior. We can only hope that life confirms Eleanor Grasso's words that "one can always find a way to manage."

The Grasso Family

SUMMARY

A. EXPECTATIONS

1. Maternal Expectations. Mrs. Grasso was fully satisfied with the prospect of having a child, especially since there had been a miscarriage and disappointment before. During the first year she revealed almost nothing of her expectations for the role of mother, but she demonstrated a child-like romanticized delight. It was not until she encountered the difficulties of her son's second year that she expressed doubts about her own ability to be a good mother. The conflict of a mother's working became an issue in the second year because of the realization that her husband was not assuming the task of supporting the family. She came to a reluctant theoretical acceptance of a breadwinning role, although it conflicted with her concept that a mother should be home with her baby.

2. Specificity of Expectations. Mrs. Grasso was inarticulate on this subject, but apparently the realities of having the baby were vastly different from her expectations. While she somewhat doubtfully accepted breast feeding, it turned out to be uncomfortable and unpleasant, so she changed to bottle feeding. Similarly, she found that babies weren't dolls and that the specifics of child care can be difficult. But she tended to take changes in her stride and readjusted as she progressed.

3. Motivational Orientation. Mrs. Grasso was predominantly child-centered in her expectations, although some shifts were observed which did not indicate basic change in motivation. From the beginning of pregnancy she was known to place a high value on motherhood. When the child came, her response was eager and warm. The period of hospitalization and the ensuing weeks were a time of "coming down to earth." She soon came to realize that there were many vicissitudes in daily caring for the baby for which she had not been prepared.

Throughout the first six months her concerns were mainly related to the well-being of the baby, and she continued to be proud of him, happy, and successful in satisfying his needs. During the second six months she began to show some signs of displeasure. Vince's hyperactivity and Mrs. Grasso's increasing difficulty in managing him, as well as economic problems, led to these negative reactions. But they were interspersed with pleasure in him and the joys of parenthood. As she herself pointed out, "I have my good days and my bad ones." To some extent Mrs. Grasso became able to adapt her expectations to the realities of a vigorous and overactive child. By the time he was one year old, she spoke about improving her own attitudes toward his behavior.

During the second year, though one would still probably call her expectations child-centered, they were more frequently related to good performance, learning, and behavioral conformity. As she continued to struggle with problems of discipline and management, she voiced expectations which were child-centered in their goal though directed toward herself. For example, she thought that she might be able to control Vince's behavior with less yelling and less physical punishment than she had come to use. Whatever shifts of expectation took place were not really shifts away from child-centeredness but a redirection of interest and concern due to the problem of economic responsibility.

4. Role of Child in Fulfilling Mother's Expectations. The pleasure and pride which Mrs. Grasso took in Vince clearly showed that he fulfilled her expectations in most areas. In one aspect, however, he apparently ran counter to her expectations of a manageable and tractable child. Vince's excessive physical output and resistance to control created a major battle in the second year.

Discipline became a constant struggle, and it was felt that one of the major problems was the mother's own inconsistency. Within the space of a few minutes her attitude could vary from fond indulgence to aggressive punishment for little reason. She was observed to be permissive on some days and restrictive on others. Nevertheless, the strength of a warm relationship remained despite the battle.

5. Paternal Expectations. Mr. Grasso also pleasurably anticipated the child, and his permissive attitudes showed consideration and tolerance for limitations of the child's ability to conform. Mr. Grasso hoped that the child would not follow his own "wild" patterns of chasing around, gambling, horse-racing, and drifting, but he set no strict standards or expectations. However, in regard to Vince's generally somewhat extreme physical activity, he was more demanding.

B. BEHAVIOR

1. Communication. There was much tender and loving physical communication between mother and son. Verbal communication, however, was used more for controlling the child's behavior than as a mode of expressing maternal feelings. Mrs. Grasso used words to teach, scold, prohibit, and threaten. But she also used them to praise and persuade. When Vince began to pick up words toward the end of his first year, his mother enjoyed teaching him to imitate adult words. She did it because it was fun and language became a game. She was proud of Vince's fast-developing vocabulary and thought him extremely bright and advanced.

2. Regularity and Flexibility of Scheduling. Mrs. Grasso put up with some sleeping irregularity, although it was quite fatiguing for her. While she liked an orderly home and strove "to get things done," it did not make her inflexible in meeting Vince's demands as they arose or changed. During the two years Mrs. Grasso maintained a flexible and permissive character in the management of routines but began to place arbitrary, specific limitations on Vince's non-routine behavior, such as his physical activity and play. These limitations became more important as he became an increasingly vigorous, active child. They were not consistently or regularly established, however, and Mrs. Grasso exhibited a good deal of variability both in her behavior and in her feelings about Vince's activities. There was conspicuous temperamental irregularity in the mother-child relationship and inconsistency in their emotional reactions to each other despite the underlying warmth and satisfaction.

3. Techniques of Management. Mrs. Grasso was permissive in certain areas of behavior and restrictive in others, with high tolerance in matters of routine care and low tolerance for Vince's hyperactivity. Permissive behavior was most generally reported, with a particularly small proportion of recorded non-permissive behavior. If Vince did not want to go to sleep by himself, one or the other parent would rock him. Both Mr. and Mrs. Grasso were particularly indulgent during periods of illness, and there was generally permissive behavior in regard to eating and sleeping. Often Mrs. Grasso told stories to get Vince to eat and provided a number of distractions. But on occasion, despite the warm interplay and affection, Mrs. Grasso refused to pick up the child when he cried, for fear of "spoiling" him.

In managing this very active child Mrs. Grasso for a long time was not ingenious in avoiding problems by removing things from Vince's reach. Thus, as he "got into everything," with damage to prized possessions, she became outraged. Towards the end of the study she began to "plan ahead" and to prevent confrontations by substituting or putting things out of reach.

4. Relation of Expectations to Behavior. Breast feeding was one of the few expectations that Mrs. Grasso had voiced during pregnancy. But from the moment of her child's birth she faced difficulties not only in carrying out this expectation but in coping with all the minutiae of child care which she had not anticipated. Once past the earliest surprises of motherhood, however, she took to the care of Vince with enjoyment and with relatively little conflict.

One is struck by the fact that most of the first-year reports of this mother's behavior were of an adaptive, permissive nature and covered every aspect of mother-child interaction. The dichotomy noted between attempts to control his vigorous play activity and her permissive ease in dealing with routine activities produced inconsistent and contradictory modes of behavior. In the second year they were more likely to be related to Vince's excessive physical activity and were either of a punishing or scolding character or involved some means of manipulating the environment to control the child.

5. Paternal Behavior. Mr. Grasso was exceptional in the considerable extent to which he shared with his wife the routine care of the baby. The fact that he was usually at home during the day made such sharing of activities possible. Reports of Mr. Grasso's part in caring for Vince began when Vince was three months old and continued for the next year and a half. He diapered and fed him, rocked him to sleep when he was ill, and played with him. There was little evidence that Mr. Grasso was as restrictive or inconsistent in handling Vince as was his wife.

When Vince got past his first year, his father occasionally took him on expeditions, such as riding in the truck. Emotional satisfactions in the father-son relationship were obviously high. By the end of the two years it was reported that Vince was not only very fond of his father but also more demonstrative toward him than toward his mother. When he was disciplined by his mother, he ran to his father for comfort. This preference caused some discomfort to Mrs. Grasso. Mr. Grasso's relation with Vince gave a general impression of child-centeredness and responsiveness to the clues provided by the child.

C. SOCIO-CULTURAL INFLUENCES

1. Socio-economic Status and Values. Vince Grasso was born into a non-striving, lower-income family, which experienced a great deal of economic insecurity. Both parents grew up in a decrepit tenement area of the city and came from families where economic pressures left little time for individual direction or attention to their children. It was thus not surprising that Mr. Grasso had drifted aimlessly with the corner gang and that Mrs. Grasso had impetuously entered marriage. Both followed the non-aspiring ways typical of most working-class youth, preferring the present satisfactions of a factory pay check to education and advancement in the occupational or social world.

Mr. Grasso's convalescence from tuberculosis included a long "borderline" period, in which it was difficult to distinguish between physical inability to work and lack of psychological motivation to do so. Mrs. Grasso vacillated between undertaking the role of wage earner and forcing her husband to do so. Towards the end of the study she hoped for a second pregnancy to free her from the task of earning the family living. At the same time, she was not very hopeful that her husband would get and keep a job.

The Grassos were a Roman Catholic family who appeared to

value their religious attachments. Mrs. Grasso grew closer to the Church during her husband's hospitalization. For her, the use of contraceptives was subject to some ambivalence and concern.

2. Extended Family. There was no appreciable conflict with the Grassos' families of origin. Both of Mr. Grasso's parents were dead, but Mrs. Grasso had a supportive relationship with his sister, who sided with her. The surface relationship of Mrs. Grasso and her mother appeared close, affectionate, and helpful, and Mrs. Grasso felt herself to be more favored than her sister. However, her repeated statement that she hoped to raise Vince better than her mother had raised her led to speculation about the underlying character of this relationship.

The maternal family lived next door, and there was a good deal of back-and-forth visiting. The grandmother kept a close eye on the Grasso household and appeared to play a role in decision-making. She served as a kind of assistant to Mrs. Grasso, and in some ways, as a model for her maternal behavior. She was a supportive grandparent, who assumed very limited responsibility for the child's care because she worked and because of her health. Throughout the first two years there was evidence of affection and pleasurable play between grandmother and grandson.

As indicated earlier, little was known of Mrs. Grasso's relationship to her father, although there was some evidence that she was protective towards him and resented derogatory remarks made about him by her mother. The fact that severe emotional problems existed between the maternal grandparents, even necessitating hospitalization for emotional illness of the maternal grandfather, was not known during the two-year study. It was revealed only in subsequent contact with the family. Undoubtedly it contributed much to Mrs. Grasso's difficulties and certainly had important implications for the nuclear family life of the Grassos.

3. Spatial Arrangements and Values. On the one hand, Mrs. Grasso organized space in the home to meet Vince's needs and surrounded him with all necessary equipment. On the other hand, she was a conscientious housekeeper, with pride in her furnishings, and found Vince's destructive explorations difficult to take. She was not consistent in removing objects from his reach to avoid struggle but tried to control his behavior. When this proved ineffective, she began, during the later period, to manipulate the environment and to remove temptation.

Mrs. Grasso was aware that the apartment was confining to Vince and that he needed more play space than was available. She desperately hoped for a new home but was thwarted by her economic circumstances. Therefore, as Vince approached two years of age, she looked forward eagerly to nursery school as a way of providing him acceptable play space outside of her own home and beyond her own responsibility. Mrs. Grasso gave the impression of not being able to handle Vince's use of household space in a way satisfying to her.

D. FAMILY RELATIONSHIPS

1. Marital. Mrs. Grasso's romantic illusions were severely jolted early in marriage by the news from her husband that he had tuberculosis and would possibly have to return to the sanatorium. Although she had a job and continued to work for a time during her pregnancy, she looked forward to the role of homemaker and was conflicted about undertaking economic responsibility, which she felt belonged to the husband. With her husband's lengthening convalescence, Mrs. Grasso became ambivalent about his health status and non-assumption of the "provider's" role.

It was difficult to assess Mr. Grasso's personality, but it seemed likely to the staff that he was using his health as a defense for not meeting the marital, economic, and family demands which would usually be assumed. Also, it appeared that marital conflict over health and economic concerns was quite pronounced, although the couple basically shared similar values, orientation, and background.

Mrs. Grasso was restrained from overtly expressing hostility or anger because of his illness, but she often expressed irritation with his habits of sleeping late, missing out on jobs, and "not getting anything done." Mr. Grasso was inclined to take things as they come, without serious regard for the future. While he did little to change their straitened circumstances, he leaned on them to discourage a second baby or plans for new housing. Nevertheless, it seemed that the Grassos had a basically warm and satisfactory relationship and had a further bond in their joy as parents.

2. Mother-Child. Though Vince was the main source of emotional satisfaction for his mother, he was not unequivocally so. The high value Mrs. Grasso placed on motherhood helped to make the mother-child relationship basically a positive, affectionate one. As we have seen, Mrs. Grasso's volatility, combined with the excessive activity of a very lively little boy, made the relationship inconsistent and highly variable. This was further influenced by an ambivalent and somewhat conflicted marital relationship.

At the behavioral level mother-child interaction shifted in quality as Mrs. Grasso encountered the day-to-day changes of life with a child. We have seen that her initial unconcern about potential child-care problems gave way to dismay as the realities made themselves known and Vince became more of a "management" problem. Despite her dissatisfactions with the child's behavior, affection for him remained a firm basis for this family's integration.

3. Father-Child. As described before, Mr. Grasso participated to a considerable extent in child-care routines and also spent much time playing with Vince. From this developed a lively and warm attachment. The situation of Mr. Grasso was marked by his assumption of many aspects of the mothering role. His continued presence in the home during the day reinforced this behavior. The father-child relationship seemed satisfying and pleasurable.

E. PERSONALITY CHARACTERISTICS

1. Handling of Anxiety and Hostility. Mrs. Grasso was unable to describe her anxiety verbally, although it was evident that she was intensely anxious over several things, especially health problems. During Vince's many bouts with respiratory infections and her own periods of ill health, the specter of tuberculosis was always in the background. She was also quite concerned about the health of her parents. But she managed to control this stress within adequate limits of behavior. Rather than say directly, "I am worried," she tried to cover up her anxiety with an offhand way of asking a multitude of questions of the study staff.

However, in expressing both affection and hostility she was more direct. When angry at Vince, she would flare up with scolding threats, and after he was twelve months old, spanking and hitting. She was a "giving" mother and expressed warmth and love, while her moments of angry hostility subsided quickly.

There were quarrels between Mr. and Mrs. Grasso, and at times this relationship appeared to be an ego-threatening one to her, but there were also apparent satisfactions. Also, she had an affectionate and satisfactory relationship with her mother as well as with a number of women friends. Little Vince was extremely important to both his parents, but he did not become the center of either of their worlds.

2. Dependency and the Sense of Security. For Mrs. Grasso the problem of finding satisfaction for dependency needs was not acute. In her relationship with her own mother, who was something of a model in establishing her own maternal role, she found support and gratification. In her marital relationship she faced problems which rose out of her husband's inability to be the economic provider of the family. But it was not necessarily a demonstration of dependency need but rather of the need for the establishment of appropriate husband and wife roles. With the study staff Mrs. Grasso alternated in her ways of expressing anxieties and the need for reassurance, sometimes resorting to offhand questions as a partial disguise for her anxiety and at other times looking for reassurance from them after occasional emotional outbursts.

3. Feelings of Adequacy or Inadequacy. Mrs. Grasso pictured herself as taking life very seriously. She did not generally question her adequacy as a mother except when she despaired over Vince's "fresh" behavior in the second year. She felt adequate in the role of homemaker, but the threat of having to assume both maternal and wage-earning roles was disturbing. This ambivalence contributed to her difficulties in managing Vince, particularly in the second year. Her vacillating feelings, however, did not operate against family integration. Indeed, she indicated that it was the "Italian way of thinking for the woman to compromise more than the man." Feelings of inadequacy in themselves were not of major consequence to Mrs. Grasso.

4. Planning and Impulsiveness. Mrs. Grasso's self-characterization as an impulsive and vacillating person was only partly borne out by her actual behavior with the child. She adapted herself to Vincent's needs in many ways, but he was an unpredictable child. His irregularity of behavior induced inconsistency and impulsiveness in his mother. The evaluation of her impulsive behavior patterns must take into account the emotional volatility and handling of tension which we have previously described. In terms of family organization, both her impulsiveness and her emotional volatility were problems, but they were not disruptive of family unity.

5. Self-Assertion. This presented no problem for Mrs. Grasso.

6. Recapitulation of Past Experiences. Recapitulation of past experiences was not prominently expressed, but in many ways Mrs. Grasso followed patterns of mothering and behavior set by her own mother.

F. EMERGENCE OF FAMILY INTEGRATION PATTERNS

1. Family Structure. The Grassos' handling of their child was characterized by a sense of togetherness on the part of all three members of the new nuclear family, and provided continuous and effective emotional satisfactions for Vince. This unity persisted despite the presence of serious health problems, economic insecurity, and some confusion of the maternal and paternal roles. There were other features of family life which made for friction: Vince's hyperactivity in a too-small apartment, absence of shared activities outside the home, the child's skill in playing father against mother in matters of discipline, and his obvious preference for his father at the end of the two years. But none of these appeared to affect materially the basic triadic emotional satisfactions. A unitary organization was achieved in the family, with basically strong relationships between husband and wife, mother and child, and father and child.

2. Division of Labor and Balance of Power. The household division of labor was rather obscured because of Mr. Grasso's constant presence in the home. It is clear, however, that Mr. Grasso, more than the other fathers, undertook a number of the duties usually associated with the wife. He helped care for the child during illness, rocked him to sleep often, and cared for him on the few occasions of Mrs. Grasso's employment. It seemed that decision-making was fairly well shared.

3. Development, Achievement and Social Behavior of Child. Vince was described as an attractive, lovable, active boy, who satisfied his parents and performed well on developmental tests. In fact, he was among those of the study children who demonstrated somewhat advanced development.

4. Prospect of Siblings. A second pregnancy was discussed on several occasions by Mrs. Grasso, who desired more children, although her husband did not initially look with favor on another child. But by the end of the two years both parents were eager for a second conception. There is some indication that Mrs. Grasso hoped a second pregnancy would once and for all eliminate her role as family wage earner.

5. Status of Family in Community. There was no pronounced extended family conflict, and relationships with grandparents and relatives were socially satisfactory. Mrs. Grasso maintained contact with girl friends from time to time, and Mr. Grasso regularly saw his buddies. In addition to her mother, Mrs. Grasso was close to her sister-in-law, whom she regularly visited. There was also involvement with a downstairs neighbor, which at times caused dissatisfaction because she "spoiled" Vince. There was little evidence that the Grassos participated in any way in the social affairs of the community.

6. Types of Parent-Child Adaptation. The Grasso family was evaluated as a unitary organization despite indications of a somewhat stressful marital situation. Nevertheless, there seemed sufficient strength in the overall dyadic relationships of husband-wife, mother-child, and father-child to characterize the family adaptation as unitary. The Grassos were essentially child-centered in orientation and permissive in management.

POSTSCRIPT

Mrs. Grasso's philosophy that "one can always find a way to manage" proved itself in the years that followed. The pattern of family life continued on a volatile, instinctual, and explosive course, interspersed by plateaus of relative stability. In his behavior and development Vince clearly demonstrated that he was both a product and a barometer of the family modus operandi.

The child's hyperactive, provocative behavior, which had already appeared in the latter part of the study, became more evident as time went on. Mrs. Grasso remained highly ambivalent in her interaction with the child: intolerant and punitive towards his transgressions, yet loving and indulgent. Her management was such as to create a state of charged suspense. Combined with a seductive type of physical interaction by both parents, it created a highly emotional atmosphere, which was sharply reflected in Vince's behavior.

In nursery school his activity was frenetic and destructive, aggressive to other children, and provocative to adults. His attention span was short, his impulsiveness predominant. Both in nursery school and in play therapy sessions there were sustained periods of willfulness, excitability, and incautious behavior to the point of endangering himself and others. But there were also periods when he was passive and subdued, seeming to want to be "good" but suffering from his uncontrollable urge to do the opposite.

Vince's peaks of difficult behavior coincided with periods of family stress that occurred with greater frequency and intensity as time went on. The marital relationship, which had hinted at problems during the two year study, began to deteriorate more overtly. Mr. Grasso's work pattern remained highly unstable, with many periods of unemployment and shifting of jobs. Financial matters became a source of much conflict. Despite this situation Mrs. Grasso was eager for a second child. After a miscarriage in Vince's second year she had a successful pregnancy, which terminated in the birth of Raymond about the time of Vince's third birthday.

Health fears generally remained high in the Grasso family. Mrs. Grasso was also beset by her parents' difficulties, which reached a climax in the eventual suicide of her father.

Mrs. Grasso found the new baby "wonderful" and attributed his placid disposition to the fact that she started him directly on bottle feeding. To Vince's disadvantage, Mrs. Grasso often compared him with his new brother, who was "more cuddly, responsive, affectionate, and enjoyable." As she lavished tenderness and attention on the baby, Vince's unmanageability became more aggravating, and she "was after him all day long."

Quarrels between the Grassos reached new heights. Mrs. Grasso investigated the possibility of a legal separation, although she "still loved Sal." Reconciliations always took place. Since they had to move from their apartment, they found a somewhat run-down house in a declining neighborhood. However, it provided each of the boys with a bedroom and a suitable back yard.

As baby Ray grew out of infancy Mrs. Grasso began to find him "hard to handle and difficult to manage" in the same ways that Vince had proved unsatisfactory. Wistfully she pointed out, "He's becoming just like Vince." Mr. Grasso commented that Ray would be "even more of a terror because he fights back" and that "she is after him all day long." Mr. Grasso's relationship with Ray was similar to that with Vince, in which he brought the child to high pitches of excitement in wild, seductive play.

As Ray started to walk and the physical contact diminished for Mrs. Grasso, a noticeable change in attitude took place. She was more critical of him and recognized that he was often the provocative aggressor against Vince. Nevertheless, she still interacted more warmly with Ray and expressed guilt "because she does not have the love for Vince that she has for Ray, although she tries hard to be fair and equal." She commented that Vince was much like his father, indifferent and unresponsive to others.

Despite a number of inadequacies in the new home, it represented a marked improvement in living conditions. Mr. Grasso engaged in home repair and spent more time with the family. Mrs. Grasso enjoyed being a devoted and creative housekeeper. Life proceeded on a more even keel. Vince's behavior began to show more moderation and impulse control. Mrs. Grasso began to find him "very good," especially as her difficulties with Ray mounted. She characterized Ray as "far worse than Vince ever was." To the study staff, Vince appeared to have become a better organized child. With the absence of his former intense excitement and hyperactivity, there was a more reasonable interaction between mother and child. It also seemed that the separation of Mrs. Grasso from her parents and their severe disturbances contributed to the relative tranquillity which she now enjoyed.

As time passed, Mr. Grasso's work history improved and the family purchased another home, this time in a desirable suburban area development, where Mrs. Grasso felt that the schools were better. With stable employment and steady income, the family's standard of living became relatively affluent and marital life lost the heated struggle of old. Mrs. Grasso radiated satisfaction in her home and family. She had a nearby job, which she found rewarding and enjoyable, but in the main her energies were concentrated on the home and the immediate family.

As a fourteen-year-old, Vince appeared lithe and supple, with a surprisingly relaxed, calm bearing and an absence of the old restlessness, tension, and excitement. He did average school work and was quite interested in sports. He had boy friends and had recently started to socialize with girls. There were definite plans for college.

The last psychological evaluation verified that Vince's frenetic fires were banked at the price of lost animation and gamin charm. He seemed to accept and be resigned to the world as it was, neither markedly anxious nor overly impelled to do anything about problem areas. Thus, time brought industry, stability, and amiability to the Grasso family. Again, only the future will determine whether Vince's appearance of control, calmness, organization, and structure of achievement will survive life's abundance of incendiary sparks.

The Cyrenski Family

PARALYSIS OF THE OLD WORLD

The boundaries of life for Rose Cyrenski were no wider than the geographical area where she was born, had stayed all her life, and wanted to stay until she died. Into her limited intellectual and emotional experience there was little penetration by a vastly intricate world, and this world made little impact upon the mediocre level of her existence.

Perhaps non-involvement in the adventure of life had had its beginnings in Rose's early family life, of which we have meager knowledge because she was the least articulate and verbal in the study group. While she was cooperative and eager to answer all questions, her lack of introspection produced little material or insight into her formative years. We could only surmise that her school days were not happy ones and that she felt excluded from the mainstream of high-school activity.

She said, "I have to admit I didn't care for school," and "It may not be a nice thing to say but I hated the homework." She described herself as "not stupid" but said she had not wanted to go to college or take any special business training, "and there's no sense going if you don't like it." A second factor was that "the students were not friendly. . . . They had their own social set, were kind of snobbish, and they kept people out." Apparently Rose was one of the "outs," and she guessed that was why she dated young men from outside school. Her mother at first objected to this but was reluctantly forced to accept it.

This was told in a matter-of-fact, smiling, and unemotional way by the chubby, round-faced, dark-eyed young woman. Although not pretty, she was attractive despite an inconspicuous scar on her large, full mouth which may have been from repair of a harelip. Mrs. Cyrenski wore a simple nondescript blue and white print smock at the first interview, which she continued to wear at practically all subsequent meetings. Her dark wavy hair was worn rather long and hung on her shoulders. Her face was friendly and mobile, her mouth well made up. On the whole, she gave the impression of health, robustness, youth, and vigor.

Rose was the seventh daughter of an immigrant Spanish family which perpetuated old customs in the new land. Her mother still raised poultry and grew vegetables because she "hated the idea of going to the store to buy them." The move to America was not an easy transition for Rose's parents. Since they could not afford passage for their family of four daughters, Rose's father came alone. After eight years of hard work he managed to save enough to transport his wife and children.

When Rose's parents were finally reunited in America, they had "a second batch" of three more children, of whom Rose was the youngest. The subject of her mother and sisters was one about which Rose Cyrenski spoke most freely and in greatest detail. Her mother was "a very small woman, very strong and always a hard worker." Even at sixty-two she still maintained the garden and also worked on a part-time job, "although she doesn't have to." One of her daughters died at the age of thirty but the others were all married. One of them lived with her children in the maternal home. Another daughter lived in New York with her two children and came to visit every three weeks. Mrs. Cyrenski said that this daughter was her mother's favorite because she had always been a "mother's girl, and spent more time at home."

Mrs. Cyrenski's mother missed her daughters and was always glad when they and their children came to visit. The ages of the grandchildren ranged from twelve years down, "three more are on the way," and "it's a riot when they all visit." She said her mother "didn't have any favorites among the grandchildren because with that many it wouldn't pay."

Mrs. Cyrenski said she made a point of visiting her mother at least twice a week because she was the youngest child and the last one to get married. Her visits were more than perfunctory. She would go early in the morning and usually remained overnight. There was always a close relationship and much talk between them.

The memories of her father were rather vague, since he died

when she was only fourteen. She described him "as very old-fashioned and terribly strict . . . but very good to us." She imagined he was strict "because they were all girls." He forbade his daughters to wear lipstick or other makeup, and they had to be in early in the evening. Mrs. Cyrenski recalled some pleasant moments with her father as the youngest child, sitting on his lap and hearing lively stories.

Then tragedy struck. Her father was accidentally run over and killed by the auto of the local police chief. The chief claimed that he was driving slowly and it was quite accidental. The family was advised by friends to sue but decided against it because "legal action would cost too much" and also they felt "it wouldn't get them anything because the chief of police was a big shot." Mrs. Cyrenski said her mother aged visibly after her husband's death, and the world outside loomed ominous to the family bereft of husband and father. Somehow they managed to get by financially because "all the girls pitched in with their earnings." Even Rose, the "baby" of the family, had her first part-time job at sixteen, and thereafter used her earnings to buy her own clothes.

For the next four years she apparently did factory work and dated sporadically. At the age of twenty Rose met her future husband in a textile mill, where they were co-workers. She reported, "It was love at first sight, and from the first I knew I wanted to marry him." They went out together "off and on for a year" and then went steady for a year. They were married when Rose was twenty-two and Stanley twenty-five.

The courtship was slow and halting at first, perhaps because neither of them made friends easily. During the courtship Stanley told her he had contracted mumps while in the Army and the doctors had warned him "he might not be able to have children . . . because the mumps had affected him 'down there' "; Mrs. Cyrenski put her hand to her groin. Stanley had asked her "if it made any difference." She had said that she would like to have babies but after all they could adopt them if they couldn't produce one themselves.

Anyway, they had tried and to her delight she had missed a period. She just "knew and felt really positive" that she was pregnant from the beginning. She said, "The first one to know about it was my mother." Then she corrected herself and said, "Of course

I told my husband first, even though I wasn't positive that I was really pregnant." They were both highly pleased that she had become pregnant so soon after marriage.

The courtship and marriage faced a formidable obstacle from the beginning, namely the elder Cyrenskis, who found it hard to welcome a Spanish daughter-in-law into their Bulgarian household. Finally, they grudgingly consented to the marriage, but for years after her marriage Mrs. Cyrenski felt unaccepted and unable to take her place in the paternal home, where her husband and his parents spoke Bulgarian, further increasing her sense of isolation and non-acceptance.

Significantly, Mrs. Cyrenski never explained why they had launched their matrimonial career in his parents' home. Undoubtedly, economic reasons were a consideration as well as strong filial ties, which were important to both of them. Further, it was similar to the pattern set by her own mother in living with her in-laws while her husband was in America. But here the parallel ended. In this case, Rose Cyrenski's husband was present and the possibility existed for an independent family existence.

In any event, from the beginning, the senior Mrs. Cyrenski made it plain that she intended to control family life. The young couple had been promised one of the two apartments in the parental home. There was a vacant modernized downstairs apartment which was supposed to be theirs on a rental basis. The elder Cyrenskis lived in the old-fashioned upstairs apartment, with ancient furniture and a wood-burning stove. But on the Sunday after his honeymoon Stanley Cyrenski had a disagreement with his parents over helping to butcher a hog. In consequence, the young couple was refused the use of the downstairs apartment. Instead they moved into the upstairs apartment with Mr. Cyrneski's parents, and for the entire period of the study both families continued to live together in a cramped inconvenient apartment while a modern one remained empty below.

The locale of the Cyrenski homestead characterized the atmosphere and boundaries of life which prevailed for the young couple and their baby-to-be. It was set in an unattractive area which hovered on the periphery of the city, neither urban nor rural, populated largely by would-be farmers whose income depended on a city job, or by "old family" immigrants, who carried on a semblance of their peasant heritage. Side by side with pasture land, truck farm, or flower garden were a variety of junk heaps and accumulations from city waste. Despite the large and tasteful flower garden at the Cyrenski home, the summer heat accentuated the potent smell of decaying foodstuffs. Around the two-story house, which was in the poorest segment of this "rurban" fringe, were a few acres of pasture and truck farm, including cows and hogs in its population.

This was the home where life began for Joey Cyrenski, shared by his paternal grandparents. The elder Cyrenskis had come to the United States from Bulgaria in their young adult years. In this homestead they worked quietly, on farm and in factory, without any appreciable change in their language or culture. After the elder Mrs. Cyrenski had had many miscarriages a "miracle" had occurred and finally a son had been born.

The coming of Stanley brought quite a change in the relationship between his parents. As the elder Mrs. Cyrenski put it, "Until you have a child you love your husband, but when the baby comes you love him so much that there isn't room for anyone else." So there was no room for Stanley's father, a silent man, who continued to work through the years, physically present but apparently emotionally removed from his wife and son. As the family history unfolded, it was obvious that he was equally removed from his grandson, for he was never mentioned in the records as one whose activities or personality were in any way involved in Joey's life.

From the moment he was born, Stanley became the focus of existence for his mother. She guarded his health zealously and hovered anxiously about him. But he was a nervous child, and his health seemed never to be very good. He was always thin, and his mother concentrated on getting him to eat and protecting him from drafts. She was ever ready to relive details of his childhood and fondly described his long curls, which she hadn't cut until he was almost five. Also, she used to dress him in girl's clothes as a toddler and enjoyed commenting that "he was pretty as a girl." She reported that he was always a dutiful son in a devout family and that he based all his decisions upon her advice.

Stanley's only separation from his parents was his three year stint in the Marine Corps during World War II, but always his satisfactions and desires remained centered upon the "home place." When he returned from the war he continued to leave most of his decisions to the judgment of his parents. His sense of responsibility and filial piety remained unchanged as he slowly began to take on the ways of a man.

The young bride tried very hard not to interfere with her mother-in-law. She knew her husband was the only child and that "naturally his mother wants to take good care of him . . . he's all she has," and "she worries about him too much because he's always been so thin." She reported with pleasure that since their marriage, "Stanley gained fifteen pounds and I gained thirteen." Then she commented, "Now my mother-in-law sees that I take good care of him."

The apartment where the two families lived was reached by a back stairway, which entered directly into the kitchen. The kitchen contained a large wood-burning stove, which dominated the room, a new washing machine, and a table with chairs. The living room was furnished with a day bed, an old organ, and Stanley's old metal baby crib, which would now be inherited by his son. The drapes, rugs, and furniture were covered with large floral designs that gave the place a cluttered and oppressive look.

The elder Mrs. Cyrenski prepared all the meals, and her daughter-in-law had little to say or do about household management. The paternal parents each had a separate bedroom, and the young people shared the one remaining bedroom. There was virtually no privacy because Stanley's mother refused to permit the bedroom doors to be closed and she was a light sleeper. Hence, the young couple had little freedom to develop their relationship. Rose Cyrenski remarked, "Stanley and I have never had a married life of our own."

During the entire course of the study Mrs. Cyrenski did not refer openly to her sexual life. It appeared to the interviewer that she was in love with her husband but that in the atmosphere of the Cyrenski home she found herself in rivalry with her mother-in-law for her husband's affections and responded by giving him the same kind of solicitous mothering he had come to expect. Not by nature an aggressive or assertive person, Rose Cyrenski tended to withdraw from unpleasant situations and to repress her anger. Yet her desires strongly needed gratification, and she looked forward with the utmost pleasure to having a baby, something of her own upon which to lavish her energy and her mothering.

Mrs. Cyrenski came to the hospital maternity clinic in the third month of pregnancy because their family physician no longer took maternity cases. Also the clinic had been used by one of her sisters for the delivery of two children. This same sister was now expecting her third child and was again using the clinic. She had told Mrs. Cyrenski that the service was very good at the clinic and that she had enjoyed all of her hospitalization here.

It was suggested that Mrs. Cyrenski discuss the study with her husband. She talked it over with him, and he said, "Anything you want to do will be all right." When asked if they planned on having a private pediatrician, Mrs. Cyrenski said that they had no doctor in mind for the baby and had planned to use the clinic at the hospital.

At the first interview Mrs. Cyrenski commented that she perspired very much and that the humid weather made her feel quite uncomfortable. So far, pregnancy had been uneventful for her, and she had had no symptoms whatsoever. She had rather expected to be nauseated but was not even slightly so. "If it's this easy I'll plan on having six babies."

Mrs. Cyrenski reported that the sister who had been using the clinic had had quite a bit of trouble with her pregnancies and with care of the children. "She has anemia, varicose veins, and large babies." Mrs. Cyrenski reported that her sister's first baby had been over eleven pounds and the second had been ten pounds. During this third pregnancy her sister had been tiring easily because the two older boys were "in the age when they are into everything. . . . They are rambunctious and strong and are really little devils." Her sister had said, "If I have another horse, I don't know what I'll do."

At the next interview Mrs. Cyrenski continued to discuss her sister's problems. Her two little boys were "fresh as ever. . . . They are pre-schoolers, and my sister almost goes crazy with them because they answer back and are so full of spunk." Mrs. Cyrenski imagined, "They are kind of spoiled . . . but I guess every mother spoils her kids a little." The youngest one wouldn't eat, and Mrs. Cyrenski explained that her sister "feels bad when he doesn't eat . . . probably most mothers feel that way." She told her sister not to pester the little boy about eating, that he would come and ask for food and say "Mommy, I'm hungry" once he got hungry.

Mrs. Cyrenski's main problem during pregnancy was her weight. She gained six pounds during the first four months and found it hard to control her weight or to stay within the diet prescribed by the obstetrician. She gave vivid accounts of her running battle with the obstetrician over weight and admitted that she "snitched" from time to time on the prescribed diet. "After all, he can't do anything but holler," she said. When he threatened to keep her in the hospital to make her lose weight, she declared, "It's bad enough to go to the hospital to have the baby, let alone to lose weight."

She stated that the obstetrician had prescribed pills, which she took. She didn't mind the pills but swallowing them was quite a chore as it was necessary to take eight at a time, three times a day. Her weight immediately decreased, but the next week it was back to its original level. She didn't understand why she gained because she ate only "one good meal a day, in the evening," but at that time she ate whatever she wanted because she couldn't go without at least one good meal a day.

The requirement of restricting her weight and dieting was not a simple one for Rose Cyrenski to meet. She felt that "a fat rounded baby was a healthy baby," and she was ambivalent about the doctor's emphasis on weight restriction, which conflicted with her own ideas of good nurturing. She rather boastfully reported that the obstetrician had teased her that "they would need a derrick to lift her to the delivery table and that she would give birth to a giant." Yet in sharp contrast with this story was the actual hospital record, which reported that she had gained only thirteen pounds during the entire pregnancy, well under the permitted maximum.

Mrs. Cyrenski expressed few expectations, anxieties, or reflections concerning her coming child. In the fifth month she felt movement and reported, "Now he really moves, and it feels good because this proves the baby is alive." The movement made her uncomfortable only because she felt that everybody was looking at her when the baby moved, although she knew this wasn't so and was "only her reactions." Later she felt that the fetus "was lumped up on one side," and kicked her with his hands and feet. She didn't find it painful and was only surprised at its strength. Sometimes it disturbed her sleep but only if she was not quite asleep.

She was tolerant of the excessive urination to which she was subject, as well as excessive defecation, although she objected to having a bowel movement at night "because one has to go downstairs to the bathroom and I'm too lazy to do that during the night." She had been attending the exercise classes for expectant mothers at the clinic and seemed to enjoy them. She had no fears about delivery and said that the doctors anticipated no difficulty and she guessed it "would be easy."

While she did not express any of the usual fears of pregnant women in relation to her own baby, she did tell of various friends and relatives who had had specific difficulties with both delivery and care of their babies. She told of a girl friend who had lost her baby after carrying it for nine months. She had not been able to deliver, and when the baby was removed from her they discovered that the cord was wrapped about its neck. Another friend had had a miscarriage in the fourth month.

It shocked and upset Mrs. Cyrenski that these friends had had such mishaps. "You never can tell what will happen," she commented, and then went on to say that she didn't want to buy too much ahead of time for the baby because she would "feel funny in case anything happened." She had bought only a few diapers and a receiving blanket up to that point and said, "After all, you can buy everything for the baby at the last minute. All you have to do is to walk into the store and pick them out."

She recounted some of the difficulties her sisters had had in breast feeding their children. One sister had not had enough milk for either of the two large babies. Another sister had felt that her first child was "spoiled" as a result of breast feeding. "She kept the child too close to her. . . . As the baby grew older, she wouldn't let her mother leave the room."

Despite her tales of certain problems with breast feeding, there was no doubt in Mrs. Cyrenski's mind that she would breast feed if she could. Since the fifth month there had been a considerable and consistent flow of colostrum. She said, "Some people say breast feeding is old-fashioned, but I will enjoy it." Other than this remark she gave no specific reason for her determination to breast feed. Taken at face value, Mrs. Cyrenski seemed to feel a confidence in herself that she intuitively understood children, knew their wants and needs, and could handle them.

In the seventh month Mrs. Cyrenski still felt fine and reported that her husband had recently secured a new job, which she had been instrumental in getting for him. She had heard of the job and had encouraged him to try for it, although he didn't think he would be accepted. She reported with pleasure, "When he did get it he was so happy, just like a little boy."

Actually, Mr. Cyrenski was now working two jobs, one in a factory and the other in a produce store, because they felt additional money was needed with the coming of the baby. Mrs. Cyrenski had hopes of saving money and some day moving to a place of their own, but she said, "I don't harp on it because Stanley gets upset." She said she missed her husband because he worked so much, and she hardly ever saw him. She had become used to being with him a great deal when they had worked together at the same factory, and now she didn't have much time with him.

She commented that her husband took money matters very seriously and recently had been upset because they had been out on strike for a few weeks at the factory. He had been worried that during the strike they would not be able to pay his parents the rent. Mrs. Cyrenski said that her husband was something of a worrier; "that's why he gets so upset when I talk about getting a place of our own."

Mrs. Cyrenski was sure that her husband wanted a boy because he would pat her stomach and ask how his son was. She had warned him not to be too set on a boy, as he might be disappointed. Mrs. Cyrenski did not say whether she herself preferred a boy or girl. "My heart isn't set on one thing or another because I don't want to be disappointed," she said. She stated, however, that both she and her husband called the coming baby "he" because " 'he' is so much easier to say than 'she.' " They had not yet decided on a girl's name but had reached an agreement on a boy's name. And then she added, "It must mean that deep down we think it is a boy rather than a girl." When asked how many children she was planning on having, Mrs. Cyrenski said she would like three or four, "but it all depends on if we can afford them."

In the eighth month Mrs. Cyrenski's main concern was her

weight gain. She was "afraid to get on the scales to see how much it is." She found that time passed rather quickly and did not drag. The interviewer noted, "As usual, Mrs. Cyrenski seemed in very good spirits and appeared accepting of all aspects of her pregnancy." Mrs. Cyrenski said she had started to make "some dresses" for the baby. Then she giggled about the possibility of putting a dress on a boy and commented, "Wouldn't it be funny to have a dress with embroidery and lace on a boy?"

She complained of the heat and again mentioned how much she perspired. However, she guessed she was nervous about her weight. Shortly after this visit Mrs. Cyrenski met the pediatrician. No arrangements had been made in advance for the appointment. Although she smiled, it was evident that she was ill-at-ease, and she sat uncomfortably on the edge of her chair without removing her coat. Her face was flushed, and there was profuse sweating of the face and hands. She asked no questions and had great difficulty in finding something to say.

In response to a question on whether she was interested in the rooming-in arrangement, she said, "I don't know." When it was described to her she only nodded and smiled. Asked how she had been feeling during her pregnancy, she said, "Good. I still can't believe that I am having a baby." Asked how she planned to feed the baby, she said without hesitation, "Breast," but seemed unable to give any reason why this had been her decision. Her constraint caused the pediatrician to wonder whether she would stay in the study.

In the ninth month Mrs. Cyrenski was scheduled to take her psychological tests. Through a misunderstanding she was kept waiting for about a half an hour. When the examiner appeared, Mrs. Cyrenski was very tense and said that she was "very much afraid of the tests." No amount of reassurance seemed to put her at ease. Perspiration was on her forehead, and she remained tense and preoccupied with her achievement throughout all the tests. She asked whether she had said "the right things" and was again told that there was no right or wrong. But even then she did not seem to accept this statement and remained doubtful about her accomplishments and distrustful toward the examiner. She departed, very glad that it was all over.

The summary of the Rorschach test stated: "This woman lives

in a very limited world intellectually as well as emotionally. However, while her intelligence seems to function on its naturally mediocre level, her affective life is disturbed by repression of anything more than the most superficial kind of emotional experience. Although stimulated by the world around her, she does not permit herself any real participation in it. She lacks empathy and shies away from any spontaneous expression of her own feelings."

The most striking fact about these interviews was the very different impression that Rose Cyrenski made on the interviewer, on the pediatrician, and on the psychological tester. Almost to the very end of pregnancy the interviewer found her "always at ease, eager to cooperate, and surprisingly astute in interpreting other people's actions, for which she finds valid, realistic, and kind reasons." The pediatrician, on the other hand, found Mrs. Cyrenski "ill-at-ease, with little to say and great difficulty in speaking." The tester found her "so tense and preoccupied that no amount of reassurance helped her."

Significantly, however, the records tell little about her deeper feelings and offer only fragmentary material about Mrs. Cyrenski and the people close to her. Whatever was reported came in a detached unemotional way. We never heard directly and could only guess how she saw herself, what were her interests, hobbies, or system of values. She did not look at her own experiences and thereby did not permit us to see them. Similarly, concerning the main figures of her environment, including her husband, mother, mother-in-law, sisters, father, we received very sketchy information in terms of their relationships with her.

During an interview early in the ninth month Mrs. Cyrenski looked rather bedraggled, having come through a rain shower. She seemed out of breath and somewhat upset. She said that she was feeling fine but guessed she was "disgusted by all the shopping done in the morning and hurrying across town to get to the clinic." She was pleased that within the last week she had gained only one pound, and she looked forward to the probability that the obstetrician would not take her to task concerning her weight gain.

Mrs. Cyrenski had spent a day with her sister's new five-week-old baby and was "amazed at how much older and better it looks than it did when it was first born." She reported laughingly, "I didn't know where to hold the baby because I didn't have a lap. My belly was so large I had to sort of put the baby on top of it, using it almost like a ledge." In the beginning she had felt a little nervous but then had found that it was easy to give the bottle. She reported that her sister was exhausted taking care of a new eight-pound baby plus two older sons, neither of whom were yet in school. She said the older boy had missed being admitted to school by just one month in age, and "It's unfair to keep a child out of school just because he's under age by a week or so." She went on to say, however, "I guess with so many children going to school these days, the school officials have to make rules which may be unreasonable."

While the interviewer was chatting with Mrs. Cyrenski in the obstetrical clinic, a mother left her small baby in a crib across the hall. The baby became fussy, and Mrs. Cyrenski fondly commented, "I guess she's getting hungry, her mother will have to feed her."

Mrs. Cyrenski missed the following obstetrical clinic appointment "because of a rain shower." It surprised the interviewer that a woman this far along in pregnancy would miss a clinic appointment because of the weather. In this last ante-partum interview Mrs. Cyrenski reported that her net gain in the past three weeks had only been one pound, and she didn't think "the doctor would dare bawl her out for gaining weight" because she was in the last weeks of her pregnancy.

She had been having some pains in her groin on and off during the past week or so and very much hoped that the baby would arrive soon and that it wouldn't be a couple of weeks late. She said that she felt less pregnant than she had felt throughout the pregnancy "because the baby seems so far down." It was interesting that for Mrs. Cyrenski pregnancy was more of a reality in the early months than as she approached delivery.

She remarked that when her husband came home each evening he said, "Are you still here?" and each morning he anticipated that this would be the day of her delivery. She wondered about the visiting hours and hoped that it could be arranged for her husband to visit at lunch time even though this was not the usual visiting hour. She thought he could visit her at noon between his two jobs.

Mrs. Cyrenski then asked what the financial arrangement would be between the pediatrician and herself. It was explained that the fee would be comparable to that of the clinic. She reported that her sister's new little baby girl had gained three pounds and "is filling out and looking like a real baby."

The interviewer asked why Mrs. Cyrenski had seemed a bit upset by the Rorschach tests. She answered, "I guess I was just scared of them. . . . I hadn't any idea they would be like that, and when I got home I remembered many answers to the questions that I just couldn't say at the time of the test." Before she left Mrs. Cyrenski remarked that they still had not thought of a girl's name but thought they might find one before she came to the hospital.

Five days later a boy was born. Mrs. Cyrenski arrived at the hospital about four hours before real labor started. The entire labor lasted twelve hours and fifty minutes — the first stage for twelve hours, the second for forty-five minutes, and the third only six minutes. The nurse characterized her as cooperative, especially after sedation.

When the baby was handed to her after delivery she held him but did not put him to her breast. She had a slight cold and thought he was too young to be exposed to it. Then she added, "I did not have anything for him." Mrs. Cyrenski did not wear any makeup a few hours after the delivery but was friendly and rather cheerful. She remarked, "Oh, I feel all right. I'm just glad it's over." She was especially pleased that the baby was a boy as her husband had wished, and they could use the name Joey which had been chosen beforehand.

Joey was not a handsome baby. His eyes were slits, his mouth large, and his chin receding. He did not look too boyish either, and one observer first guessed "definitely feminine" and then switched to "possibly male." When informed of the baby's gender, the observer said she would "characterize him more as 'neuter.' "

On the whole, the observers felt at ease with Joey and able to handle him without too much caution or anxiety. His movements were well coordinated and relatively purposeful. Comment was made on his dark, straight hair, which was "neat in its arrangement," and his long, well-formed hands. The summary was that "he was too serious and mature looking to be called 'cute,' and that it was gratifying that a four-hour-old baby could look so thoroughly well, so physically strong . . . a very nice . . . a very satisfactory baby."

Although Joey impressed the observers as a quiet, rather placid baby, he fell within the exact median of the study group as a whole. One knew what to expect of him, that he would neither reach a climax of activity nor a complete absence of movement. This predictability of activity was interpreted as "evenness of temperament," a quality which would make Joey easy to take and would prove very satisfactory to his mother.

He reacted to approximately half of the acoustic and tactile stimulations. Sound was more effective if it happened suddenly than if it was continuous. His lower extremities seemed more sensitive to touch than the upper ones, and rhythmic touch stimulation appeared to comfort him. When uncovered, he tended to get more excited but quieted down when the blanket was replaced.

In nine out of ten observations the observers tended to believe that Joey was asleep, and there were few clues to enable them to differentiate between sleeping and waking. Actually, he seemed to respond more to stimulation in the so-called sleeping observations than in the one in which he was described as awake. This lack of differentiation between sleep and wakefulness was surprising in an infant who appeared so mature by his weight and by the general impression he gave.

The observation of Joey awake showed one feature which was distinct from when he was asleep — the lack of startle. During observations in so-called sleeping periods frequent startles were observed, which seemed rather unspecific and not related to particular stimulus. The startles almost always began by the extension of all his extremities when tensing and the flexing of his extremities while relaxing, a departure from the usual startle, which begins by flexion of the legs and not by extension.

Joey's episodes of crying were short ones, but this did not mean that he never looked tense or ill-at-ease during the observations. He often frowned quite distinctly, became red in the face, and tightly flexed both his legs and arms, forming a real ball, the prototype of the fetal position. This seemed to have a comforting effect on him. His hand-mouth contact was effected through self-stimulation by hand to face. His hand was so widely spread over his face that it covered it almost completely. Occasionally his fingers directly entered the mouth, then he sucked them and was comforted. With Joey there was not one but many fingers in his mouth at a time.

It appeared that the essential feature of Joey's oral stimulation was the tactile stimulation of his face. This implied that feeding, especially if it was breast feeding, could easily have the secondary effect of pleasurable stimulation to the facial skin. It was noticed that Joey established hand-face contact always with his left hand when in supine and with his right hand when in prone. Such ease in change of the mouth-contacting hand was surprising but understandable. Joey's preferred position was prone, where the right hand was best fitted for the hand-face contact. But his mother preferred face-to-face contact and placed him mostly in supine, forcing his head "to look at her." This significantly demonstrated the mother's determination to assure constant contact with her infant, and it also demonstrated that the infant's motor preferences were susceptible to influence by factors around him. It indicated that Mrs. Cyrenski would try to manage Joey in such a way as to establish the maximum unity between them and it seemed that she would be successful in this endeavor.

Although Mrs. Cyrenski found Joey's delivery "very painful," she still maintained that she would like two or three more children. She was very pleased with Joey from the start, and the nurses noted that she took excellent care of the baby. During the hospital stay Joey nursed every three and a half to four hours, taking about one hour on one breast. It was noted that Mrs. Cyrenski's milk flowed so freely and abundantly that Joey had to be encouraged to suck, since it required little effort on his part to get food. At home his feedings became more frequent, every hour and a half to two hours during the day, plus a midnight feeding, taking one breast at each feeding.

Mrs. Cyrenski's experience as a new mother during the next months was inextricably tied up with her mother-in-law. The grandmother was a light sleeper and would become irritated if Mrs. Cyrenski didn't immediately awaken when Joey cried. Mrs. Cyrenski asked for some medicine to sleep less soundly. Her mother-in-law could not tolerate Joey's crying at all, and therefore both of them were wont to hold him practically all of his waking hours.

With the passage of time Mrs. Cyrenski confessed to loneliness. She said she had no one to talk to except her mother-in-law, and "you can't make conversation forever with a mother-in-law." The fact was that except for the baby Rose Cyrenski was usually alone.

Her husband worked two jobs, and it was usually well after midnight before he returned, often too tired to do anything except go to bed. Although he had little involvement with his son's care and even less comprehension of an infant's needs, Mr. Cyrenski relished the fact that he had a son. A week after Joey's birth his father was ready to buy a sled for him.

The family owned two cars, but Mrs. Cyrenski could not drive. Thus, friends and relatives seemed far away. Since they rarely telephoned her, she rarely talked with them. Even visits to her mother became restricted to an occasional Sunday evening. In her loneliness, it was perhaps natural that she should take special pleasure in holding her infant son. But it began to appear to the research staff that the enjoyment Mrs. Cyrenski received from her son was more than the ordinary maternal pleasure in nurturing a helpless infant. There were obvious signs that breast feeding gave her intense erotic pleasure, and similar satisfaction seemed to come from close bodily contact with her child.

At five and a half weeks Joey was reported to show little interest in sucking or even swallowing what dripped into his mouth. Mrs. Cyrenski later reported that after ten or fifteen minutes of nursing he did not appear to be hungry but played with the nipple, taking and letting it go repeatedly, and finally just holding onto the breast until he fell asleep. Mrs. Cyrenski experienced this "play" with considerable pleasure. "It makes me feel so funny," she said, "when he puts his hands to the breast and hits or pats it." She hoped his teeth would be delayed so that she might continue nursing.

Around two and a half months Joey was given teaspoons of cereal mixed with water and a tablespoon of applesauce every day, with the breast as "dessert." A month later Mrs. Cyrenski reported that he enjoyed being tied into his high chair with a diaper while he ate these and additional foods three times a day, with breast feeding four times a day and also at midnight. His sleeping pattern was fairly consistent, with an early morning nap, a long nap before lunch, and then one in the afternoon. His bowel movements were reported to occur every other day at first and then every three or four days. He did not cry when wet or soiled.

The interviewer noted that when Joey was three and a half months old, his crib was no longer in the living room but was now in the Cyrenskis' bedroom. Mrs. Cyrenski explained that she wanted the baby near her so she would be sure to hear him if he cried and thus keep her mother-in-law from being disturbed. Despite her concentrated care, however, the elder Mrs. Cyrenski was not satisfied. Although the older woman undertook all the household tasks herself and left her daughter-in-law free to give her undivided attention to Joey, she could not refrain from making invidious comparisons with the way in which she herself had mothered Joey's father.

It was not surprising, therefore, that Mrs. Cyrenski became anxious about Joey's welfare and hovered about him. She even felt guilty if she found him wet in his crib. If he was put to bed without his nightcap, his grandmother was sure this would result in his catching cold. As if to bear out the older woman's prophecy, Joey had a slight cold at one month, with some difficulty in breathing, and another cold at three months, with nasal discharge and a slight cough. A week later a severe cough and "a rattle in his chest" were reported, but on examination he appeared to be normal. A few days later he vomited and had a slight fever plus acute otitis media. After dosing with penicillin and the application of olive oil to his ears he recovered from the infection.

At the first two well-baby clinic examinations the pediatrician described Joey as "a large, alert, and content infant who is fairly inactive." And Mrs. Cyrenski's reports during the four-month period substantiated this passive aspect of Joey. The only report by her of more vigorous movement was that Joey would bounce actively when held with his abdomen against his mother's chest.

The third well-baby clinic disclosed a smiling baby in whatever social situation he was seen. But there were marked differences in his smile. With the examiner the smile was exclusively centered around the mouth, with little participation by the eyes, and he vocalized little as long as the examiner's face was animated. His vocalizing increased only when the examiner's contact lessened. His smile to the mother, on the other hand, was a smile in which the whole face participated, including the eyes. There was no doubt that she was the preferred object and that focus was upon her. The nearer she was, and the more intense the contact, the more he vocalized. When in contact with either the examiner or his mother Joey's general motor activity decreased.

When Joey saw his own face in the mirror his joy and laughter were so intense that he was irresistible to the observers. The positive emotion expressed toward his mirror-image was quite unusual for a child of his age and indicated a pleasure-provoking element in the perception of facial expressions. Joey now preferred the supine position, showing greater peacefulness and more vocalization than in prone. The reason for this preference seemed to be that it allowed visual contact with his mother.

In the supine position Joey used his legs as a grasping force and as objects to be grasped. The legs apparently served as a stimulated part of himself and the outside world, towards which he actively moved. In this context every observer was struck with how subtly Joey's mother constantly played with his legs.

When Joey put his hand into his mouth it included the thumb and at least two other fingers. The mouth movements were of the regular sucking kind, but the hands played a complicated role. As one hand was drawn into the mouth the other hand grasped the wrist of the mouthed hand and pulled it from the mouth. Thus, when mouth-hand contact was established, the second hand was used to assume the regulating function of "giving and withdrawing" sucking pleasure. It also bore out the mother's report that Joey grasped the breast very vigorously with both hands and directed his water bottle with both hands.

The two-handed mouthing pattern interfered with Joey's ability to respond to an offered toy. The toy was not a sufficiently strong stimulus to interrupt the two-handed mouthing but neither could it be ignored. Joey's reaction was to bend forward, kick his legs, and increase the pulling-out and pushing-in actions of his hands. But his eyes focused constantly on the toy. It seemed as if this child was in conflict between the urge to gratify his sucking need and his urge to get in contact with the outside world.

Joey was not much of a grasper. The object had to be near his hand to be grasped, and it had to be to his liking. It appeared that Joey was right-handed for three reasons: first, he was more skillful and varied with that hand; secondly, when he grasped an object with the left hand he kept trying to transfer it to the right hand; and thirdly, the right hand was used more frequently in his two-handed mouthing pattern.

Joey showed little reaction to sound and the ringing of the bell. Even the noise of the rattle or the human voice evoked little interest, let alone pleasure. In this context it was observed that his mother never talked to Joey without first catching his glance and fondling him, while her voice remained monotonous and soft. The pediatrician reported that even on the phone Mrs. Cyrenski spoke so softly as to be hardly audible, for fear of disturbing Joey or waking him up. It seemed likely that these were some of the factors in Joey's lack of response to sound.

However, Joey did babble in different ways for different situations. As pointed out, his vocalization was the least when he was most involved with the human partner, and it was greatest when away from social contact. In terms of inanimate objects, his vocalization was in direct proportion to the difficulties the object offered. He vocalized little, if at all, when the object was easily grasped and manipulated. He vocalized most when the grasping and manipulation became impossible. Thus, it might be inferred in Joey's case that with "perfect understanding," he felt no need to communicate, but that under stress there was more incentive for communication.

At his chronological age of 4 months Joey had a developmental age of 5 months and 15 days on the Viennese test. His performance was of excellent quality throughout.

When Joey was given an immunization Mrs. Cyrenski held him on her lap but looked away. Joey started to cry only at the moment of the injection but the crying terminated in a few seconds when his mother pressed him against her body. However, a few moments later, in a sort of delayed action, he started a screaming protest that lasted quite long.

There was little change in the Cyrenskis' living pattern between Joey's fourth and sixth months. In the warm weather the whole family cooked and ate their meals in the "summer kitchen," a building set back some distance from the house. Rose Cyrenski no longer felt it necessary as a married woman to buy new clothes or to make herself attractive to her husband. Where other women would have insisted on finding other living quarters, she was content with feeble protests and daydreams about her "dream house."

Her main object of interest was Joey. She said she felt she knew "what every little thing means," and the interviewer reported that she did seem to interpret his wants correctly, was spontaneous in her comments to him, and showed considerable warmth. This "attitude of concerned motherliness" also extended to her husband, as she described his recent dental extractions, his intense fear of the operation, and his being upset by the loss of teeth at so early an age. Mr. Cyrenski had not been feeling very well lately, which his wife blamed on difficulty in acclimating himself to the night shift. She complained that they "really had very little time together," and she looked forward to going off somewhere for a vacation, even if they "had to take Joey, this happy ball of trouble."

Joey grew, and as the months progressed he began to leave his infant ways behind. It was this growth that was to provide Mrs. Cyrenski with the first serious problems of parenthood. When Joey was only three months old, his mother had already dreaded the prospect of his first teeth because they might interfere with breast feeding. When Joey was five and a half months old, her fears were confirmed when he bit her breast. Although for the next several months this biting continued sporadically, sometimes drawing blood, the gratifications that both mother and child achieved from breast feeding were so intense that no serious attempt was made to wean Joey.

He now had three meals of solids per day, was nursed after each, and also had the breast around midnight and upon awakening in the morning. He loved fruit and hurried through his cereal or vegetable to have it. He disliked peas, bean or liver soup (as did his mother). He also enjoyed milk or water from a cup and orange juice or tea in a small glass.

With four teeth Joey was biting the breast a good deal, and Mrs. Cyrenski was forced to think about weaning. She said, "he bites only when he gets nervous." On one occasion he bit so hard that she "wanted to choke him." She pulled him away and looked angrily at him, to which he responded with laughter. At six and a half months (and six teeth) he was reported to be biting harder. Mrs. Cyrenski had an infected nipple and had to use only one breast for some days. Joey would clamp down on the breast with his teeth and fall asleep that way. When she tried to withdraw the nipple the biting grip became more firm, and she had to wedge his mouth open with her fingers. It rather surprised the research staff that these sharp discomforts did nothing to dissuade Mrs. Cyrenski from continuing breast feeding.

During all of Joey's waking hours either Mrs. Cyrenski or her mother-in-law held the child, and when Joey was in his mother's lap she typically held him close to her bosom. The boy learned to go to sleep at his mother's breast, and if he was not hungry he was always rocked to sleep.

Joey did not sleep through the night, and Mrs Cyrenski wondered "if he ever would." Often she nursed him in her bed at 3 A.M., and she frequently fell asleep with Joey beside her through the rest of the night. Though she said she got cramped because she couldn't move her position for fear of hurting him, she obviously enjoyed it, describing their closeness as "just like leaves of a book." Joey usually woke up at 5 A.M., and his "singing" aroused the whole family. He usually had a two-to-three hour nap in the morning and a one-hour nap in the afternoon.

At a clinic visit in the fifth month the pediatrician noted that Joey showed some interest in the materials presented but turned easily to mouthing his hands and feet when an object was removed. A great deal of mouthing was also reported a month later. The pediatrician described Joey as "a large attractive baby, with advanced physical growth, who appears somewhat older than his age."

In the sixth month Mrs. Cyrenski called to say that Joey felt hot and seemed irritable. The pediatrician found that the room temperature was 90 degrees and that Joey was overdressed. He had a 102.8 degree temperature and an acute pharyngitis. Penicillin was given, and the following day his fever disappeared.

From Mrs. Cyrenski's meager reports it was learned that Joey expected to be held frequently. The only picture of an active Joey was when he was in contact with his mother, and here the scene was both so intimate and such a struggle that the interviewer was prompted to describe her own uncomfortableness during that home visit in the sixth month. There was considerable affectionate interplay and constant interaction between Joey's body and Mrs. Cyrenski's, alternately meeting and being pressed close together or with Joey pulling and straining away from his mother. He frequently looked as though he were trying to "devour his mother's face with his widely opened mouth."

Joey was at one moment radiant and the next fussy, his face screwed up in a puzzled, fretful expression. He showed constant motor activity, arms clawing the air, entire body squirming, giving the impression of a struggle to get loose from the restraining arm of his mother. It sometimes seemed that he rebelled against this smothering physical contact, and there were moments when all his mother's caresses would no longer quiet his angry wails.

The well-baby clinic evaluative observation disclosed that Joey made little effort to sit up. When put in a sitting position, he sat very badly and showed no inclination to stand up. During the whole visit it was clear that Joey kept track of his mother and moved his head about in order to keep her fully in focus. His grasping patterns were quite advanced, but he hardly moved at all. His legs moved only in supine, and there was no incipient creeping or crawling in prone. This gave the general impression of muscle tonus lack. Of all the boys in the study Joey seemed to have the "softest" body.

His vocalization was considerable, most of it directed toward his mother. It was far from friendly, however, and reminded one of grunting, grumbling, or scolding. His angry vocalization seemed to indicate that if an adult was holding something, he expected to get it, and his relationship to the adult was passive rather than active.

Nevertheless, he performed well. On the Gesell test at the age of 6 months and 29 days he had attained a general maturity level of 32 weeks and a developmental quotient of 110. On the Viennese test he was given a developmental age of 7 months and 27 days, with a developmental quotient of 118.5.

Mr. Cyrenski had a two-weeks vacation, which he spent working around the yard and garden. His hobby was flowers, and Mrs. Cyrenski also began to be interested in plants. She was described as looking even heavier than in mid-pregnancy and felt so self-conscious about her appearance in a bathing suit that she wouldn't take Joey to the beach. She said she would like to diet but wondered if this would affect breast feeding. She wished she and her husband could be together more. He had to commute sixty miles a day and found it difficult to stay awake while driving.

At eight months Joey's appetite was reported to be excellent. He had cereal, fruit, and a breast feeding for breakfast; vegetable, fruit, and a breast feeding at lunch; more cereal, vegetable, fruit and a breast feeding at supper. Before bedtime at 9 P.M. he was again breast-fed, and he usually awoke at 2:30 A.M. for nursing.

Mrs. Cyrenski was very reluctant to wean Joey, as breast feeding offered her so much pleasure. On the occasions when she had refused him the breast, "the way he looked at her" made her feel extremely guilty. He would make a characteristic whimpering sound and search with both hands and mouth for the breast. She felt as though she were depriving him by refusing. She now associated his severe biting merely with teething, and since it had let up a bit she delayed the start of weaning despite the pediatrician's recommendation.

In the seventh month at the well-baby clinic Joey was rather unsmiling throughout, but occasionally he smiled radiantly at his mother. A week later the home visitor was favored with an immediate smile, which even surprised his mother, since he had been rather cautious lately with strangers. He did cry, however, when his mother left the room.

At eight months Joey pushed himself about the house in something resembling a Taylor Tot. He also spent some time outside on an old mattress placed in the back yard, but for the most part he was held by both his mother and grandmother during his waking hours, with little opportunity to creep. By nine and a half months he had developed a peculiar kind of crawl, hitching himself along with one foot and one knee in a sitting position.

He preferred toys that made noise and could even be content with a cereal box containing some object that rattled. Around this time Mrs. Cyrenski found that he loved a tub bath when she gave him his first one. He was not in the least afraid of the water, as she had always thought he would be.

During this period the interviewer described what she called "an extremely seductive interplay" between mother and son. As Mrs. Cyrenski held Joey standing on her lap, he would sway in towards her body, burrowing into and mouthing her face, arms, and bosom. He frequently bit her face and shoulders. Mrs. Cyrenski laughingly told him not to, but as he swayed she would draw him closer, laugh with enjoyment, and nestle his body against her. The interviewer found it "more suggestive of two adults making love than of a mother with her baby."

At nine months Joey's schedule remained essentially the same except that breast feeding was somewhat diminished. Bowel movements had changed from two per day to one per day, most frequently after breakfast and sometimes after supper. The paternal grandmother could encourage Joey to urinate into a small container held before him by making a certain noise, but he would not do this for his mother. Mrs. Cyrenski remarked that when Joey was undressed "he pulled at his penis." She felt, "This is all right because he doesn't know what he's doing." During weighing at the clinic Joey handled his penis frequently and had an erection. When he was nine and a half months old, Mrs. Cyrenski again reported that he usually handled his genitals when undressed.

The kind of problems which so typically annoy the parents of infants did not appear prominent in the Cyrenski family. Feeding was never a problem. Although his mother had once wondered whether Joey would ever sleep through the night, by nine and a half months this pattern was well established. Neither was elimination a source of intense concern, although Mrs. Cyrenski gave this matter the same watchful attention that characterized all her care of her son.

Illness and the fear of sickness, however, were major sources of anxiety in the Cyrenski family. The grandmother blamed her daughter-in-law for every illness Joey had. It was her view — successfully imposed upon the rest of the family—that illness was the direct result of parental neglect. Thus, overlooking the fact that her house was ill-heated, she blamed Joey's frequent colds and earaches upon the fact that his mother had not bundled the child enough or had left him outside too long. The elder Mrs. Cyrenski said of her daughter-in-law that she was completely incompetent to raise a child. Her constant interference and the anxiety she aroused in Mrs. Cyrenski prompted the pediatrician to recommend some firm measures to deal with the elder Mrs. Cyrenski.

When the threat of illness did materialize, Mrs. Cyrenski was beside herself with guilt and anxiety. Even a minor cold would keep her up all night with the baby. This pattern with respect to illness extended to Joey's father, too. Both his wife and his mother were constantly alarmed over his poor appetite and the threat of sickness. "Poor boy, he works too hard," his mother commiserated. "Poor Stanley, he's so tired," his wife sympathized.

At the observation evaluation Joey was very much at ease in his mother's arms but had no difficulty in separating from her. He turned immediately to the mirror at the end of the crib, grinned, and "vocalized with the zest and animal-like tone of Tarzan." When he was offered a ball "he leaped for it like a kangaroo" but was quite ready to give it up at his mother's second request to give it to her.

Joey looked like a husky, big baby, with an immaculate white skin and a peaceful, good-natured face. The only feature which seemed disturbing at this visit was a certain hypotonicity. He was not as muscular as the other boys in the study, nor even as the girls, for that matter. At his attempt to stand up he did not get further than kneeling on one occasion, and then he tumbled as he tried it a second time. The pediatrician helped him and pulled him up to standing. He did not resist when she sat him down again, nor did he express any displeasure when his own efforts to stand up had failed. For a child of this age as well developed as Joey, he showed a very low desire to stand up.

At the age of 41 weeks he performed at a general maturity level of 47½ weeks on the Gesell test, with a developmental quotient of 115.6. On the Viennese test he scored a developmental age of 1 year, 9 days, with a developmental quotient of 129.9.

Joey demonstrated an unusually clear hand preference. Except for those objects which were too large to be grasped or lifted with one hand, he manipulated almost every offered object with the right hand, with which he was far more skillful. However, when his right hand was filled, he used the left with no awkwardness. In contrast to his poor body coordination, the cooperation of Joey's hands seemed far advanced.

Banging was still his main occupation with toys, but he did not mouth them nearly as frequently as before. His response to the toys was friendly, and he accepted them graciously but without too much eagerness. The only toy to which he gave a more enthusiastic welcome was the bell, but even then he did not resist when the pediatrician removed it.

In terms of mother-observation the pages are very unrevealing. Mrs. Cyrenski remained most unobtrusive. When Joey was unhappy she comforted him, when he almost fell on trying to stand up she rushed to his rescue, when the pediatrician failed to get the ball from Joey she succeeded. Although she remained in the background, she was by no means a bored spectator. According to the observer, "She responded to her child's moods of anxiety, irritation, or pleasure as if they were her own. But when he became intently absorbed in material she looked and acted deserted. In repose her face was sad."

Around this period Joey had two major outings, a visit to a sick relative in Maryland and a reunion party of Mrs. Cyrenski's family. Shortly thereafter the pediatrician was called because Joey had a temperature of 100 degrees and couldn't be comforted. Examination was negative except for a slight infection of the left ear. At the home call the pediatrician described the kitchen and pantry as dirty and untidy, the toys as old and unattractive. The house had a drab, bleak, and grimy appearance inside and out.

Mrs. Cyrenski complained of her increased loneliness and dissatisfaction with the living arrangements, the fact that she had virtually no privacy. She felt that her husband's family "never truly wanted" her and she often felt they were talking about her. When she spoke of this to her husband, he became very hurt and upset, and "then he doesn't eat." In a sad, resigned way she stated that the only solution she could see "to keep peace" was for her to get a job and let her mother-in-law take over Joey.

One afternoon Mrs. Cyrenski omitted the afternoon breast feeding. That night when Joey awoke and cried she tried to nurse him, but he refused his mother and could be comforted only by his grandmother. Mrs. Cyrenski interpreted this as a reaction to her denying him the breast earlier. As a result she felt that the only way to wean Joey was to stop altogether. She said she just could not go through his denying her again.

She realized that she could not continue nursing Joey indefinitely, but she also knew it would be extemely difficult for her to stop. While nursing him she knew that he needed her and that she was doing something for him that no one else could. But it was also becoming clear to her that he needed her less and less, and this was disturbing since he was really the only person she had at this point. She rationalized, "How can I stop when he keeps asking for it?" But then she added, "I'll have to do it quickly and stop altogether." She was torn between the perception that it had to be done and her desire to continue this gratification as long as possible.

Two weeks later Mrs. Cyrenski had still not attempted to wean Joey, and she feared what the pediatrician would think at the next clinic visit if he were still not weaned. The day before the clinic visit at the end of the tenth month Mrs. Cyrenski stopped nursing altogether. She said her breasts felt very tight and uncomfortable. Several times the pediatrician observed that she touched her breasts, and she cautioned Joey not to touch them as she held him.

The ensuing weeks were "terrible," and she was miserable from her deprivation and guilt because she hadn't "given Joey what he wanted." She managed to live through the period "from day to day." A month after the trauma of weaning she reported that Joey had "kept asking for the breast and acting as though he'd lost something." He would awaken at night but refused milk by cup. Now he still "asked" occasionally but seemed to have settled for the cup.

By the end of this period Joey was waking at 7 A.M. He was always rocked to sleep in the evening and slept through the night. He still slept in his father's old crib, though it was now too small for him and its sides were very low. His father had slept in the crib until he was two. Mrs. Cyrenski feared that Joey would fall out, so she pinned the blanket to the mattress to keep him more secure. She still changed Joey's diaper before she went to bed, and the pediatrician suggested that she desist, but Mrs. Cyrenski said she felt guilty if she didn't.

Joey had become afraid of strange people and places. His reaction was to give the adult a sober look, screw his face into a grimace, and turn to his mother's shoulder with an angry-sounding wail, usually without tears. The wailing lasted as long as the visitor remained. Joey was sometimes mistaken for a girl, since his curls were still uncut and the study members frequently remarked on his effeminate quality. Mrs. Cyrenski hated to cut the long thick curls, and in this her mother-in-law was in full accord.

The pediatrician also noted that Joey appeared flabby and had a generalized poor muscular tonus. However, Mrs. Cyrenski reported that he was more active now and crawled a great deal. Yet a month later she remarked to the home visitor, "Joey wants to be picked up every minute." He had also developed the habit of loud screaming when he didn't get his own way. His screaming invariably aroused the elder Mrs. Cyrenski, who thought her daughter-in-law should pick him up when he cried. But Mrs. Cyrenski was now beginning to feel that Joey didn't walk because he was held too much.

Joey was reported to be "crazy about his father." He would go to his father's bed, throw himself on him, and hug him. Mrs. Cyrenski felt "a little bit jealous" of it. Joey's contact with his mother remained "rough and seemingly erotic," according to the interviewer. At one visit he repeatedly ran his hand up and down the back of her leg, which she obviously enjoyed. As he fondled her breasts, she smiled at him radiantly. Next to her on the sofa he pressed his body hard against her, pushing her head roughly against the wall. She protested with laughter.

As Joey approached his first birthday he increasingly lost his attractiveness to the research staff. The pleasing appearance of infancy gave place to the picture of a pale and petulant child, the product of what the staff felt to be an environment overhung by "an air of brooding ill health." Joey's evaluation observation at one year of age corroborated this impression. His flesh looked flabby and whitish-gray in color, as if he had had no fresh air and had been fed solely on carbohydrates. His facial expression was even more disturbing, like "the expression of a middle-aged suffering woman."

He left his mother's lap only once, in order to get the spinning top, and it was noticed that he could walk a little. He rarely sat erect. Always he curved his back, his arms, and even his fingers around an object. Most of the time he leaned against his mother and pressed his whole self "into" her, rubbing himself against her in an ever so slight, ever so slow motion. He looked sleepy, but his mood was not one of pleasurable relaxation. He grunted and grumbled constantly in the most angry tone, which increased in vigor when some reason for anger occurred.

Generally speaking, he was not too interested in objects, rarely smiled at them, and never speeded up in order to approach them. His way of contacting objects was to "press" them as if they were elastic and could be squeezed, bringing to mind his experiencing of the breast. His mouth was also used frequently to suck the objects. Surprisingly enough, the mouthing was immediately interrupted when his mother said, "Stop, Joey," in a low voice and without any detectable anger. Joey's angriness was his most sustained mood during the evaluation, and his mother seemed incapable of soothing his anger.

Nevertheless, his developmental picture was far better than appearances indicated. At the chronological age of 12 months and 11 days he rated a general maturity level on the Gesell test of 14½ months and a developmental quotient of 116. On the Viennese test he scored a developmental age of 1 year, 5 months, 7½ days, with a developmental quotient of 139.5. His weakest area was language, but generally there was an improvement in performance. Outstanding in the behavioral picture was "the indolence, lack of tonus, and a continuous undertone of anger."

Rose Cyrenski realized that her son's behavior was not wholly pleasing to outsiders and that the situation did not follow commonly expected norms for child-rearing. Increasingly she began to describe Joey as "spoiled" and blamed his grandmother's insistence that he be held so constantly. Although she reacted to Joey's demandingness, Rose Cyrenski was little involved with his social and intellectual development.

Indeed, the home situation was hardly calculated to foster such development. Throughout the entire study period there was a marked paucity of toys in the household. Sometimes Mrs. Cyrenski tried to distract him with adult magazines, but there were no children's books available to him. Although Joey was "crazy" about his father, the latter was never observed to play with him in an appropriate way during their infrequent contacts. And his mother's conversation and attempts at play seemed to the observer to be peculiarly remote from the interests of a one-year-old child.

Mrs. Cyrenski pointed out that their living arrangements prevented her from raising Joey as she would like, but she saw little hope of improving the situation. Her mother-in-law still interfered with Joey's care and contradicted Mrs. Cyrenski's prohibitions. The elder Mrs. Cyrenski insisted that Joey's hair not be cut, and she proposed making dresses for Joey and alternately dressing him as a girl and then as a boy. Mrs. Cyrenski adamantly refused this suggestion but was less successful in validating his maleness by an appropriate haircut. Both she and her mother-in-law hated to make this sartorial break with infancy. Again procrastination ensued.

The study visitors were impressed by the gloom and oppressiveness of the Cyrenskis' apartment and were made uncomfortable by the heat and odor of the place. The shades and venetian blinds were ordinarily drawn, no windows were open, and the pervasive smell of the open garbage pail at the door penetrated throughout the house. The air was extremely warm, stale, and sour.

Mrs. Cyrenski reported that her mother-in-law "hollered" at her, called her a "dope" and "lazy." She felt unable to "stand up for herself," as she had always been shy and unsure. The elder Mrs. Cyrenski made all her dissatisfactions with her daughter-in-law known to Stanley, and Rose observed, "She is nice to me when Stanley is here, and he can't understand how she treats me when he is gone." During Joey's infancy Mr. Cyrenski had usually taken his wife's side in an argument, but now he refused to listen to his wife's complaints. Again she complained bitterly of the lack of privacy and their cramped sleeping arrangements. Sexual relations had virtually ceased, as they had to be so quiet about everything.

Mrs. Cyrenski looked very slovenly. She said she would like to diet but felt she needed "someone like a doctor to hound her to stick to it." She also knew she should see a doctor about an ear ailment but postponed it because she "had always been embarrassed by examinations."

Joey had several illnesses between twelve and seventeen months. First he was extremely fussy while cutting a molar, then he was reported to have a cold and running nose but no fever. A month later he had another cold, with nasal discharge, for four or five days, followed by a discharge from his eyes. Upon examination he was found to have a generalized upper respiratory tract infection, which was extensive but not acute. Penicillin was given, fluids and steam inhalations recommended. A month later another cold was reported, which was followed by a temperature of 103 degrees. He was again found to have an upper respiratory tract infection, with pharyngitis and acute ear infection. Mr. Cyrenski had also not been feeling well and had a slight cold and sore throat. Four days later penicillin was given to all members of the household. Somewhat later it was reported that Joey's face was swollen from gnat bites and that he was uncomfortable.

Usually Joey's appetite was excellent except when he suffered from a cold. He drank about a quart of milk per day and had a daily egg at the pediatrician's suggestion. He loved tea, preferring it "straight" from a small glass, which he held well without spilling. At sixteen months the interviewer watched Mrs. Cyrenski feed him. He sat on his mother's lap and she pinned his right arm against her. She allowed him to make one or two attempts to feed himself, but when he had difficulty with the fork or tried to use his fingers she again immobilized his arm and did the feeding.

Joey usually took a three-hour afternoon nap and slept through the night from 8 or 9 P.M to 7 A.M. When he was disturbed by nasal congestion Mrs. Cyrenski took him to bed with her although she knew "you are not supposed to do this." For several nights he woke up at 2:30 A.M. and after some milk usually went back to sleep. Mrs. Cyrenski generally rocked him to sleep while he enjoyed pinching small folds of her skin.

The pediatrician had suggested that Joey have a separate bedroom, but Mrs. Cyrenski "didn't see how it could be managed." The only available place was the alcove. "That would be too cold for him, and I wouldn't be able to hear him if he cried out." As for a larger crib, that was also out of the question, since the bedroom was too small.

Joey had one bowel movement a day, either on awakening or before evening bedtime. He usually grunted and sometimes squatted as he passed the stool. He did not object to a wet or soiled diaper, but when asked if he was wet he would grab the front of his diaper over the genital region. He strenuously objected to being put in supine for a diaper change, so Mrs. Cyrenski would change him in standing position.

At sixteen months Joey was reported to urinate into the toilet with help, but no attempt was made at bowel training. A month later Mrs. Cyrenski said, "I guess I should be doing something about it." He had a small toidy chair in the bedroom, but it was so inconvenient that it was seldom used. Mrs. Cyrenski hadn't thought of putting it in the bathroom. Joey once or twice referred to his bowel movement as "doo-doo."

The observations during this period were in direct contradiction to Mrs. Cyrenski's reports of Joey. She said he was "driving her crazy" with his activity. He was into everything in the house and also loved the garden, especially "tearing worms apart." He "danced" to music and liked to bounce on the rocking chair. But the observation reports said that Joey hardly moved away from his mother at all, and that indeed he seemed almost unable to move. He lay on or across her lap in an inert and limp manner or stood completely silent for minutes at a time, with his head under the folds of her dress pressed into her groin.

Mrs. Cyrenski reported that Joey was very interested in the sight of her body, and though she turned away from him while dressing, he ran around to look at her. He became extremely angry and red in the face if thwarted and let out piercing screams. She said, "He's too young to spank, and he really doesn't understand when he does something wrong." She added, "I can't keep a straight face when scolding him because he usually laughs at me, so I give in." Although Mrs. Cyrenski's attempts at discipline were ineffectual, Joey seemed to respect his father's prohibitions.

By this time Joey's curls were very long. This, in combination with a pale pasty complexion and general flabbiness, gave the appearance of unattractiveness and ill health. He could walk steadily and well but did not climb. His only words were "mama" and "dada." It was reported by his mother that he also could say "by-by" and "all gone" and that he tried to repeat words.

As Joey became more mobile and desired to explore, there was an increased number of quarrels between the two women of the house. His grandmother complained that he constantly upset things, and Rose Cyrenski felt that these complaints were unjustified. During the first year of Joey's life his mother felt she dared not have another child because of the additional expense, which would affect her aspirations for a home of her own. But during the second year she said that the grandmother "did not want another child, one was trouble enough." She felt, too, that everything she tried to get Joey to do was negated by her mother-in-law.

In any event, her own disciplinary efforts were inconclusive. She was inconsistent, now permissive, now forbidding, and she found it almost impossible to implement a command. She tried to reason with her son but found him stubborn. Instead of being firm, her prohibitions ended either in indulgent laughter or desperate capitulation. So Joey was observed more than once carrying paring knives unopposed or disregarding his mother's orders to put them down.

Conflict over discipline was but one aspect of a generally unsatisfactory state of affairs, however. For Rose Cyrenski, each day of her son's growth seemed to take him inexorably away from her. Although she could hardly bear the thought of leaving Joey in his grandmother's care, she also was distressed at her own diminishing satisfaction with him. Therefore, in the second year of her son's life, unhappy with living arrangements, a critical mother-in-law, and a child who was leaving the happy period of infancy, she began seriously to consider taking a job. Characteristically, however, this step was repeatedly postponed. In the meantime, life continued in its tense and unsatisfactory manner.

The evaluation observation at the well-baby clinic in Joey's seventeenth month created strong impressions on the study staff. One report said, "Joey at this point gives no clear picture of being a boy nor does he look like a girl. His long blond hair, softly curled is girlish in appearance, but the flabby tonus of his body and his awkward movements do not give any impression of feminine charm. He seems almost like a castrate — neither male nor female in any positive or identifiable way. The overall impression is one of generalized impotence." A further report said, "When undressed for the physical examination, his body was revealed as 'lumpy.' . . . Before the physical he fingered his penis and pulled at the skin of his scrotum. It was a shock to this observer to see him actually possessing a male genital." The mother's observer added, "Is this . . . mother emasculating this little boy?"

Through the first part of the observation Joey hardly moved at all and stood as if glued to the spot, holding his mother's skirt. Mostly he hid his face in her lap. When one saw his face it was apprehensive and unhappy. He registered little change when toys were offered. Occasionally he looked at the pediatrician but mostly watched his mother or stared into empty space. The only response related to the offering of toys was his vocalization, an ugly, grating "ahhhhhh," with rising and then lowering pitch. The pediatrician estimated this unbearably long period of utmost passivity as "at least twenty minutes."

Mrs. Cyrenski said, "He always likes the bell most of all," and it was the bell that finally induced Joey to give up his completely passive resistance. While he handled the bell he remained serious and absent-minded. After this, however, Joey touched other test objects that were offered to him. But his concentration on any test object was never deeper than on the bell. The only toy that secured an emotional response from Joey was the rubber cat with the protruding tongue. He kept his eye on the cat every minute of the demonstration and then turned to his mother with a vapid smile, which finally widened. After another short furtive look at the cat he leaned far back and vocalized "a brittle, grating, and rather loud 'aaau.'" He never attempted to reach toward or to grasp the cat.

For a child almost one and a half years old, Joey's vocalizations were inarticulate and unrecognizable. They were mostly unstructured enunciations of a purely vowel character, which Joey's observer called "petulant," "ugly," "guttural," or "grating." The paucity of his vocabulary was astonishing. On one occasion the word "no" was understood and also the word "dog" was heard. Although his mother tried to make Joey say all sorts of words during the observation, her reports about his verbal performances at home were meager. Allegedly he said "lo-lo" for "hello" and played a counting game. If we understood this game correctly, it consisted of the mother's counting up to two or three and Joey's grunting in between.

Again Joey's developmental picture was far better than one could hope. At the chronological age of 17 months and 10 days he showed a developmental age of 21 months and 22½ days, with a developmental quotient of 125.48 on the Viennese test.

The mother's observer characterized Mrs. Cyrenski as "not well combed nor possibly well washed." She also noted that Mrs. Cyrenski interfered with the testing procedure by handling the testing objects for Joey and demonstrating how they should be used. Mainly she was impressed by the mother's constant physical contact with Joey.

If Joey did not lean against his mother, she leaned against him. She held his hands and played with them. The observer wrote, "When they are not in such contact the mother bends so low that neither her face nor her hands are often out of the child's vision and awareness." All this physical contact on Mrs. Cyrenski's part was accompanied by smiles or laughter, but the expression underneath was one of "a child-like discontent." What was so disquieting to all members of the staff was "not the feeling of an overprotective mother but the feeling of an outspoken sexual relation between mother and child which was hard to look at."

It was strongly felt that Mrs. Cyrenski was constantly seducing Joey. He answered with complete passivity. It was hard to judge whether absorption in the sexual game kept his interest from anything else or whether his passivity was a direct answer to the mother's desire. In any event, the complete lack of independence of body and mind in this one-and-a-half year old child was "torturing to witness."

In Joey's eighteenth month the whole family was busy with the haying season. Joey was left to play by himself outside while the adults worked. His "sandpile" was a heap of gravel too coarse to mold, shape, or dig in. A month later the Cyrenskis again visited Maryland to see their critically ill relative, who died shortly thereafter. This death made Mr. Cyrenski ill. He was so upset that he couldn't eat. A month later he was again sick when he heard that a friend had died. Because of his ill health he gave up the 9 A.M. to 12 noon part-time job.

The burden of two jobs had left its mark on Stanley Cyrenski. His nerves had become ragged, and he had lost weight. His wife told him to "slow down" on the full-time job, but he was unable to do so. Thus, when his faculty for doing ten hours labor in eight won him a promotion his wife insisted on his giving up the second job. At this time the opportunity for a better full-time job presented itself, but Stanley decided against taking it because he feared that he had a hernia. Two doctors reassured him that this was not true, but Mr. Cyrenski felt that it was safer to stay with his old company (and their disability insurance) "just in case."

With the elimination of one job, Joey's father was able to spend more time with him than ever before. His attention, however, was not undivided. He worked about the grounds, allowing his son either to watch or to play alone nearby. Under these new circumstances the staff came into contact with Mr. Cyrenski at well-baby clinics and other occasions. They found him warm and friendly in his relationship with his son and much less emotionally involved than was his wife. The protectiveness of his own mother, the competition between her and Rose Cyrenski, and the continuation of his own filial role made Mr. Cyrenski appear a sibling to Joey in some respects rather than a father. Thus, when questioned by the staff about Joey, his replies seemed almost invariably to be not merely about his son but about his own childhood. His wife also seemed to sense his childish role. On one occasion she prepared baskets of Easter eggs for both Joey and his father.

In Joey's twenty-first month his mother finally made the break and started to work. She found herself a precision job in a factory and worked from 7 A.M. until 3:30 P.M. Although she could hardly bear the thought of leaving Joey in his grandmother's care, she was also distressed at her own diminishing satisfaction with him. On her first day of work Mrs. Cyrenski was almost in tears because it was so hard to leave Joey. The elder Mrs. Cyrenski reported that Joey "went slowly about the house calling 'mommy, mommy' all day." When Mrs. Cyrenski returned, he threw his arms about her and refused to let her out of his sight.

At first Mrs. Cyrenski's separation from her baby was as difficult as weaning had been, but gradually Joey's reaction to the separation came to be mainly his eager greeting when she returned. Mrs. Cyrenski found her job pleasant and hoped to make friends there. She enjoyed being away from her mother-in-law and found her co-workers genial. For the first time since Joey was born she began to feel in contact with the outer world, and this made life more bearable. Observers reported some diminution in the almost seductive physical contact between mother and son.

Yet it is significant that Joey's behavior problems seemed most marked when his mother was home. His grandmother, who seldom took him out of the house, claimed that "Joey was as good as gold" all day and was very easy to manage. Mrs. Cyrenski felt that he must store up his energy for her when she came home, because then he was very active and quite difficult to manage.

During this same month Joey had a cold for two or three days but no fever. Since he was now in the care of his grandmother, the interviewer remarked to Mrs. Cyrenski that this was one cold for which her mother-in-law couldn't blame her. But Mrs. Cyrenski still took the blame. She said she had caught it at work and given it to Joey. She reported vaguely about Joey's feeding schedule. He ate table foods almost entirely and loved meat in any form. He refused milk except at breakfast and drank soda, tea, or coffee during the day. During the summer months he was especially fond of the berry patch and ate as much as a cup of blackberries at a time. At twenty-two months he fed himself well with a fork.

Joey still took a late afternoon nap and usually woke up about the time his mother returned from work, at which time "all hell breaks loose." At 8 or 9 P.M. Mrs. Cyrenski rocked him to sleep, and he usually did not wake until morning. Joey had started taking a teddy bear and a rag doll to bed with him, which his parents would remove after he fell asleep for fear that he might suffocate or be harmed by them.

Mrs. Cyrenski said that Joey occasionally grasped his diaper over the genital to indicate he was wet. She reported that she had tried to put him on his toidy seat for one bowel movement, but when he cried she had stopped. Lately Joey had told his mother either during or after a bowel movement, but if he was put on the toilet he just sat and then passed his stool when taken off. At this time Mr. Cyrenski reported that for the last several months they had "been trying to break him" but that "he is hard to break." At times Joey indicated that he was dirty by using a Bulgarian word that means "anything that stinks."

Joey appeared to be getting used to the home visitor. His response was not nearly so negative, and he even gave her a smile occasionally. He still spent much of the time passively on his mother's lap or next to her, but the physical contact was more and more initiated or perpetuated by Mrs. Cyrenski than by Joey. When he was allowed to have some freedom he seemed like a different and better-natured child. He moved freely about the room, vocalized more, and even smiled.

It was a pleasure for the interviewer to discover in the middle of the twenty-first month that Joey had had his hair cut. This was a difficult thing for both Mrs. Cyrenski and her mother-in-law, and it had been handled with typical delay. As Joey's locks grew longer and longer he continued to be mistaken for a girl by the few strangers who saw him. This suited his grandmother well. She had kept her own son in curls until he entered school. Mrs. Cyrenski, too, was ambivalent about the matter. She said she hated to have his hair cut because "they were such pretty curls," and she procrastinated indefinitely. The haircut was finally accomplished in Sampson and Delilah style. While Joey slept, Mrs. Cyrenski held him down and his grandmother cut. It took three naps to complete the job.

Actually, it made less of a change than everyone had expected. Joey now looked less like a girl than before, but still there was nothing masculine about him. The absence of curls around his neck accentuated the flabbiness of his flesh, and his general pallor and look of ill health were still striking. Joey was reported during this period to say "man," "all gone," and "soda" without the "d." He climbed stairs easily, handled a cup well, turned pages singly, and had about fourteen single words in his vocabulary. He made no attempt to help in dressing or undressing himself. It was reported that he was putting several words together and had echoed two or three words in either English or Bulgarian.

When Joey was twenty-two months old, his appearance still made an unusually strong impression on the staff. "His head is covered with unruly, badly combed and badly cut, straight, sandy 'stubbles.' . . . Despite his little boy's suit Joey is far from looking masculine. . . . One would like to see his ghastly greyish white skin exposed to air, sun, and light." There was a particularly effeminate quality about Joey's hands and facial expression. The hand movements were gracefully delicate and completely without vigor, the frown between his eyes reminded one of feminine fretting, and the mouth had the expression of a wailing woman. "There was something in his appearance that was uncannily suggestive of bisexual association, which was hard to take."

The first twenty-five minutes of the observation were exasperating for all participants because the examiner and Joey's father fought a constant, losing battle to engage Joey in an activity or even to catch his attention. The lack of activity was not merely negativism but suggested deeper psychological roots. He related to nobody and to nothing, nor did he focus on any living or inanimate object in the room. His eyes did not move at all, and his head-turning in the direction of an object was never sufficient to get it into real focus. It was postulated that Joey tended to avoid visual contact with his environment because he had not reached the stage of any "give-and-take" reciprocal contact. One could also speculate further that the lack of activity in reaching a goal was a negativism due to already experienced disappointment, or the loss of a love-object from which he had not recovered. One could argue that nobody would resist finding out about another person or object unless one had already experienced that the "finding out" was disappointing.

In contrast to the unmoving character of Joey's eyes, there was quite a bit of movement around his mouth, which drooped sadly at the corners. His soft, colorless, well-modulated lips never parted except when he spoke, and this rarely happened. But frequently there was a rather strange and fierce baring of the teeth, which was accomplished by pulling the lips away from the teeth so completely that the lower lip formed a triangle. An observer with a Freudian analytic background hypothesized that Joey's teeth-baring, combined with the lack of vigor around the mouth, seemed to contain two conflictful aspects: his desire to destroy an element of the outside world and his necessity to bridge the gap between self and that element of the outside world.

There was the further psychoanalytic speculation that because of his late weaning Joey had come to identify the breast as both belonging to his own body scheme and yet partly representative of the outside world. He was weaned at the end of his first year, when the distinction between "I" and "you" should have been fairly well established. But in this case such differentiation may have been blurred by the ever-accessible breast. Thus, the object he wanted to destroy was not really an outside object but one inside himself, which he need not approach for attacking, but one that he must not release by opening his mouth.

He might also have identified with the mother's conflict about "holding and letting go," each impulse being so far from autonomy that each was destructive to the other. Joey would thus reproduce in his mouth movements the mother's struggle to hold that which would be destroyed in letting go.

Joey hardly verbalized at all, and even his vocalizations were meager. Except for episodes of screaming, the groaning and moaning sounds appeared at rare intervals. The words he used were few. His skimpy verbal output was limited to protests ("no"), demands ("keys," "mommy") or to a combination of both ("mine"). In striking contrast to this limited verbal output was the occasional subtlety of his verbal intake or understanding. When his father discovered that he had brought a sheet instead of a second diaper, Joey offered brown paper towels, which he had picked up from the table, as a diaper substitute. When Joey held his book turned the wrong way, and his father commented about it, Joey turned the book around immediately. It was quite evident that verbal output was limited so as to preclude any sharing of verbal communication. His intake or understanding, however, was on a level to permit him to "hoard" other people's communication as his mental property.

In contrast to the inertia of Joey's body and extremities his fingers were in constant, slow, but extremely delicate and superbly coordinated motion. The transition from one movement to the next took from six to seven seconds, and if one tried to imitate the speed of these finger movements it would have appeared like a slow-motion film. During all his finger play the fingers were stretched only once, curled only twice. In all other positions they were loosely flexed and performed via the "knuckle-joint" which gave the impression of loosely bent straws that moved like puppets on a string. There was rarely an instance in which two fingers moved simultaneously. The movement of one followed the movement of the other with a most subtle timing, as if one finger took over the movement from the other. These finger movements were carried out by the two hands simultaneously.

During most of this time Joey played with his father's keys, which seemed to be only accessories to the finger movements and not an object of motivation in themselves. Nevertheless, they were not dropped, and he "held" them by the accidental coordination of his finger play. A transition from the keys to a celluloid doll astonishingly brought no change in the finger technique whatsoever. They languidly continued their slow and graceful motions around the doll, as formerly around the keys. Then the grasp loosened and the doll slid to the floor; this was as much a part of the movement as the holding on to it. Joey did not throw or drop the object more actively than he held it.

There were two pieces of evidence in the observation that Joey was destructive with objects in a way which would lead to separation from them, but at the same time he could not bear the burden of his own destruction and separation impulses. In one instance, he twisted the leg of the celluloid doll, and in the other he piled up blocks and rings in a way that made his product bound to crumble. After each of these incidents he wet his pants. The second wetting episode was too near the first to be accounted for physiologically.

Joey looked neither the least bit pleased nor the least bit guilty after each episode of wetting his pants. It would appear that his difficulty in showing aggression of a separating nature was clearly demonstrated by the disguised way in which he performed it and by the manner in which he reacted to it.

At the next home visit, when the question of nursery school for Joey was raised, Mrs. Cyrenski said she thought it was a very good idea but that "he might be frightened of the other children." Joey was still timid with strange people, but if they didn't immediately approach or talk to him he could gradually accept them.

Mrs. Cyrenski described Joey as "getting into everything, opening drawers, and taking everything out." She said that spanking didn't seem to do any good, although "I don't really spank him so that it would hurt." She felt that it worked best to try and reason with him. "At times he will listen and be quite good, but at other times he goes right ahead with what he's doing anyway."

At the final evaluation of this study the parents reported that Joey was definitely indicating his need to have a bowel movement before having it in his diaper. He was more likely to advise in advance about this than about the need to urinate. The impression of Joey on this examination was that "for the first time he looked like a little boy with some independence from his mother. He did not cry or whine, nor was there facial grimacing." Joey made several spontaneous comments about what he saw or heard and correctly identified the sights and sounds by name.

His language had advanced in production and clarity. It was used for communication and in some instances it sounded almost "assertive." He had a greater freedom of gross motor activity and seemed to operate without the immobilizing dependence on his parents. This indicated that Joey might now be ready to enter the nursery school group, and the Cyrenskis seemed to welcome the possibility. At his chronological age of 2 years and 13 days Joey scored a developmental age of 2 years, 6 months, and 18 days on the Viennese test, with a developmental quotient of 125.

Possibly the release of Joey's mother from her "captivity" by going to work may prove to temper the "brooding ill health" of the Cyrenski home. And one can hope that the time is not far off when Rose and Stanley Cyrenski will take the step towards a home of their own, away from the paternal parents. Yet these are the judgments of a culture whose values are in many respects alien to those of Joey's family. The ease with which he acculturates to the norms of urban American society will probably measure the accuracy of these judgments. And of this we can now have no final knowledge.

The Cyrenski Family

SUMMARY

A. EXPECTATIONS

1. Maternal Expectations. Mrs. Cyrenski was fairly inarticulate about the concept of herself as a mother, but it was obvious that she placed a high value on motherhood and child-bearing. Words and behavior expressed her happiness with pregnancy, there were no anxious questions or predominant fears, and she was physically comfortable. There was no conflict about outside employment as opposed to maternal interests until the second year. Then it appeared as an escape from a pressing family situation and some growing discontent that the child was becoming more independent of her. It was as if she were leaving her son because of his growing separation from her.

2. Specificity of Expectations. Very few expectations were overtly expressed except the desire to breast feed the baby. Mrs. Cyrenski referred to difficulties experienced by one sister in disciplining or controlling her two little boys, who "were wild as devils." And she reported that another sister's baby had been "spoiled" by breast feeding, but it did not alter her own determination to nurse. She seemed quite confident in her ability to understand the needs of babies and to handle them intuitively. Perhaps she expressed no specific expectations about the child because of her general inarticulateness.

3. Motivational Orientation. Mrs. Cyrenski was predominantly child-centered, in accord with her unequivocal pleasure in the prospect of a child and her experiences with the infant. However, as Joey grew older and she was deprived of some of the gratification she had had in his infancy, she began to relinquish some of her absorption in the child. Her reluctance to wean him was evidence of an exceedingly slow and painful process to decrease the close physical contact with her son. But since the inevitable had to be faced, and as the stressful family situation became more intolerable, Mrs. Cyrenski began to shift somewhat from her extreme child-centeredness. Nevertheless, throughout the entire study she remained essentially a child-centered mother.

4. Role of Child in Fulfilling Mother's Expectations. Joey Cyrenski eventually displayed growing physical activity, which jarred the expectations of eternal infancy held by his mother. However, the development of independent body movement in the first two years was slow, and in the early months particularly his passivity and indolence were such as to fit the "helpless infant" maternal expectations. When he finally began to protest against prolonged infantilization, it was not with active physical protest but with crying and whining. Joey became a querulous child, and his efforts were less direct or positive than those of the other boys in the study.

The mother who was so perceptive and even intuitive toward the infant's needs was quite vague and unperceptive about clues relating to change in developmental status. It was not until Joey was almost two years of age that his mother began to realize that social, adaptive, language, and motor development were less than optimal. She then justified herself by blaming her mother-in-law for some of these problems. This characterized not only her generally immature relationship with Joey but also other relationships in the existing family structure.

5. Paternal Expectations. Mr. Cyrenski expressed great pleasure in anticipation of the child, heightened perhaps by the fact that he had been told he might be sterile because of having had mumps. Because Stanley Cyrenski's filial ties with his own parents had remained immature and unbroken since childhood, he was unable to separate the filial role from those of husband and father. He demonstrated no strong identification with an independent paternal image and related more as a sibling. Toward the end of the study it was observed that he had a warm interest in the child, although he was far less emotionally involved than his wife.

B. BEHAVIOR

1. Communication. In terms of both verbal and physical communication Mrs. Cyrenski was in a class by herself. In sharp contrast to other child-centered mothers, Rose Cyrenski produced almost no report of talking to Joey, but there was considerable evidence that she comforted and reassured him. When she did talk to him there was no attempt to adapt her words to the limitations of his ability to understand her. This may partly have been because of her general inarticulateness and incapacity to express herself. Mainly Rose Cyrenski was ever quick and intuitive in response to her child's clues relating to mood and affect. She spared no effort to accommodate him in these respects.

Their extraordinary close physical interaction was the main avenue of communication between Mrs. Cyrenski and Joey during the first year, undoubtedly heightened by the prolonged breast feeding. This intense physical interaction became an intuitive "oneness" between mother and child to the point where she even assumed that her baby would automatically like or dislike what she did, which oddly enough seemed to be so. But as Joey became more independent, at around one year, this strong physical communication became less effective and less characteristic.

The second year saw considerable increase in the use of language as Joey started to reach for independence. There were some half-hearted and ineffectual attempts to discipline and reprove him. Joey developed no words during this period but vocalized in a way usually described as whimpering or angry demanding, screaming, and crying.

Mrs. Cyrenski showed little perception of Joey's developmental clues in regard to more independence, and Joey often missed his mother's clues relating to anxiety, apprehension, or consolation. With the decrease of close physical communication between mother and child there was also heightened conflict between them, but typically this resulted in capitulation by Joey's mother. In the second year the interaction between them increasingly took the form of seductive and intense rough play.

2. *Regularity and Flexibility of Scheduling.* Emphasis on the child's "demand" schedule determined Mrs. Cyrenski's management of his eating, sleeping, and all other activities. Regularity was never defined as a problem, and she flexibly responded to what she understood as his expression of a need. Joey ate when he was hungry, slept when he was sleepy, was rocked, carried, and comforted

whenever he cried. On his part, Joey was a fairly regular baby. Mrs. Cyrenski made no attempt to set up a schedule for him, but by the beginning of the second year mother and child had established a notably regular feeding routine and Joey's sleeping pattern was only a little less so. There was no regulation to be observed in other activities such as playing, comforting, holding, and rocking. During Joey's first year these activities were the constant practice of all the adults in the household. Joey's mother was freed of the usual household responsibility for cooking, marketing, and management because these had been assumed by the elder Mrs. Cyrenski. Rose Cyrenski applied herself to Joey's care virtually twenty-four hours a day.

3. Techniques of Management. Mrs. Cyrenski's behavior and techniques of management were preponderantly permissive during the first year. Most of the reports centered on feeding and physical activities. She permissively tolerated all kinds of behavior by Joey, including biting, kicking, and pulling her hair. She showed little ingenuity in providing substitution or diverting him from such activities. On the contrary, she seemed to encourage these displays. Occasionally she reached a saturation point. Once he bit her so hard that she "felt like choking him." But she was not consistent in her prohibitions or demands on Joey and usually capitulated to him.

Some forms of restriction were seen, mainly for the purpose of maintaining his infantile status and discouraging independent movement away from her. Thus, she kept him pressed close to her when it was obvious that he wanted to escape from such smothering encirclement. Or she pinioned his arm against her while feeding him so that he was not free to attempt self-feeding.

In the second year the proportion of non-permissive reports increased as Joey became more mobile and independent. With the fading of the intense physical relationship there was an increase of verbal prohibitions and scolding. But Mrs. Cyrenski still remained unsuccessful in her disciplinary efforts, and Joey was more apt to respect his father's and grandmother's prohibitions than his mother's.

4. Relation of Expectations to Behavior. There seemed to be no need for Rose Cyrenski to express in detail any expectations about her child. Her behavior showed that the core of relationship was the intense unity of the two, the instinctive mothering of the helpless infant. This was the foundation of her expectations, a dependent infant for whom she was the all-nurturing force. And it led to behavior which tried in vain to maintain the dependent relationship and the gratifications derived from such a close and captive relationship.

After the first few months, however, Mrs. Cyrenski became aware of the inevitably changing circumstances, which aroused new expectations. Her own wishes and needs for an infant struggled against the pressure of his growth and change. Her deep satisfaction with the earliest months gave way to frustration. She responded by an increase in controlling and restrictive behavior and finally by resignedly going back to work and relinquishing Joey to the care of his grandmother.

5. Paternal Behavior. There was little evidence of Mr. Cyrenski's participation in care of the child. Since Rose Cyrenski's sole role in the household seemed to be child care, she applied herself so completely to the task that there was little need or opportunity for her husband to become involved. Finally, Mr. Cyrenski himself was given so much attention and mothering by both women in the house that it made him appear more of a sibling to Joey than a father.

As in most of the other families, however, a growing relationship was noticed between father and son as the son moved from infancy to childhood. This was facilitated by the fact that Mr. Cyrenski had abandoned his part-time job during Joey's second year, which gave him opportunity to spend more time with his son. By then, also, Mrs. Cyrenski had taken a job and was out of the house a good part of the day. A number of her duties in relation to Joey were therefore assumed by her husband. This included taking Joey to the well-baby clinics and observations. The staff had the opportunity at those times to see that the relationship between Mr. Cyrenski and his son was warm and friendly, but that he was not as emotionally involved as his wife.

C. SOCIO-CULTURAL INFLUENCES

1. Socio-economic Status and Values. The Cyrenski family showed little interest in social advancement and little evidence of concern for the future beyond the maintenance of their current level of economic security. Neither was interested in higher education or training for work beyond ordinary factory skills. Mrs. Cyrenski did encourage her husband to handle two jobs in order to save money for a house of their own, but this goal was more a "dream" fantasy than a realizable goal. Mrs. Cyrenski's escape into work was less a move toward advancement than flight from frustration within the family circle and a search for satisfaction through personal contact with others.

2. Extended Family. The role of the paternal extended family was so strong that it prevented the achievement of dyadic togetherness by husband and wife. Even their privacy was violated by the paternal grandmother's insistence that bedroom doors remain open at night. The dominance of the elder Cyrenskis was such as to work against the creation of independent and flexible personalities, either for their son or their grandson, to say nothing of the alien daughter-in-law.

There was overt competition between mother and grandmother in making decisions about how Joey should be raised and how his father should be looked after. The perpetuation of the filial role in both young parents effectively prevented the establishment of a triadic family during the period of the study.

Mrs. Cyrenski's contacts with her own family were relatively slight because of isolation and distance. But what contact there was appeared to be warm and supportive to her.

3. Spatial Arrangements and Values. Joey Cyrenski slept in his parents' bedroom for the full two years of the study. The bedroom was crowded and had barely space for the crib. There was no alternative place for him to sleep. There was only a cold alcove available, which none of the adults felt was an appropriate place for the baby. Aside from the limited sleeping space, the gloomy crowdedness of the close, dark apartment permitted Joey little in the way of exploratory freedom. What opportunities he had were largely provided out-of-doors.

The Cyrenskis lived under severe spatial handicaps in the house. Problems of management were exacerbated when the child was at the crawling, exploratory age and also when he embarked upon the toddling phase of his development. However, the use of space was also an indication of the interpersonal relationships. For example, the denial to the young family of the desirable downstairs apartment was a definite refusal by the elder Mrs. Cyrenski to allow them an independent existence. The acceptance and toleration of this situation by the young couple implied a passivity and immaturity on their part, related to their own personality characteristics.

D. FAMILY RELATIONSHIPS

1. Marital. Mrs. Cyrenski had frequently felt out of place and not really a part of most social groups in which she participated. In some ways, her adult life seemed to recapitulate her school adjustment problem of "not belonging." The different cultural characteristics of the family into which she had married, plus their speaking in a language she did not understand, accentuated her feeling of separation.

Her own early family life encouraged tendencies in Mrs. Cyrenski to withdraw from situations which demanded self-assertion and to repress angry or hostile feelings. Sensitive and lonely, she had married into a family where she was forced into rivalry with her mother-in-law for both husband and child. Her husband was a dependent, immature, hypochondriacal, and unassertive man who did not provide the strength of personality which his wife needed in the emergent family setting. He had a tremendous need to be mothered, and this his wife was inclined to do. But in this she was also forced to compete with her mother-in-law, for whom she was no match.

While the marriage did not seem to suffer from intense strife, neither did it appear entirely happy. The paternal grandmother continued to rule the household authoritatively, and the young married couple never really had much opportunity to achieve an independent marital development. Even their sexual life virtually ceased because of lack of privacy. Mrs. Cyrenski finally surrendered to the paternal grandmother and sought more satisfying social relationships by working outside the home. It was not tension between Mr. and Mrs. Cyrenski but rather frustration from failure to achieve an independent marital relationship that was the crux of their problem.

2. *Mother-Child.* Of all the study mothers, Mrs. Cyrenski was the most absorbed in her child. Conflict with the paternal grandmother was constant, and the immaturity of her husband did not permit him to be an effective source of support to her in this struggle. She tended to withdraw from possible conflict situations and to submerge her feelings of hostility. Furthermore, she was physically and emotionally isolated from her own family and her friends. Driven as she was by loneliness and a need to foster dependence, it was not surprising that Joey was called upon to fill an emotional "vacuum."

The characteristics of this mother-child relationship have already been described. It was marked by an intense physical closeness, bordering on the erotic, shown in constant handling of the child and an intuitive anticipation of his infant needs. As Joey grew older, this relationship was changed into a struggle to keep him in infancy. It was, of course, a losing battle, as was her effort to gain some independence from her mother-in-law. As she turned to work outside the home, Joey ceased to be the all-absorbing center of her life. At the end of two years she had a somewhat less intense, though still loving and satisfying, relationship with him.

3. *Father-Child.* There was only the slightest involvement by Mr. Cyrenski in day-to-day care of the child, plus some minimal play interaction. The sibling quality of the relationship impressed the observers as an identification of son and self. One cannot say that there was a strong dyadic relationship between father and son, only that there was warmth, friendliness, and an absence of conflict. The absence of conflict probably accounted for the fact that Joey was more responsive to his father's prohibitions than to his mother's.

E. PERSONALITY CHARACTERISTICS

1. Handling of Anxiety and Hostility. The staff believed that Rose Cyrenski had unusually strong hostile and aggressive feelings but that these were suppressed except for rare temporary explosions. She confided her discouragement, sorrow, resentment, and resignation to the staff, but she rarely expressed these feelings to her husband or the grandparents. On the rare occasions when she did express such feelings to her husband, he rather unsympathetically told her not to worry about them. She would then become depressed and cry. She seldom became overtly angry nor did she take action about the unsatisfactory extended family situation. Often the anger welled up inside but was only indirectly expressed in the form of unrealistic and exaggerated fears concerning Joey's health and activities.

There was some speculation that Mrs. Cyrenski's erotic closeness with Joey was, in part, a displacement from angry feelings toward her husband and the paternal grandparents. Trapped in a struggle with the paternal grandmother over control of Stanley, Rose Cyrenski reacted by struggling to control little Joey. Mr. Cyrenski expressed his own considerable anxieties in a great deal of hypochondriacal somatic complaints and fantasies about health and illness.

Rose Cyrenski's childhood home had been one of poverty, which increased after her father died. She characterized her family of origin as undemonstrative and lacking in affection. She had found her school years unhappy and lacking in the ties of friendship. She had been very shy and had thought she was rejected by her peers because she had had no pretty clothes. Although she had shared a bedroom with her sister, there had been little sisterly companionship. Thus, submissiveness to her mother-in-law's dominance was to some extent the continuation of a childhood reluctance to share her feelings and thoughts with others. In many respects, hers was a lifetime difficulty in establishing intimate relationships with others.

We have seen that the warm emotional tenor of the marital relationship was threatened by the dominance of Mrs. Cyrenski's mother-in-law. In the course of this struggle, and because of her inability to establish an independent place in the extended family, Mrs. Cyrenski found her deep pleasure in her new son the chief source of emotional gratification.

2. Dependency and the Sense of Security. Rose Cyrenski's need to be dependent might have been much less acute had she not experienced competition and conflict in the paternal grandparents' house. As the youngest child in her family of origin, Rose was the last to marry. She saw her mother fairly frequently during pregnancy. After Joey's birth the contact between her and her mother was largely by telephone, and she became increasingly lonely with no one to talk to except her mother-in-law for much of the time. She had few friends, no intimates.

It was important for Mrs. Cyrenski's sense of security to feel that there was someone who completely relied upon her for the satisfaction of needs. Ordinarily this might have been achieved via her husband and child. But the care of her husband was denied her. Deprived of a husband who fully "belonged" and needed her, she turned to her infant. But here again her mother-in-law contested her exclusive possession.

3. Feelings of Adequacy or Inadequacy. There was no clear demonstration that Mrs. Cyrenski had feelings of inadequacy. During pregnancy she raised no matters about possible inadequacy. In fact, she appeared quite confident about her approaching motherhood. Her care of the child substantiated this confidence. Aside from physical care, however, the relationship with Joey raised questions about the integrity of her feelings of adequacy. Her verbal communication with him has been described as ineffectual. It was vague and not sustained by enforcing her instructions to him. Also, she was unable to set a structure and limits within which Joey could behave. Perhaps feelings of inadequacy may be partly responsible. One staff observation hypothesized that the seductiveness of the mother-child relationship was related to the question of adequacy in that it probably strengthened Mrs. Cyrenski's feelings of adequacy.

4. Planning and Impulsiveness. Mrs. Cyrenski was not called upon to plan in family life with her parents-in-law. For the most part planning was accomplished by the paternal grandmother. There was also no evidence of impulsive behavior on Mrs. Cyrenski's part. She showed some planning prowess in helping her husband to get a better job and in encouraging him to work two jobs so that they could save money for a home of their own. But there was no continuing evidence of strong planning motivations.

5. Self-Assertion. Mrs. Cyrenski was characterized as having self-assertion difficulties in adult relationships. These difficulties began in her early years, when she tended to withdraw from conflict-producing situations and to repress her anger and hostility. These feelings were bottled up except for rare temporary explosions. Especially in dealings with her mother-in-law Mrs. Cyrenski could not assert her own prerogatives or establish for herself a definitive position in the household. Similarly, with her husband, she feebly attempted to assert herself but easily abnegated "because it would only upset him and he wouldn't eat."

6. Recapitulation of Past Experiences. There was strong reaction by Mrs. Cyrenski to perceived childhood deprivations. She recalled her strict father and the difficulties his restrictions had made for his daughters. She remembered her unhappy school experiences and the feelings of "not belonging and being snubbed." She described the "struggle to get by" financially after her father had been accidentally killed. But there was no verbal expression by Mrs. Cyrenski to the effect that things would be "different" for her baby and no strong indication of striving to alter Joey's environment.

F. EMERGENCE OF FAMILY INTEGRATION PATTERNS

1. Family Structure. The Cyrenskis were least successful of all the families in achieving an identity as a triadic nuclear family. The rivalry between Mrs. Cyrenski and her mother-in-law for the central place in Mr. Cyrenski's life extended to Joey also. The peculiar psychological constellation of the group intensified their individual traits — a domineering mother-in-law, an immature husband, a weak and abnegating wife. These combined to make a strong triadic unit impossible and also formed a strait jacket around Joey Cyrenski.

In the second year Mrs. Cyrenski's growing dissatisfaction with her relationship to Joey contributed still further to the weakening of nuclear family feeling. It probably influenced her to give up the struggle and permit her mother-in-law to control the situation while she looked outside the family for some emotional satisfaction.

Mrs. Cyrenski's isolation was accentuated by the changes that occurred during the two-year period. At the time of Joey's birth there was pleasure and pride in the mother-father-child constellation on the part of both parents. But this began to fade with the failure to establish a triadic unity under the circumstances in which the Cyrenskis lived.

The marital relationship was not characterized by undue strife and appeared to have the potential for satisfaction were it not for the fact that Mrs. Cyrenski and her mother-in-law were in competition for Stanley's love. In this family the matriarchal authoritarianism of the paternal grandmother, in combination with Mrs. Cyrenski's reticence and her husband's immaturity, made a nuclear family identity impossible. The family emerged as segmental.

2. *Division of Labor and Balance of Power.* The family division of labor was actually between Mrs. Cyrenski and her mother-in-law, with Mr. Cyrenski playing little or no part in it. The older woman managed the house, cooked the meals, and dominated all aspects of family life. Mrs. Cyrenski's main responsibility was the child. One could say that the balance of power rested with the elder Mrs. Cyrenski and that neither Rose nor Stanley Cyrenski wielded any significant power authority, either within the household or their immediate family.

3. *Development, Achievement, and Social Behavior of Child.* Although Joey was an extremely passive and inactive child whose verbal output was quite limited, his actual developmental scores were higher than one would expect. In a more stimulating intellectual environment one might wonder about Joey's potential for even greater development. The personality and cultural factors which surrounded him and which operated outside the norms and

influences of the urban scene seemed to the staff to be dangerous to the child's optimal development.

For a long time Mrs. Cyrenski seemed unaware and unperturbed by his unattractive social behavior, his gross motor lethargy, and his inadequate communication. She was far more concerned about the problems connected with his developing independence and growing away from infancy, the stage in which he provided her with the greatest satisfaction.

4. Prospect of Siblings. Mrs. Cyrenski at first desired to have several children, and she spoke of her wish for a second child when Joey was only two months old. The stress of life in the paternal home dampened her enthusiasm, especially since the paternal grandmother was opposed to another child, saying "one child was trouble enough." In any event, no second pregnancy occurred. We do not know whether the grandmother's dominance prevailed or whether Mrs. Cyrenski's discontent with her situation was the deciding factor.

5. Status of Family in Community. There is little doubt that the community environment provided by the elder Cyrenskis was extremely limited and quite remote from the general stream of American culture. In their isolation the grandparents succeeded in maintaining much of their old Bulgarian peasant atmosphere. They were devout, hard-working, puritanical, and familistic, but their traditionalism made it impossible for them to accept either contemporary ideas or a Spanish daughter-in-law.

There was a severe lack of friends or social relations of any kind in the gloomy atmosphere of the paternal extended family. Except for contact with this study there was no evidence of any community involvement or participation.

6. Types of Parent-Child Adaptation. The Cyrenskis were clearly characterized as child-centered and highly responsive to the emotional and physical needs of their child. Permissiveness was predominant throughout the study, even though there was a noticeable change towards less permissiveness in the second year. Since the triadic family unit was not established and the twosome relationships between mother-father, mother-child, and father-child did not wholly or satisfactorily develop, the family functioned as a segmental structure. It was therefore designated as a segmental, child-centered, and permissive family.

POSTSCRIPT

Contact with the Cyrenski family continued for only six months following the study. Since Mrs. Cyrenski worked days and her husband worked nights, Joey sporadically attended nursery school, accompanied by his father. Mr. Cyrenski was quite protective and anxious with Joey, frequently asking, "Are you afraid?" He gave the impression of a sibling eager to share attention and activity. Joey approached the nursery school experience timidly, but there was evidence that he enjoyed it and would adjust appropriately.

Mrs. Cyrenski remained on her job, which provided practically her only social contact with the outside world. She indicated that she would probably go on working indefinitely, as they were "scarcely getting ahead financially." Her interaction with Joey was notably less physical, mainly because the child became more independent and removed himself from the close contact. Mrs. Cyrenski suffered a sore thumb, which the shop nurse allegedly diagnosed as a vitamin E deficiency that "comes from lack of sexual intercourse." Mr. Cyrenski's term of address for his wife was "sis." In a word, this may tell much of the marital relationship.

Joey's speech improved, and he became able to express himself understandably. He engaged moderately well in activity and play. Mrs. Cyrenski reported that he was often teasing and provocative at home but that discipline was ineffective because she "had to laugh back at him." Furthermore, so many adults were telling him what to do that he didn't listen to anyone. Toilet training seemed under reasonable control. Apart from several respiratory infections Joey's health remained good.

In the final contact Joey still looked like a pale and rather flabby child, whose hair was jaggedly sheared from his grandmother's latest ministrations and who was clothed in a cut-down velveteen jumper of indeterminate age and origin. His environment remained meager and impoverished in terms of Joey's own enrichment or his family's development.

It appeared that the Cyrenski family would continue under the paternal grandmother's hegemony, and that neither husband nor wife would have the will to change it. Her resignation was well expressed in Rose Cyrenski's words, "As long as I have to live here, I might as well keep the peace."

The Harris Family

SAVING GRACE OF PARENTHOOD

Irene Harris' search for happiness and contentment was perpetually haunted by her sense of rejection and deprivation. Overlooked in her timidity and undemanding in her desires, she was ever the little girl vainly yearning for the treasures of life that would inevitably be denied. And so it came to pass that she was even barred from the precious solace of the Roman Catholic Church.

"I need a church very much. I went past the church on the green and I saw the doors standing open and I wanted to go in but I did not dare." The words burst forth emotionally from the rather reticent, attractive twenty-nine-year-old brunette with large dark expressive eyes and a ready smile. This ambiguity toward the church epitomized the irresolution of Mrs. Harris's wishes and desires, sense of rejection and fears, anger and feelings of deprivation. "It is one thing that is on my mind all the time, and I don't know what to do about it."

The rejection and deprivation started early for Irene Harris. Her Italian-born parents had had little education beyond "what was called second grade." Her parents came to this country in their early twenties, married here, and were numbered among the thousands of uneducated Italian villagers who arrived in the early twentieth century to tend the clanking machinery of American factory lofts. There was the constant problem of finding enough money to finance bed and board, and there were the recurrent bewilderments of life in alien America.

Their two children came quickly, first Irene and then Dominick sixteen months later. This undoubtedly complicated the life of a working mother. From an early age the two children roamed the streets together, their environment the brick walks of the Italian section. Despite her inability to exercise constant maternal supervision, Irene's mother played a dominant role in her family. She bossed her husband constantly and berated him for bringing home so little money. He remained "a shy and retiring sort of person, not interested in contacts with people."

Italian was always spoken in this lonely family, estranged from its neighbors and from the American community. Irene herself did not learn English until she started school. Lenient and indulgent to her children, the mother nevertheless inculcated a sense of dependency in them, so strong that Mrs. Harris said neither she nor her brother had ever been able to overcome it.

The early insecurities of life left their mark on Irene. Though she was one of the street gang and had many girl friends, she suffered always from timidity and uncertainty, never taking the lead in any activity if she could avoid it. And thus she came to feel that somehow she could only be a follower, often overlooked and deprived, unable to demand or expect anything. But there was always the haven of the Church, where "for a few pennies" she could find comfort, peace, security, and the sacred blessings. It became a refuge for the child, who was never close to her mother, an answer to the yearnings for reassurance and protection.

Those early years brought physical and emotional burdens. Irene developed pulmonary tuberculosis infection "sometime during her childhood," and the scars were discovered in a routine high-school survey. She still had to be checked at regular intervals, which was "a great chore." In contrast to her girl friends, who began menstruation at about eleven or twelve years of age, Irene did not start until about fourteen. She had received no preparation on this from her mother but "knew all about it" from her friends.

When Irene finally menstruated, her mother "gave her instructions in how to care for herself" and explained to her that she "was a lady now and had to be careful and not be too familiar with boys." Irene was not frightened or upset by this first period, but she did not have another for several months. From then on, she was quite irregular and "would sometimes miss anywhere from one to three months." When she was about fifteen years old, her mother took her to a doctor, who gave her some injections, but "that did not make any difference."

After she finished high school Irene worked as a receptionist in an insurance agency, where she led an uneventful career for six years. Shortly after the outbreak of World War II she met and married Eddie, a career man in the Navy. Life at home now became punctuated by exciting and happy "shore leaves" with him at one or another of America's seaports. Her love for him was such that she "would never be able to love another person as much as that." But Eddie was an irresponsible sort of person "who did not think of marriage in any serious terms and never had an idea of their having a home together." He was such a poor correspondent that he sometimes failed even to write of an approaching mainland interlude. Irene explained, "We were both probably too young, and my parents should never have allowed me to be married."

Although she very much wanted a child with Eddie and they used no kind of contraceptives, she was never able to become pregnant. This convinced her that she could never conceive. She and Eddie were finally divorced.

Alone and bitter, Irene met Herb Harris about a year after the divorce. He was thirty-seven years old, almost ten years her senior. He too had been married before and was responsible for supporting two children from that marriage. After a courtship of several months they planned to be married. Irene "had no idea" of her pregnancy at the time they had a small wedding in September, with only their parents present. Premaritally she had not used contraceptive precautions since she was under the impression that she could not conceive.

This pair, once disillusioned in marriage, buried their old wounds and embarked on matrimony once again. In each other their illusions took tangible form. Mrs. Harris thought her husband "wonderful," an adult responsible man with a good job and a secure future. He, in turn, loved her exceedingly well. But in reaching out for new happiness Mrs. Harris had had to sacrifice old securities. Her remarriage barred her from a main source of peace and comfort, the Roman Catholic Church. This rejection remained a specter to haunt the marriage from its very inception.

Already three months pregnant at the time of her marriage, Mrs. Harris became a clinic obstetrical patient because "Herb supports his children and it makes a difference financially." She said that she was familiar with the hospital and maternity services from hearsay and that she knew about the rooming-in plan, which she very much wanted for herself. Her response to the projected study was that she would like it very much but of course would want to talk it over with her husband.

Mrs. Harris selected a straight chair in the interview because "her back bothered" her. She mentioned her surprise when the obstetrician told her that she was practically five months pregnant. Since she had never been regular in her menstrual periods, she had not thought anything of it when she had missed. One month ago she had had acute abdominal pain and had been taken to the hospital. They had performed a laparotomy, suspecting that she had a tubular pregnancy. However, they found that she had a normal uterine pregnancy and would have a baby. "They didn't tell me that I was this far along."

When asked how long she had been married, Mrs. Harris wrinkled her nose, made a face, and said, "Only three months. . . . I guess we got started on this baby early." The pregnancy was quite a surprise and required an adjustment of their plans. They had just moved into their own "rental" but planned to buy a house. This would now have to be put off, even though Mr. Harris had "a very good job as an auto salesman" and made "a very good salary."

In response to a question as to whether Mrs. Harris had ever had any experience with babies, she told of having liked and taken care of babies when she was in high school but not having had much to do with them since. Her younger brother was also married and had "a lovely baby boy." Her husband's brother and two sisters were also all married and had families. She said her husband was "delighted about the idea of a baby." There was a general air of happiness about her as she spoke of her husband and family.

She reported that a young couple had moved in next door and that the girl was expecting in February. Mrs. Harris had been borrowing books from her on natural childbirth and child-rearing. She referred to the coming baby as "he," but in respect to preference she said that she really didn't care, but that her husband would probably prefer a boy, "as most men do." She had always thought she would like to have a little girl and supposed that perhaps she would have two children.

In the second interview Mrs. Harris described her four-room apartment, in which one room had not yet been furnished and had been set aside for the baby. There was a questioning note in her voice as she said that she thought a separate room was better for the baby.

She said she felt fine but had gained seven pounds without realizing it, as she had not really "felt larger." It meant that she had to be very careful with diet from now on, and this would be hard, as she always loved food and had a healthy appetite. She hoped she would have the same doctor who had taken care of her when she had had the laparotomy operation.

Mrs. Harris seemed very enthusiastic about herself, her pregnancy, and everything that was happening. Her back pain had not bothered her recently, and she supposed "the exercise classes were going to be good to get my muscles in better condition." She seemed very interested in the idea of talking to the pediatrician from the research group and said she had been giving considerable thought to her delivery and the plans for it, although she was not apprehensive. Nevertheless, she told about a woman she had known who had become mentally disturbed after the birth of her baby. And she also recalled that some women screamed in delivery and she hoped she would not be like that. When asked about help after the baby was born, she did not seem to anticipate the need of help but said, "If I do, my mother will come and help me out."

At the next interview Mrs. Harris was pleasant and smiling but seemed to prefer not to talk. She said she was glad not to have gained in the past two weeks and that she was trying hard to eat carefully. She felt fine and said she felt fortunate not to have been nauseated. She looked forward to "the baby's really being here" but had not purchased any layette because "it is not a very good idea to have too many things ready because something might happen."

The interview in the seventh month of pregnancy again disclosed a withholding quality in Mrs. Harris's talk, although she was as pleasant as ever. She reported that she felt fine but then told about recent hemorrhoids, which "were most painful and uncomfortable . . . like a sharp thorn." She had called the doctor, who prescribed some medication. It gave only temporary relief, and she was going to ask him if anything further might be done to alleviate the pain. "Perhaps it has something to do with gaining more weight, which increased the pressure of the fetus." At any rate she had gained even more weight and knew "the doctor was not going to like that." She didn't blame him because "it's for my own good that the doctor insisted on it."

When the questionnaire was introduced, Mrs. Harris began to speak in a more lively fashion, especially concerning her husband. She mentioned that he belonged to the "Toastmasters' Club," made up mostly of salesmen and businessmen "who practiced making speeches." She said that her husband was a very good speaker but that she couldn't speak to a group at all. Mr. Harris also read as many as three or four books a week, but she read so slowly that it took her weeks to finish one book.

She took pride in the fact that her husband liked to engage in all kinds of sports, such as hiking, hunting, bowling, and various water sports. "He has a small boat which he made himself. He's very handy with tools. He's made quite a few things for the house." Mrs. Harris deprecated her own abilities in anything other than cooking and sewing, which she thought she did rather well. She thought that probably both she and her husband were very good at using their hands to make and do things, and said that they both liked swimming a great deal. What she really enjoyed was "dusting, housework, and keeping the house the way I like it."

When the tests were mentioned, Irene wanted to know if her husband would also be tested, as she was uncertain how he would feel about that. She agreed to the tests for herself but warned that "Herb's evenings are very much taken up with various activities." She was impatient to leave, as she did not want to get home too late to get dinner."

Mrs. Harris returned the following week and was now somewhat resentful about the doctor's emphasis on weight because "what can make the baby grow if I don't gain?" Nevertheless, she thought that his observation that her legs were swollen was valid, and she was pleased that the swelling had gone down. She had been especially careful of her salt intake.

As she talked, Mrs. Harris moved uncomfortably about in her chair, trying to find a suitable position. She said, "There seems to be such an upward pushing on the part of the fetus that I keep wanting to stretch out taller and taller." Her appearance did not seem very large, but she felt "very big and heavy" and wondered how she could "possibly stand the next two months."

Mrs. Harris asked how often she would have to bring the baby to the well-baby clinic and what it would cost. Financial planning was important, she explained, because her husband planned to buy a house. It was in an outlying area, and possibly it would be too much for her to manage the trip often. The house they had in mind was in the process of being built. It had four rooms downstairs and space for two more rooms upstairs. She mentioned again that "Herb is clever and handy," and she felt they would have a minimum of expense in fixing up a new place.

In discussing the baby's due date, Mrs. Harris said that she had always kept an accurate calendar of all her menstrual periods because of her irregular menstruation. This irregularity had not really bothered her in the past because she had always wanted to become pregnant but in the future, she thought, it might be more of a worry. While she would like to have a second child, she wouldn't want another right away.

In the eighth month Mrs. Harris broke one appointment "because of a cold." However, from the numerous excuses in regard to appointments with the pediatrician and the psychological tester, it appeared that she was reluctant to have these appointments. Finally, she said she wondered if she needed to see the pediatrician at all because she had been told "all I need to know." The interviewer asked if the many interviews and questions disturbed her. Mrs. Harris admitted that she did not understand "why you need to know so much." After the matter was discussed in terms of the research project she seemed to understand the importance of knowing as much as possible about the parents and background of a baby "to understand how it is developing."

When she returned the questionnaire Mrs. Harris made reference to some of the questions. She mentioned that she regarded herself as "a friendly person but not the kind who goes out easily and makes friends." Apropos of this, she referred to the girl in the downstairs apartment and indicated a considerable feeling of rejection. The girl had visited her and had borrowed things, but she had never been invited to the girl's apartment nor did she feel free to return the visits. She had the feeling that the girl had withdrawn from contact with her and did not want to talk with her. This led to discussion about her feeling of insecurity with people because she was not sure she was "wanted."

The talk then focused on religion. With considerable feeling Mrs. Harris said that both she and her husband "have been thrown out by our churches" because of the divorces and remarriage. Mr. Harris was an Episcopalian, but it seemed "the Episcopal church is even more strict than the Catholic church in regard to remarriage." The baby could not be baptized in either of their churches, and while neither she nor her husband "had any religion now," she felt that all children should be baptized and she didn't know how this could be arranged.

It made her angry to think that if she had "a considerable amount of money," she might be able to get an "indulgence." She felt that this was very unfair. She described a visit to her priest before she had remarried. He had not talked very pleasantly and had said that the Church did not recognize her divorce and that if she married again she would be "cut off completely." Because of that talk she knew that "it would do no good to go back to him since he was so final about this decision."

When she and her husband planned marriage they both agreed that they wanted to be married by a minister and not by a Justice of the Peace. They had gone to a Congregational Church and spoken to the pastor, who "talked very nicely" to them for about two hours. He discussed the question of their marriage and asked how they both would feel about being cut off from their own churches. Also, he raised the question about what they would do in regard to children. Since she had been sure she could not have children, they had assumed it would be no problem to them.

The interviewer suggested that she talk to the Congregational minister and then decide on the baptism after the baby was born. But Mrs. Harris was very emphatic that she would not want to wait a month or two for the baptism and that it was something that must be done immediately. There was considerable hesitation in her manner as she said, "I don't think my husband would object to baptism, but I know he feels bitter toward his own church for taking such a definite stand about his remarriage."

An appointment towards the end of the eighth pregnancy month found Mrs. Harris again rather reluctant to talk. Her husband was sick at home, and she felt very bad about leaving him. She was unsure whether she could keep the appointment with the pediatrician and did not feel that there was anything special she needed to discuss. She had continued in the exercise class, which she liked very much and had found very helpful. In fact, she said, she would not have known about preparing her breasts for breast feeding except from what she learned in the exercise class because the obstetrician had not mentioned it.

She said that she knew "some girls have trouble breast feeding," but since it seemed to be a good idea for the baby, she hoped that she would be able to carry through with it. Mention was made of the new house, and Mrs. Harris said that it was now in the process of construction. She seemed most enthusiastic about the new home, mentioning that they would be able to choose their own paint colors, have flowers, and perhaps even a little garden. There was some mention of transportation difficulties from the new house to the hospital. When it was suggested that transportation could be arranged, Mrs. Harris seemed quite relieved and more enthusiastic about talking with the pediatrician.

In the ninth month of pregnancy Mrs. Harris had her pediatric interview. The pediatrician found her a pleasant, attractive young woman, somewhat ill at ease during most of the interview. The rooming-in form was filled out, much to Mrs. Harris's satisfaction. She asked whether there would be someone to show her how to take care of the baby and was reassured on that score. She estimated her date of confinement "in about three weeks" and said she planned to breast feed because "it is better for the baby."

At this point the pediatrician introduced the question of her old tuberculosis in relation to breast feeding. Mrs. Harris became visibly more agitated when it was explained that some specialists in chest disease automatically excluded breast feeding, while others thought it perfectly all right. The pediatrician asked if she had discussed this with her physician, and Mrs. Harris said that he had told her, "Just go ahead and forget you ever had tuberculosis."

She seemed uncertain about accepting the pediatrician's offer to check for her, and there was no doubt that she preferred it not to be done. In fact, it seemed that Mrs. Harris wanted to repress the entire question of her old infection. She complained that while the doctor had told her to forget it, he nevertheless had asked her to return for regular examinations. She saw this as a contradiction in advice and said, "I want to forget it, but they won't let me." The pediatrician felt that the old tuberculosis was of more concern than

Mrs. Harris admitted and that "it may be evident later in relation to the baby." In general, her impression was that Mrs. Harris looked forward to the baby with considerable pleasure.

In the next prenatal interview some clues were presented for the first time that Mr. Harris was not quite a pillar of perfection and that home life was not without its dissatisfactions. Mrs. Harris mentioned with some resentment that her husband complained about "Italian food, which he used to like very much when he came to my mother's home." He also had been scolding her for eating rich desserts, "not just because of the weight gain but because he thinks it caused the breaking out on my face."

Mrs. Harris asked about having a private pediatrician "when the baby is ill" and wondered if such a pediatrician "would want to know all that you know about the baby." She was assured that cooperative plans would be worked out with any private pediatrician and that the study would also want to be informed of what happened during a baby's illness. Mrs. Harris said that her husband objected to going to a pediatrician suggested by the study as "he knows a number of pediatricians with whom he had car dealings, and he thinks we should choose one of these men." She was told that she was free to choose whomever she would like and that the study group would be cooperative in every possible way.

Mrs. Harris reported that the house was coming along fast and might be finished in May. They had been advised by the contracting company to select kitchen linoleum and would later select their wallpaper. She was somewhat hesitant in saying, "I really preferred blue in the kitchen, but Herb wanted green, so we settled on green." She explained that she had wanted blue because she had made two pairs of red curtains, which would have gone with the blue, and she "wanted to be able to use them someplace."

The house was located about a half mile from the shore, and Mrs. Harris was delighted "to be so close to the water." There was, however, some concern about its distance from good shopping stores. She was presently situated close to a large market, where she could "pick up bargain specials," and she was afraid it would cost them a great deal more if she were unable to do that. She planned to shop once a week, when her husband would drive her in the car, but she very much preferred shopping alone "because Herb gets very impatient if he has to wait at all." Mr. Harris had suggested that she brush up on her driving and had offered to buy some kind of small car for her own use, but she said she had never cared very much about driving.

In response to a question as to whether they had settled on a baby's name, Mrs. Harris said with a smile, "If it is a boy, of course he would have to be Junior." Mr. Harris had heard the name Heather on television some time ago, and "this seemed to have stayed in his mind as the name he wants for a girl." Mrs. Harris had thought she would like to name the baby Luciana because she liked it and also because it was her mother's name. But Mr. Harris's attitude was that "he does not believe in catering to families." He felt they had their own lives to live and didn't always need to consider what their families wanted. Mrs. Harris said she didn't feel that way.

Again Mrs. Harris spoke of the baby's baptism and the fact that she had done nothing about it yet. She came out with the statement, "A Catholic baptism is what I really would prefer. . . . Any other baptism would not be the same. . . . But I know this is the one thing to which Herb would object, although he would not object to some other type of baptism." She felt unable to make any arrangements unless she first talked to him. "It's not that I'm afraid of him, he's really not the kind of person that anyone would be afraid of, but this matter of religion is a very sensitive point, and it would be upsetting if I should mention it." Again she repeated that he was "such a wonderful person" and that he gave her "all the things" that she had always felt she wanted in marriage.

In this connection, she evaluated her first husband "who really did not think of marriage in any serious terms." "Now I just forget about the fact that I was ever married before and only think about my present marriage." Then she stressed "how dependable Herb is" and seemed to be assuring herself that it was possible for her to talk with him about the baptism.

The interviewer pointed out that a prior Congregational baptism did not preclude a later Roman Catholic baptism. Mrs. Harris said, "That's what Herb implied, and he might be able to accept some non-Catholic baptism now with the idea that later on the child could choose its own religion."

Some time in her ninth month Mrs. Harris came for psychological testing. She said she felt "funny" about the test and wanted it explained a little more. She also wanted to know if the tester was a psychologist or a psychiatrist, because she had told her husband that she was going to be tested by a psychiatrist and he said she had probably gotten it all wrong, and that it would be a psychologist. She added that she was "always getting words mixed up."

The reference to her husband brought to mind an association with the baptism of the baby, and she said she finally had been able to talk to her husband about this. He had said that he knew of a Congregational Church in the area to which they planned to move, and they could wait until then to baptize the baby. While Mrs. Harris seemed acquiescent, she commented that she hoped it would not be delayed too long because in the Catholic Church babies are usually baptized by the time they are a month old. It seemed that she would be satisfied "as long as some kind of baptism was arranged."

The bitterness and hostility surrounding her rejection by the Church was revealed by Irene Harris in the comment that "in the Catholic Church every sermon is about money." She said "It costs so much every time you go to church. . . . I know that churches have to have money, but when I was a little girl the children were only expected to take a few pennies to church. Now anything less than a quarter isn't even considered. . . . It costs a family two or three dollars every time they go to church." The interviewer explained that there was only one collection during the service in the Congregational Church. Mrs. Harris broke in rather angrily to say she did not see why there had to be so many different churches and different ways of acting in church, "because if there is only one God, then things ought to be the same way in all churches."

At the next interview Mrs. Harris looked rather tired and was quite subdued as she talked. She had speculated that she might even be in the hospital this day, since her delivery date was just two days away. She told of recent pains and sensations which she thought indicated that her time was getting near.

She wanted to know if the interviewer had anything to say about the psychological tests which she had taken. They had taken much longer than she had expected, and she did not think it was because she had been especially slow on the testing. She felt she knew some of the things pretty well but "could not even begin to think about the mathematical problems." This had surprised her because she had always been "pretty good at math in school."

She commented that "everything else is about the same now" and that she was "just waiting for the birth of the baby to be over with." "It's not that I'm dreading it so much. . . . It's just that there seems to be nothing to do until that is through." She hoped her labor would not be too long, although she knew that the first baby sometimes took quite a while. In terms of help after delivery, she mentioned that she intended to have diaper service and that her mother would be able to come over during the day if she needed her. "In fact, my mother wanted me to come and stay with her for two weeks after the baby is born, but Herb won't hear of such a thing."

Then Mrs. Harris began to talk about her husband's relationship to both their families. He firmly believed that married couples should be independent of their parents, and for him independence implied the absence of contact. Mrs. Harris said, "My mother would be perfectly willing to come and stay at our house, but Herb keeps saying that 'we don't want a lot of strangers around.'" For her part, she would like to have her mother with her even when she is in the hospital during labor, but her husband objected to this. He said that she was married now and had a husband, so she need have nothing more to do with her family. She had never been close to her mother, but she did feel that at a time like this her mother would like to be a bit closer to her.

In the discussion Mrs. Harris wavered back and forth between the kind of relationship she would like to have with her parents and loyalty to her husband, whose "ideas were completely different." She spoke enviously of her brother's wife, who was "so close" to her parents "with much visiting back and forth." At this point she mentioned that Mr. Harris had never invited her parents to have a meal with them, nor had he invited his own parents to even visit their home. Just recently for the first time he had said that they "might plan to have her folks over for dinner sometime" but now it was too close to the baby's delivery.

Mrs. Harris talked to her mother by phone every day, and her husband's mother usually called her too. She said, "Herb likes my parents, but he just does not see family relationships the same way

I do." To the interviewer's question as to whether Mr. Harris's "different ideas" might have anything to do with his first marriage, Mrs. Harris immediately said, "Oh, I know it does."

She did not know too many details about that first marriage and said she didn't want to know. But she did say she knew they had lived with his first wife's parents for a time and she was quite sure that his present feelings about interference from families came from that. Then she assured the interviewer, "I'm not complaining about Herb because he really is a wonderful person."

At the next interview a week later Mrs. Harris said that she had so much hoped it would be all over by this time, although she had been feeling perfectly fine and only had a pressure discomfort. She knew that many women did not have their babies on the expected date. Her mother had been three weeks late with Mrs. Harris's brother, and a girl friend's baby had been two weeks late. She said, "It might be better if the obstetrician did not mention the earliest possible date because you do build up a climax waiting for that early date."

The scale showed that she had gained two pounds in the past week, and she "didn't see how that could have happened" because she had been "very careful." At any rate, she hoped not to gain any more, especially at this point. "The sitting around and waiting" was difficult for her, she said as she "can't plan on anything" and was afraid to go anywhere alone, since the "water might break" or she might suddenly begin having contractions. Actually, she had not "just been sitting around" but had been very active doing extra chores and getting her summer clothes in order. She said that Mr. Harris called her three or four times a day but she had "nothing to tell him."

A week later Mrs. Harris called a greeting, "Well, here I am again." She was more resigned to the fact that the birth was delayed but wished very much that it would be over. She referred constantly to the baby as "he," and the interviewer commented that evidently she had decided what sex it was going to be. She smiled and said she wished it would be a boy but that everyone had been telling her it was going to be a girl.

Mrs. Harris looked very well, and her complexion was more clear than it had been during most of her pregnancy. She said that her bag was all packed and that everything was prepared for the baby and herself when she returned home from the hospital. She hoped that the next time she saw the interviewer it "would be in the maternity ward."

Still another week passed, and Irene Harris shook her head, saying, "We've decided to give up expecting that the baby will arrive any time soon at all." They guessed "that the doctors miscalculated," and now she had decided "to just go along as though not expecting the baby at practically any moment." Her husband had also resigned himself and no longer called her several times a day.

She reported that the house might be ready for occupancy sooner than she had thought. This was not an unmixed blessing, for she "would have liked to have a little time to get used to the new baby before being in the midst of moving." Again Mrs. Harris referred to the possibility that her mother would come in each day to help after the baby was born and said this would be a better plan than going to her mother's home. There was still no arrangement for anyone to stay with her full-time when she returned from the hospital.

A few days after this interview Irene Harris gave birth to a baby girl. She was named Heather, the name Herb Harris had selected from a television program. The delivery was not highly traumatic. Labor lasted six and a quarter hours, during which Mrs. Harris was talkative and cooperative at the beginning but less so at the end. At first she refused an offer of Demerol, but three-quarters of an hour later she accepted it. She had heard the doctor discussing the cord, which was around the baby's neck, and worried whether the baby was all right. Also, she felt dissatisfied with her performance in labor. When seen by the pediatrician a few hours after delivery Mrs. Harris presented a picture far removed from maternal bliss.

The baby's condition at birth was not too good. She cried only when strongly stimulated, her color was poor, and oxygen was given periodically, whereupon the color improved. When the baby was put to the breast Mrs. Harris needed reassurance and help with the handling. The two observers of the newborn infant did not agree in guessing the baby's sex. One found her looks "boyish" and continued to call the infant "he" even after learning the correct sex. The other observer found her "definitely feminine." There was a measure of accuracy in both observations. The femininity was expressed in Heather's mobile cupid-bow mouth, while there was something boyish in the vigor of her movements, sturdiness of build, and the oval shape of her face surrounded by thin, dark hair. The observers were in definite agreement, however, about the maturity of the infant. Although they stressed her healthy looks and strong little legs, they were even more impressed by her advanced behavior, commenting, "She looks much, much older."

They were surprised that a newborn behaved as Heather did, with patterns that appeared outstandingly well coordinated, purposeful, almost intentional. This impression was substantiated on two scores. Her response to the surrounding world was better than usual in the newborn, and the intensity and diversification of those responses were on a higher level. Her organism seemed to be sensitized for "surprises." She responded to an interruption of stimulation just as well as to the sudden start of stimulation. And when stimulation went on for a certain time there was an accumulation of impact, calling forth an ever increased variety of response. This ranged from a frown and mouth movement to organized motor discharge of the whole body, accompanied by crying. The longer the stimulation lasted, the more massive was the response. These two features provided Heather's organism with a positive adaptation to the outside world.

In her tension discharge Heather was well organized and quite predictable. As a rule, the movements of newborns are difficult to describe because every part of them moves in an unrelated manner. But Heather's movements appeared coordinated and purposeful to the adult's eye. It seemed as if she pushed herself away from the crib's side when her foot touched it by a coordinated movement pattern of the trunk, legs, and arms, which displaced the weight so adequately that locomotion resulted.

A capacity to raise her head from a supporting surface was demonstrated as Heather freely changed her head positions. She showed skill in achieving hand-mouth contact with the appropriate hand. When her head was turned to the left she succeeded in putting her left hand into her mouth, and when the head was turned right hand-mouth contact was with the right hand. During her stay at the hospital Heather's hand-mouth contact became even more skillful. When she was in supine with her head turned to the right she found it possible to contact her mouth with the left hand and vice versa. Such hand-mouth coordination and contact showed greater freedom than in other newborns and an innate tendency to coordinate instinctual patterns.

Heather's crying sounds were vigorous, angry, and so characteristic that one recognized them from the corridor and tended to interpret them as "a cry of demand or of protest." Upon being picked up, held securely, and stroked, she quieted magically. Stroking without holding did not provide the same effect. It implied a basic social need for contact with the adult human, and possibly a certain demandingness which might present difficulties. Heather was greatly peaceful in sleep, and her sleep was very clearly defined. No stimulation could wake her, and the whole body and face appeared relaxed and satisfied, with frequent mouth movements. Thus, in sleep, Heather seemed to find a comforting refuge from life's difficulties.

In view of Heather's promising responses and adaptation it was surprising that the study group found it harder to make predictions for her development than with the other study children. There was the feeling that if Heather did not get the responses she needed she might withdraw into sleep, and that only if her social demands were satisfied would it be possible for her to make use of this better-than-usual adaptation at birth. The study group felt that Heather might not be an easy baby with which to contend.

After a month in their city apartment the Harrises moved to the new home, which was in a fairly unsettled suburban area. The five-room, freshly painted Cape Cod house was furnished with temporary secondhand furniture except for the bedroom suite, which the Harrises had bought when they married. In the baby's room the used crib and chest were brightly decorated with colored decals, and Mr. Harris had put up useful shelves. He had also been busy during the summer months fixing up the yard and getting a lawn started. But financial pressures made them plan to sell their English bicycles and the portable boat for money to use on other things.

In the new home Irene Harris's parents came to dinner for the first time, and her mother continued to visit two or three times a week because she was "just crazy about Heather." Mrs. Harris was radiant in her motherhood and enjoyed her daughter thoroughly, while Mr. Harris was the typical "new father." Neither of them could resist holding Heather and "wanting to give her every love and attention." In fact, Mrs. Harris neglected her housework to make contact with the baby, and Mr. Harris made enough noise in the morning to wake Heather so that he could play with her before going off.

One anxiety continued to prey on Irene Harris. The baby had still not been baptized. Her preference was still for a Roman Catholic baptism, but at least her husband had agreed to see the Congregational minister. However, he had "refused to be rushed into it." In the first month Mrs. Harris expressed some concern about Heather's slight spitting up after feeding, and at the end of three months the baby was still spitting up a mouthful or two of milk one or more times daily. Her husband had told her to "check this" with the pediatrician, who reassured Mrs. Harris that it was probably just a case of over-filling. The pediatrician noted on her record at this time that Mr. Harris seemed to stir up his wife about a number of things which otherwise would not worry her.

In the hospital the staff had found Mrs. Harris considerably variable in her nursing ability from one feeding to the next. Sometimes she was quite awkward and held the baby in uncomfortable positions for both of them. At other times she was skillful and adept. But at home all seemed to be going well and Heather was wholly breast-fed, to her parents' great satisfaction. There was little regularity in Heather's feeding during the first few weeks except for the 1, 5, and 8 A.M. nursings. She demanded the breast every two hours and sometimes oftener, but if held and talked to she was able to wait quietly as long as fifteen or twenty minutes before a feeding.

Mrs. Harris hoped Heather would soon give up night feeding, as she felt "lonely and exposed" in the new isolated house when she got up to nurse. During this period Heather slept soundly, cried when she awakened but quieted when picked up. At two months Heather still refused a bottle but would take a little water from a jigger. Mrs. Harris wondered if her increased need for food meant she was ready for solids. The pediatrician agreed that this might be preferable to suggesting a formula, since breast feeding obviously meant a great deal to the whole family.

Both mother and staff described Heather as an extremely happy, good-natured, and responsive child, to whom social stimulation meant a great deal. She reacted with smiles and vocalizing to the adult's voice, more to her mother's than to the examiner's. It was reported that she laughed aloud, pulled the sheet over her head, and also her shirt and dress. She seemed more interested in the human face than most children her age, and it was hard to distract her even with specific material from watching the adult's face. At six weeks, Mrs. Harris reported, Heather noticed the decals on her crib and reached out to them.

In the ninth week Mrs. Harris said that Heather was content to amuse herself a good part of the time and did not demand to be picked up so frequently. She seemed very interested in her own hands, cooed, chuckled, and talked to her toys. Her prone behavior was quite advanced, and she could raise and hold her head high for several minutes. She focused on and followed visual stimulation, reached out her arms at sight of an object, and smiled at her own mirror image. There was some discrimination between mother and stranger. By ten weeks of age Heather usually slept through the night from 8 P.M. to 6 A.M. and woke very happy and good-natured.

At the end of the third month Heather gave a strong impression of independence, with little of the vulnerability commonly associated with tiny infants. The pediatrician did not need to comfort or fuss over her, nor was the mother's help required. Similarly, the mother did not act as if her baby urgently needed her ministrations. While Mrs. Harris was obviously enchanted with her baby and immediately wiped her mouth when she spit up, she did not hover anxiously about her. She said in a warm, loving tone, "You stink," and concentrated on conversation around the spitting up.

This quality of independence in Heather seemed to stem from the amazing social response for an infant so young. She vocalized repeatedly to the adult's conversation even if not directly engaged, and she smiled spontaneously and frequently with or without direct social stimulation. She seemed to thrive in a social atmosphere and was strongly aware of the presence of human partners. While she had started to discriminate between her mother and strangers, her reaction to strangers was not of an anxious nature.

Her body mastery was excellent. She succeeded in actually turning over to the prone position, held her head up high with chest off the mattress, and seemed to be visually concentrating on the observation screen. The fact that Heather at less than four months could change and adjust her position to her own liking was impressive. It contributed to the adult's feeling that she could take care of herself and that one need not hover over her constantly. Heather was very advanced for her age, the evaluation concluded, and both her social and motor responses were more characteristic of a child of six to seven months than of a baby not quite four months old.

Around this time events in the Harris household began to take a turn for the worse. Mr. Harris left the firm where he had been working as a salesman because he feared that competition with the boss's son would block future advancement. He took a position with another agency that seemed to offer him a better future, but his pay was entirely on a commission basis, which was inadequate to support his family. During most of Heather's first year of life, her family was in serious financial difficulty. To compensate, Mr. Harris took on a factory job from 3 to 11 P.M. and worked as a salesman from 9 A.M. until 1 P.M. and all day Saturday. The factory job was to his liking because he did not have to talk with people. He became increasingly withdrawn and resistant to outside social contacts. Thus, Mrs. Harris found the usual immobility common to all new parents exaggerated by her husband's refusal to go out. Since she valued sociability highly, it became a new issue which divided husband and wife.

Mr. Harris's new schedule created other complications as well. Mrs. Harris was afraid to be alone in the evenings and frequently invited her mother and friends to visit. Her husband disapproved of so much contact, so she was forced to conceal it from him. Also, she found the neighborhood not at all friendly because Mr. Harris had antagonized some neighborhood teenagers who had trespassed on his lawn. They retaliated with pranks on the property. Finally, the new families moving into the neighborhood seemed quite undesirable. They did not emulate Mr. Harris's heroic efforts with his lawn, and they allowed their trash to blow across his neatly kept property. Within six months the Harrises were not on speaking terms with their neighbors. This was very upsetting to Mrs. Harris, who said she hated the place and wished to move. They were considering selling the house.

During this period a Visiting Nurse paid a call on Mrs. Harris and recommended a chest X-ray, which aroused Mrs. Harris's old anxiety about tuberculosis and its relation to breast feeding. She was apprehensive because she now felt she should tell her husband about her past medical record, which she had not mentioned before. It troubled her that she was not free to make her own decisions and had to contend with her husband's very different attitudes towards family and social life.

She attributed his attitude to the fact that her husband had "no bond with his family." He intensely disliked his father, a solitary, withdrawn carpenter, and he characterized his mother as "an unloving gadabout." His turbulent home life had been resolved by living with a favorite aunt during high-school days and then fending for himself at an early age. Like his wife, Mr. Harris felt that by comparison with others, particularly his brother, he had always been deprived. His reaction was to "go it alone." Since Mr. Harris was "so crazy about Heather," his wife couldn't understand why "he wanted no more children." Sometimes she felt that he said this just to hurt her.

At the home visit in Heather's fifth month Mrs. Harris seemed less upset. The X-ray proved that there was nothing to worry about, and Mr. Harris had not seemed at all concerned about her medical past. Heather had been thriving, and there were no illnesses.

Some stranger anxiety was seen at this age, with shyness and crying at the first approaches of a stranger, but after a while she would warm up into her charming smile. Some separation difficulty was noted in that she seemed to grow attached to a toy and cried if it was taken away.

As Heather approached the age of six months Mrs. Harris attempted to stop breast feeding during the day and nursed only at night or when she wanted Heather to nap. The spitting up of small amounts had continued, but this seemed to be of no great concern. By six months Heather was taking only one or two brief naps, and her mother felt that "Heather hardly gets any sleep during the day."

The next clinic evaluation brought comments from one observer that Heather was "very charming, very pretty, her body nicely formed, and lots of fun to watch." She sat steadily and unsupported, assumed a standing position, supported most of her weight in standing, turned from supine to prone, from prone to kneeling, from kneeling to sitting, and crawled. The evaluation placed Heather's body mastery on the level of a ten-month-old child.

There were some small signs of grasping inhibition, possibly related to newness of the situation. It was expressed by a hesitation to grasp the objects that were offered to her. However, when the examiner actually handed her the object it seemed to provide a permissive sanction. This led the evaluator to conclude, "Heather indicated a surprisingly high stage in the development of her object relationships." She also showed ingenuity in adapting to her environment. If she was not presented with an object, she managed to find something to serve as an object of interest. These included a piece of yellow paper, the door knob, a safety pin, and a curtain. The report said, "Her approach toward the world was not only highly receptive but also highly productive. . . . The reality principle is surprisingly effective in Heather's world, considering that she is only six months and fourteen days."

Heather's ability to imitate the activity of an adult was less impressive. She performed a movement which was similar to that demonstrated, but at no point did she really imitate an activity performed with objects. Also, her reactions were fairly bland and suggested a scarcity of emotional expression. Although she vocalized in a general way, the vocalization was not specific to any highlights of success or failure, excitement, pleasure or frustration. When she fussed she was easily comforted; when she caught her hand in the cup she did not show signs of deep disturbance. It appeared to the staff that Heather did not need to rely on great emotional expression because the relationship with her mother counteracted the negative impacts of the world and provided her with a positive reliable source of gratification and security on a permanent basis.

Heather's movements were quite purposeful, and she used the appropriate parts of the body for them. There was an almost equal and dexterous use of both hands. The right hand was used for intentional grasping and manipulation of objects, while the left hand was predominantly used for mouthing, storing of objects, or unsuccessful attempts at grasping.

Heather's mouthing of objects was quite minimal, and there was no mouthing of any part of her own body. Most of her mouthing was with objects that did not seem to have the function for sucking but rather for oral touching and retaining. That autoerotic elements were nonexistent in Heather might be attributed to the fact that there existed a good balance between gratification from the outside world and self-satisfaction in her own movements in contacting and enjoying the world. In summary, the evaluation showed that Heather was a child with a high frustration threshold and high functioning level resulting from a well integrated and interiorized picture of the mother.

Heather's exposure to her first Christmas tree at eight months elicited some immediate fear and avoidance. Then she became intrigued with its sparkle and loved to crawl around it. At Mrs. Harris's insistence the Harrises spent both Christmas and New Year's Day at her mother's. Heather was finally baptized sometime around Christmas. Because of his wife's constant urging, Mr. Harris finally told her to contact the minister herself. Both parents attended an instruction session and were satisfied with it. Mrs. Harris reported that at the baptism "Heather was without doubt the best of the seven babies present." Some of the babies cried, but Heather "held a little conversation with the minister and seemed to enjoy every minute of it."

At a home visit when Heather was just nine months old the interviewer met Mrs. Harris's mother, whom she described as "obese and with very rapid Italian-accented speech." The grandmother tried to show off Heather and definitely competed with Mrs. Harris for possession of her. She pressed on the interviewer many details of her aches and pains and blood pressure and opinions on raising children. She described how difficult it was to visit her daughter and grandchild, and how much this meant to her. Mrs. Harris tried valiantly to shush her mother but to no avail.

Mr. Harris had been toying with the idea of leaving his sales work and working full-time at the factory. However, his wife opposed this because full-time factory work would keep him away from home longer hours. She said she was willing to forego the possibility of greater income rather than to be alone more. The interviewer felt that some status for Mrs. Harris was possibly involved in the selling position.

Heather continued to bring great pride to her parents. Her mother claimed that she did not want a great deal of attention, but "babies need attention and love, and it hasn't spoiled her." Mrs. Harris pointedly contrasted Heather's accomplishments with those of her sister-in-law's boy, who was older but much slower. She added that she had "had to quit talking of Heather's progress, since people won't believe all the things that Heather can do." Mrs. Harris did not seem driven to push her daughter toward further achievements.

Physically Heather presented no problems. She had a cold around eight months, which bothered her little. She had no apparent discomfort from the two teeth that erupted. A recurrent rash on her buttocks and genital area cleared within twenty-four hours after use of a boric acid ointment.

Mrs. Harris reported on Heather's eagerness and enthusiasm for food, saying, "She's just a little pig." She ate three meals a day, snacked on cookies and milk in between, and had gradually taken to whole milk from the cup. Up to about seven months she demanded the breast at night, sometimes waking two or three times. But often she did very little sucking at these night feedings, and Mrs. Harris felt that it was more for comfort than anything else. The pediatrician had the impression that Mrs. Harris was ready to stop breast feeding if Heather started to bite, which she did not do.

By seven months Heather solved the problem herself, suddenly and undramatically. On a day which had been busy with many guests she took no nap, and when put to bed that night she showed no desire for breast feeding and hadn't shown any interest since. She was reported to have only occasional night awakenings. Daytime naps were abandoned except for one fifteen-to-thirty minute nap late in the day, only if she was exhausted. However, if she was placed outside in her carriage she did take a longer nap.

With strangers Heather had an initial aloofness, then warmed up to responsive and friendly behavior. Mrs. Harris was concerned that fear of strangers would affect her. She described Heather as "happy all the time," said she cared little for toys but loved to explore "all sorts of things around the house." She vocalized a great deal, had whole phrases of sounds in tone, and had started to develop a jargon. At close to nine months she was observed to walk with evident enjoyment of the balancing and motion.

At 9 months and 13 days Heather's gross motor development was at the 15-month level, her fine motor development at the 13-month level, her adaptive performance at the 13½-month level, and her language and personal-social skills at the 12-month level. On the Viennese test her developmental age was 1 year, 1 month, and 27 days, with a developmental quotient of 147. The quality of her performance was excellent.

Stranger anxiety remained evident. She did not move in the direction of a toy offered by the stranger but would take it from a "neutral" position, such as a table top or floor so long as it did not increase the distance from her mother. She could overcome her reluctance to accept a toy from the examiner if she was in bodily contact with her mother. The mere touching of her mother's knee gave her more security, and her movements became sure and swift.

Heather's babbling was quite diversified and expressive. She used a number of consonants and was reported to say "dada." Her skill in "sizing up the situation immediately" and reacting accordingly was demonstrably well above her age level. This was also true for her motor development. She could walk without support and bend down while standing to pick up things that had fallen. In none of this exceptional performance did she give the impression of exaggerated effort.

The study group speculated whether this acceleration of development was a predictable outcome for a baby who had shown a high level of functioning at birth and whether this optimum functioning level reduced the mother's anxiety, thereby creating favorable conditions for a good mother-child relationship.

In one developmental matter Heather's progress was rather less than satisfactory. She had several periods when her night sleep was interrupted by wakening for cuddling and play. At its most acute phase she would wake up as many as six times a night and require one and one-half hours rocking to get back to sleep. She never slept beyond 6:30 A.M. The ups and downs of this sleep problem never caused negative feelings towards her on the part of her parents despite their reported loss of sleep. After a few feeble attempts to let her "cry it out" Mrs. Harris's attitude became one of resignation. Once, when Heather's sleeping was least satisfactory, her mother called her "pesty." In handling the situation her parents capitulated to her demands for attention.

During the ninth and tenth months Mrs. Harris was completely worn out by the sleeping problem. Heather hardly slept at all during the day and at night slept only until 4 or 5 A.M. Then she awoke in the best of spirits, ready to play. Mrs. Harris used all her ingenuity to get her back to sleep but to no avail. Mr. Harris blamed the sleeping problem and Heather's recurrent buttock rash on his wife's weekly visit to her mother. He claimed that something Heather ate at her grandmother's was the cause of the rash and the sleeping upsets.

But these visits and sewing lessons were just about all the social contacts which Mrs. Harris had. Relationships with their neighbors remained tense, with continuing harassments by the teenage boys. Both parents hoped that Heather would not learn to behave in the manner of the local children. Mr. Harris had done a great deal of work to inprove his grounds and had also erected a wire fence to protect their property from the drifting trash of the less well kept yards. The selling job had shown some improvement, and Mr. Harris thought they could manage on that income alone. So he planned to leave the factory job as soon as his replacement was trained.

During this period Mrs. Harris expressed her boredom and blamed her husband for a number of small things. Although he smoked, he objected to her doing so. She had to "sneak in" cigarettes. He thought it "dreadful" for her to complain about being home all the time and implied that she was bored with Heather. Mrs. Harris said she wanted more children, but her husband still refused. "As a surprise" he had bought her a new stove, but Mrs. Harris said it would have been nice if she could have picked it out herself.

There was also an increasing antagonism between herself and her brother's wife, Lucy. Mrs. Harris said that her sister-in-law "made life hell" for her brother. She described Lucy as a willful woman who dominated her husband and who was "moody, sweet, and generous one day, selfish and belligerent the next." It was especially provoking to Mrs. Harris that her sister-in-law insisted Heather was being "spoiled." With some triumph Mrs. Harris said that Lucy's son, who was older than Heather, "looked retarded when compared to her." For more than six months during the study Mrs. Harris and Lucy were not on speaking terms. As for Herb Harris, he had nothing to do with Lucy at all, as might be expected.

At a home visit when Mr. Harris was available he talked a great deal of himself and his feelings, with frequent reference to his short and stocky build. As he described putting up the fence alone, he emphasized that he was "the type of person who works and plays better by himself rather than in a team." He spoke at length about his brother "who always got the best of everything," to Mr. Harris's disadvantage.

While in the army Mr. Harris had worked for four years with the testing and placement division and had become quite familiar with psychological tests. He was interested in the kinds of tests Heather had been given. The interviewer reported "an expression of intense hostility and feeling of deprivation in relation to his brother, his boyhood, and his later years. . . . There was no reference to his previous marriage, to other financial responsibilities, or to the fact that he had fathered two babies prior to Heather."

On Heather's first birthday she received two small burns on each of her wrists from placing them on top of the radiator. Although they were red and blistered, no infection developed. Her appetite was excellent, and she enjoyed a wide variety of foods. Her milk intake had decreased somewhat, but she nevertheless consumed about fifteen to twenty ounces a day. Her evening meal consisted almost entirely of regular table foods, which she enjoyed very much.

There had been no consistent effort to train Heather, and she gave no signs of noticing wet or soiled diapers. Mrs. Harris said she knew when to change diapers only by the length of time from the last changing. She reported that many times she had placed Heather on the toilet with no results and then Heather ran nude from bathroom to bedroom, leaving a trail of urine and feces. Though she did not consider it toilet training, Mrs. Harris had been placing Heather on the toilet intermittently for some four or six weeks. Heather had a potty chair but didn't use it except to stand in the pot, and her mother felt that she didn't yet understand what it was for.

By her first birthday Heather was reported to be quite friendly with people but had developed a fear of dogs ever since one had approached her abruptly. She delighted in producing noises and squeals, along with a soft continuous jargon. She loved being cleaned up; laughed, crowed, and vocalized as her mother wiped her dry. Her interest in toys was not great, but she played with anything at hand and was constantly moving. At one year she was reported to remember things from previous visits, such as the piano in the home of one relative or a candy jar in her grandmother's home.

At 1 year and 7 days Heather scored a general maturity level of 14 months and 3 weeks, with a developmental quotient of 121. On the Viennese test she rated a developmental age of 1 year, 6 months, and 18 days, with a developmental quotient of 152. The clinic evaluation showed that Heather did not have any special difficulty in adapting to the test situation but though her performance was high, it was nevertheless rather scattered, or below her level. There seemed to be two reasons for this behavior. First, after Heather had learned and mastered a performance she lost interest in it. Secondly, she functioned according to her own rhythms, i.e., solving a problem at the time this problem appealed to her, regardless of outside stimulation.

The least advanced level of Heather's behavior was the imitative one. She made no effort to duplicate the adult's activity, although she used her social charm to get the adult to reproduce activities which were pleasurable to her. Heather was especially astute in observation and memory. She remembered the rubber cat with the protruding tongue. When the tongue was missing, she looked for it long after the usual time, giving the impression that she would remember that cat and its tongue indefinitely. This independence of memory despite intervening diversions was a developmental step which hardly ever happens before the third year. It may have been a prime factor in her advanced behavior.

Spatial concepts were also highly developed, and Heather was aware of direction without having to control it with her eyes. She also had a correct anticipation of the spatial order pertaining to the structure of the outside world and her own body. She was well able to relate the two spatial systems.

Heather's continuous soft sounds and jargon remarkably resembled Mrs. Harris's continuous, soft, and monotonous talk in the observation booth. One had the impression that one should understand what Heather was saying. But despite the elaborate jargon, which resembled the adult's language in melody and intonation, she actually had only three real words. The study members found it interesting that this extremely advanced child, who seemed to have the smoothest relationship with her mother, had an elaborate jargon but so few words.

The Harrises' home situation continued to deteriorate. They needed money so badly that Mr. Harris had given up the auto sales job and was working full-time at the factory, sometimes even on Saturday and Sunday. His 4 P.M. to 1 A.M. shift left his wife alone in her most anxious hours, and she found it impossible to go to sleep until he returned. Furthermore, the entire neighborhood was being troubled with the teenagers' depredations, and the police had brought court action against the boys. They were also investigating reports of a prowler, which completely terrified Mrs. Harris.

During the following months the situation became even more drastic. They planned to sell their home and move into an extra room in the maternal grandmother's four-room apartment. Mr. Harris gave up his factory job and commuted to a town forty miles distant for training in automotive repair, a prerequisite for becoming a district salesman for an automotive firm. The job would require traveling over a large portion of the state. Although he was currently on a salary, the financial situation would continue to be pressing until he could earn commissions. Mrs. Harris was quite concerned with how her husband would respond to living with relatives. Further, she anticipated difficulties with her brother's family, who also lived in the same house. There was already rivalry between his son and Heather.

Mrs. Harris seized an opportunity to speak to the pediatrician, saying, "You are a doctor, and I know your line is children, but I want to get your opinion." She had been having some mild abdominal cramps and some vaginal discharge and hoped it was a sign of pregnancy. She wanted another baby so that Heather would have a playmate and also for other reasons which she couldn't explain, saying only, "I should have had Heather when I was 21." Her husband was opposed to having another child, and she didn't think she could persuade him.

At the next home visit Mrs. Harris casually mentioned to the interviewer that she was quite sure she was pregnant. She had had some slight nausea, a feeling of not wanting certain foods, and some breast changes. But any delight in this possibility was mitigated by the proposed change of plans, living conditions, and money problems.

It was learned that they had received considerable financial help from Mrs. Harris's mother as well as most of Heather's clothing and toys. Mrs. Harris expressed intense hostility towards her husband over this. She said she realized his work made many demands on him and that she "tried to be understanding and sweet," but recently she had reached her limit and told him she was "tired of being sweet, that he should think of her and Heather occasionally."

The only thing that tempered this difficult period was the Harrises' open pride in their daughter and her accomplishments. "We think she's wonderful," they said.

At 13 months and 11 days Heather earned a general maturity level of 15 months, 1 week and a developmental quotient of 112.5 on the Gesell test. On the Viennese her developmental age was 1 year, 6 months, 27 days, with a developmental quotient of 141.39.

Heather fed herself foods that she could pick up with her fingers, and she was interested in using a fork. When told it was time to eat she pulled her high chair to the table and got her bib. The only real problem was her irregular and sporadic sleeping pattern. She awakened from two to six times a night, not going back to sleep unless her mother lay down with her. Her father was no longer a satisfactory substitute, and only close physical contact with her mother seemed to facilitate sleep. A temporary mild sedation was suggested which might help Heather to sleep through the night, but Mrs. Harris exclaimed, "It's not right to give a little baby drugs." The pediatrician noted, "I can see no solution but a gradual withholding of maternal handling."

Heather still gave no sign that she had soiled herself or was about to, and her mother felt that since her bowel movements were so frequent (about two to four a day) there was no point in trying to anticipate them. Hence, she put Heather on the toilet only irregularly. Heather did not use her own potty chair, although she seemed to know now what it was for. When her mother went to the bathroom Heather would stand beside her, tear off paper and hand it to her. She even would try to wipe her mother.

In the fourteenth month at the well-baby clinic it was noticed that Heather bit her fingers and mouthed or chewed test objects. She was also observed to rub her feet together repeatedly in an excited fashion when playing with the clay. During this period there was a return of stranger (or separation) anxiety. Her reaction was to be initially frightened of strangers and withdraw behind her mother's skirts with sober observation of the intruder. She seemed to need a great deal of physical contact with her mother and returned often to her. In addition to dogs there were a number of objects that frightened her, such as the mop, carpet sweeper, broom, kitchen spray and shower, trucks, and the ironing board.

The list of things that she enjoyed, however, was far longer. She had tremendous delight in copying her mother's every job and imitated mixing something with her own spoon and pan. When Mrs. Harris did some washing in the sink Heather brought a chair over and was practically in the washing herself. She plied her mother with all sorts of articles when Mrs. Harris tried to take a bath. She loved the out-of-doors, played in the sand and in the flower beds (much to her father's despair). She put grass and small stones in her mouth but spit them out when prohibited and then ran away laughing at her mother. Most of her activities were accompanied by a constant jargon with considerable inflection, gestures, and smiles. She had started to use many more words and some combinations, such as "all gone," "see kitty," "got it," etc.

At the evaluation in the middle of her sixteenth month it was observed that Heather had changed the least of all the study children. She still impressed observers by her vivacity, the astute glances of her slightly slanted eyes, and the mobility of her soft and strong mouth. She was still attractive though not pretty. While she hesitated in her approach to strangers, she nevertheless communicated better with the stranger than any other child. She smiled radiantly at the examiner and even her withdrawal had a coquettish tinge to it. All adults felt the charm of Heather's coy invitation toward friendliness.

Much of the routine testing was eliminated because everyone agreed that Heather would easily solve the problems, as she always had. On the other hand, the examiner introduced certain new variations of the test situation to demonstrate Heather's personal way of functioning. In many instances Heather quickly guessed what was expected of her in a special situation, and she guessed correctly. The six observers behind the screen followed her behavior with much enthusiasm and relaxed laughter, highly gratified when "she won." In contrast to other of the study children, Heather's actions gave understandable clues to what was going on in her.

Heather left no doubt which test items she would tackle and which she would not. Her interest seemed uniquely determined by the specific nature of the task. If she was interested, she applied herself at once with great competence and glee. Her competence did not depend on how she felt physically, for she had a severe cold and her nose dripped at times. Neither did fatigue seem to interfere with her performance during the unusually long examination.

If Heather were not interested, she returned the material to the examiner firmly, purposefully, and with neutrality, as matter-of-factly as it had been handed to her. Once the material was rejected Heather refused to accept it when offered a second time. Occasionally she deigned to solve a problem in which she was not really interested, like putting the round piece in the round hole of the formboard. However, she gave the impression of a token performance only as evidence of social compliance and "to humor the examiner." She seemed already to know the "bribe value" of obedience and positive performance.

Heather not only completed the task of filling the cup with the cubes but she spotted another cube of different color among the test materials and tried to put that into the cup also. She made three different attempts to decide between her tendency to "complete the task" and to "have only completely alike objects in the cup." Once she put the "alien cube" into the cup and hid it with the others. Once she tried to add it as the very last piece. Then she put it aside and later asked the examiner to add it to the other cubes. This elaboration was over and beyond the requirement of the test and revealed Heather's high level of functioning as well as her intellectual independence from adult guidance. The evaluation report said that Heather had "started on her own conceptual discovery of the world around her. This developmental step is usually found in children in their third year."

The Harrises lived for one week with the maternal grandmother but returned to their own home because they saw no prospect of selling their house immediately. The experiment was not highly successful. The maternal grandmother was not well and required rest and quiet, but she became even more active while Heather was around. There was not enough room in the apartment, and relatives interfered with Heather's care. Heather would not sleep at all except with her mother. Mrs. Harris felt that this was so because she did not have her own crib. Things improved somewhat when they returned home.

Mr. Harris was pleased with his job and worked hard all day. In the evenings he worked in the basement office he had set up at home, doing his bookkeeping and scheduling appointments. Apparently the job had its ups and downs. Often he came home either elated or depressed, but always too tired to take his wife or Heather out anywhere. Financially they were still dependent on Mrs. Harris's mother for assistance.

From Heather's sixteenth to twenty-first month the majority of Mrs. Harris's conversations with study members focused on her marital difficulties. In the first months of this period she was mild in direct criticism of her husband, but when he was present at one of these interviews she attacked him with sarcastic and hostile remarks, discouraging his attempts to be enthusiastic about his work.

When Heather was eighteen months old the lid blew off. Three little incidents precipitated a major crisis: Mr. Harris's impatience with Heather's fussy response to a cold, his anger when her play interrupted his morning sleep, and a fight over a Sunday ride during which Mrs. Harris frightened Heather. For days Mr. and Mrs. Harris spoke to each other only when it was absolutely necessary; their sexual relationship was interrupted, and thoughts of divorce were aired.

By the end of Heather's nineteenth month the conflict was even more exacerbated. Mrs. Harris complained bitterly about her husband, his lack of consideration and social decencies, and his selfishness. They had spent at least two weeks not speaking to each other, merely being polite. Their sexual relations had ceased, and Mrs. Harris had threatened to leave him.

Just as Heather had inadvertently touched off this crisis so also the child's importance to her parents brought peace to their household. The prospect of losing Heather made the thought of divorce intolerable for both, and thoughts of her welfare helped them seek a rapprochement. It was Mr. Harris who made the first advances.

After they had talked things over at length, followed by efforts on the part of each to please the other, Mr. Harris began to pay more attention to Heather's care. This only made Mrs. Harris suspicious that he was trying to win her affection. Although Mrs. Harris did not believe there had been a fundamental change in her husband, a modicum of harmony was achieved. Mr. Harris helped his wife with Heather's care and some of the household chores, and he was more considerate toward her family.

To further threaten this tenuously balanced situation, Mrs. Harris's pregnancy had been confirmed. She looked quite unwell, with large dark circles under her eyes, and her skin appeared sallow and muddy. This pregnancy was considerably more difficult than the first, with vomiting and more of a weight problem. Because of Heather she could not get the increased sleep she craved. Backache and feelings of "heaviness" were constant. In her fifth month of pregnancy she said that the pregnancy was "just beginning to be a reality" to her and she "couldn't imagine loving another baby" as much as she did Heather. Thus, her strongest feeling about the pregnancy was to wish it would be over. Both parents continued to be extremely pleased with their daughter and were trying to prepare her for the new baby.

Heather had diarrhea in her eighteenth month, accompanied by nasal discharge and a decrease in appetite. With paregoric and dietary changes she recovered within three days. A week later Mrs. Harris reported that Heather had a slight cough and a temperature of 100.2. The pediatrician found a slight redness of the throat and recommended appropriate treatment. The mild diaper rash on her buttocks also continued. Heather's appetite during this period was reported as irregular. On some days she ate well and at others refused a meal or ate only small amounts. Breakfast was usually her best meal.

She began to hold a spoon in her left hand and soon was feeding herself with the spoon at lunch and supper. She handled a large glass well and drank twenty-to-thirty ounces of milk per day. Wine was among her favorite beverages, and she had as much as half a glass at a time.

During this period there was less sleeping difficulty. Heather was put down at 6:30 P.M. and required no attention other than insistence on her yellow blanket and occasionally a small paper book. She was still an early riser, waking at 4:30 and 5:00 A.M., which was hard on her parents. At mid-day she napped for one or two hours.

From the time she had burned herself on the hot air register Heather had developed a fear of the toilet, which was situated near the bathroom air vent. By eighteen-and-one-half months the fear seemed to have disappeared, but she still did not use the toilet when placed on it. Mrs. Harris was now more concerned that Heather should have bowel and bladder control before the new baby arrived, as "two sets of diapers would be too much to wash."

So she had been putting Heather on the toilet seat more frequently. Heather used it for urination but not for stool. Occasionally her mother called her a "bad girl" when she soiled her diaper.

It was reported that she had begun to bite and chew a great number of things. At the clinic it was also observed that she mouthed her hand when she heard a baby crying, but little, if any, thumbsucking was evident. At two clinic visits Heather placed her hand to her genital several times. Her mother pulled her hand away on one occasion, and reported that Heather "did this often."

During this period Heather was characterized as being much more friendly and responsive to strangers, both by report and observation. She did not become upset when her mother left the room, and she initiated many contacts with the visitor. She was described by the pediatrician as having an "infinite amount of charm and grace."

Heather's fears were more in control at this time. She had lost her fear of the ironing board, and dogs frightened her only when close. Her father wanted to get her a puppy so that she would become more accustomed to animals, but Mrs. Harris's own fear of dogs prohibited it.

Although Heather enjoyed playing with her cousin George, when she heard him approaching she clung to her toys and clothing, yelling, "Mine, mine, mine." This behavior continued frequently for the next two months even when the little boy was absent. She also invented a game of hide and seek with herself, standing in the corner and calling, "Heather, Heather."

At the clinic evaluation in the twenty-first month there were some rather marked changes in Heather. Unlike her former coyly smiling hesitancy with the stranger, her glance was now concentrated, unsmiling, and scrutinizing. It held no obvious anxiety but gave the impression of a penetrating examination. Then an expression of displeasure passed over her face, and she went to her mother to be picked up. It took quite a while before she could be induced to sit on the little chair at the examining table, and it was some time before she became her old smiling self.

Heather's interest in the book was half-hearted and there was even less interest in the cubes. She put one on top of the other sloppily so that they had to tumble. Finally she brushed them from the table with a delicate but determined gesture. She hardly paid any attention to the formboard and did not concentrate on its solution. In all of her performances it seemed that she simply obliged the examiner in turning toward the material but made no real attempt at problem-solving. On the Gesell test she scored a general maturity level of 23 months and a developmental quotient of 108.5.

She became preoccupied with trying to find what was hidden in the chest of drawers and kept saying, "More, more." It looked as if she was dissatisfied with what she had and hoped to find pleasure from something new. But the new thing seemed to become as uninteresting to her as the old one. The drive to ferret out the "hidden" things inside the chest of drawers might possibly have had some association with her mother's pregnancy, an effort to find out what was "inside."

Mrs. Harris looked very pregnant, and Heather's capacity for keen observation would make it likely that she was well aware of the change. Once she approached her mother and patted her stomach asking, "Where is the baby?" She also gave indirect evidence of knowing about the coming baby in the way she played with the doll. Unlike earlier records of elaborate make-believe doll feeding, this time she hardly fed the doll at all. Instead she insisted that the nipple be taken off the bottle and pretended to drink from it herself. She presented the milk bottle to the doll's mouth only on her mother's request and then moved the doll toward the bottle rather than the bottle toward the doll. She bit the nipple repeatedly, although her mother told her not to.

There was a form of incipient joking in her behavior, giving the impression that it was used as a defensive measure against a threatening problem. For example, in throwing the ball to the adult she aimed carefully but then threw it in a different direction so that the adult could not possibly catch it. She laughed loudly when the ball was missed. When asked to name the four pictures on the Gesell test card she named three and gave the card back. When the card was returned with a renewed request to point to the fourth picture she deliberately pointed to the empty back of the card and giggled.

Another indication of fears was her refusal of the furry toy monkey and elephant with the explicit words, "Afraid — take it away." The observers were struck by the ability of a child under two years of age to verbalize inner reactions. It seemed that Heather's preoccupation with the "inside" had created a need and a capacity for introspection and that verbalization was a way of reducing this fear.

Although she moved less than at former observations, Heather still retained her graceful, smooth, swift, skillful, and rhythmical movements. Nevertheless, she was not as fearless as she had once been in her motor performances. When the doll was put in the crib she first tried to climb up to it but soon gave up. She pushed the chair nearer the crib, attempted to stand on it, but hesitated and indicated that she needed the mother's help. Four months ago she had carried out such a project without any need of help. This demonstrated that Heather had learned caution and the realization that some of her achievements were potentially dangerous. It may also have been related to the psychological separation from her mother which had been taking place. As gratifications became independent of her mother, Heather became more aware of inherent dangers.

The impressions of this observation were that something had happened in Heather's happy life, either the discovery of her mother's pregnancy or her mother's preoccupation with the pregnancy. It served to reduce Heather's fearlessness and increased her tendency to select activities. It cancelled her investment in "uninteresting occupations" and led to a low test score in the elements of adaptive behavior.

On the other hand, it seemed to have increased her faculty to observe and to puzzle about the fellow human being. She was able to tease consciously and had the capacity to recognize and name the inner state of anxiety such as fear of the animals. It seemed that the increased conflicts she was experiencing had made Heather's individuality more marked and that these difficulties of life had changed her from just a toddler to a little girl.

Between Heather's twenty-first and twenty-fourth months her parents shifted their living arrangements a great deal. While Mr. Harris was away on a four-day business trip Heather and her mother stayed with the maternal grandparents. When they returned home a buyer was found for their house, and plans to move became more definite. Unable to stabilize their financial situation enough to buy a suitable duplex, the Harrises decided to move in for a year with the maternal grandparents. They shared the second-floor apartment of the two-family house, while the ground-floor rooms were occupied by the family of Mrs. Harris's brother.

The upstairs apartment had a small living room, large kitchen, and a very small room which was allotted to Heather and the future baby. The dining room was converted to a bedroom for the Harrises, but Mr. Harris usually slept in the partly furnished attic room when he was at home. The main bedroom was used by the garrulous grandmother and her silent, henpecked husband, who scarcely seemed to count. It appeared to the interviewer and to the pediatrician that it was a very crowded, inadequate, and uncomfortable arrangement for four adults and two children.

Mrs. Harris foresaw difficulties in the arrangement, especially with her sister-in-law, but she thought they could manage. She expected no difficulty with her mother, whom she described as "a wonderful person." Mr. Harris spoke of the move with undisguised regret at giving up the house and yard over which he had worked so hard. The interviewer felt that for him to sell the property was a difficult concession to his wife.

In the latter stage of her pregnancy Mrs. Harris continued to feel miserable and fatigued, regretful but not really concerned about her large weight gain. Both sides of the family wanted a boy, and characteristically the Harrises could not agree on a girl's name.

Twice Mrs. Harris was admitted to the hospital with false labor and then sent home. Finally after some vigorous housework Mrs. Harris was indeed in labor. She made three different trips to the delivery room before she at last delivered an eight and one-half pound boy. The pediatrician remarked, "She went through labor and delivery with as little evidence of discomfort and pain as I have ever seen." The baby Jimmy was described as "a quite self-contained and poised" infant.

Heather seemed to understand that her mother went to the hospital to "buy a baby." While at the maternal grandmother's, she said the words "hospital," "brother," and "baby" but would not repeat "Jimmy." She kept her yellow blanket with her almost constantly and occasionally cried for her mother, especially when her daddy came home. But apparently she knew that her mother would return, talked about it, and "helped" her father put up the infant's crib.

On the day of discharge from the hospital Mrs. Harris became annoyed with her family about a number of minor things. For one, Mr. Harris had brought her clothes in wrinkled condition, whereupon she complained, "Nobody thinks about me; my mother didn't even iron my slip." For another, she was obviously concerned about meeting Heather, whom she had failed to call on the phone during the hospital stay. Both parents were apprehensive about the homecoming, but the pediatrician had the feeling that they were unable to share their feelings.

Just two weeks short of her second birthday Heather met her new brother Jimmy. In those cramped conditions the first night home was "terrible." Heather ignored her mother but seemed to like the baby. However, when Mrs. Harris first nursed Jimmy, Heather began to cry, pushed at Jimmy, and said, "No baby, no baby." Heather cried, Jimmy cried, and Mrs. Harris cried. In the days that followed, Mrs. Harris was extremely disappointed in her lack of milk and felt that Heather was "acting impossible."

If her grandmother tried to care for her, Heather insisted on her mother and vice versa. When put to bed she cried, kicked, and bit, whereupon her mother spanked her. After ten days she started some tentative approaches to her brother, touched his eyes with her fingers, sometimes patted him. Mrs. Harris said this was "more of a hit" than a pat and described Heather as "being fresh."

Convalescence and the adjustment to infant routines were complicated by the constant hum of human activity in crowded rooms. Mr. Harris was manifestly uncomfortable and unhappy, and his wife even more so. Heather showed the strain in willfulness and excessive tears. Under the circumstances, it was not surprising that Mr. and Mrs. Harris quarreled.

Mr. Harris took Heather back to their house for a few days before the house had to be vacated. Efforts were renewed to find another house. But the only prospect within reason did not appear too hopeful. Two weeks later the Harrises had another fight and several days of not speaking. Mr. Harris had objected to his wife's impatience and anger in disciplining Heather, which set off innumerable complaints she had of him, especially blame for the predicament of their present living situation.

At the final well-baby clinic evaluation the examiner and observers were nostalgic about the Heather that they remembered from former periods. In looking over earlier snapshots of her, they admitted that she was not so pretty now as before and that the overwhelming charm which greeted and embraced the whole world in these pictures was now not so evident. Their remarks wistfully concluded that, "Heather is still very charming."

In her play Heather did not ignore the adults but verbally enlisted their help and attention to what she was doing. Her language was well developed, and she used whole sentences. Her vocabulary was rich, including many words which were surprising from a two-year-old. Because she spoke so softly the staff had difficulties in hearing her. Yet Mrs. Harris heard and understood every word. With her constant flow of soft chatter it seemed that Heather kept in contact with her mother and included her in the intimate world of her experiencing.

There were several surprises at this clinic visit. First, Heather imitated the examiner precisely in wiping the test table, crumpling the wet towel, and putting it on the radiator. This contrasted with her former lack of imitation. Secondly, she spontaneously and carefully built with blocks, something she had formerly resisted. But most astonishing was her sudden failure to solve problems. In earlier periods she had tackled and succeeded in tasks which seemed unsolvable at her age level. But at this evaluation she found it difficult even to put the lid on the saucepan or to perform with the formboard which was an easy task for a two-year-old. Her observer was puzzled by these failures and noted that "she seemed confused and unable to solve the problem."

The feeling now prevailed that Heather performed as any two-year-old would, sometimes succeeding and sometimes failing. But she had lost her highly individualistic way of approaching, choosing, and solving problems. By beginning to act in a more conventional manner she no longer appeared so strikingly gifted or able to solve every problem which she tackled. While she still performed in a more charming manner than some children did, and while contact with her mother was warmer and more intense than that of many of her agemates, the exceptional radiance and individuality seemed to have dissipated. This may be why the observers kept assuring themselves that Heather "was still charming," although any impartial and new observer would have no doubt of it.

One could speculate that this was a natural depreciation of glamorized gift and personal charm, which look so dramatic in the first two years of life, just as defects, deviations, or disturbances may appear exaggerated. Or perhaps Heather's role as the integrating force between her parents was a burden too great for any child. Beset as the Harrises were with serious problems of job, income, domicile, and marital strife, there was no denying that Heather constituted their greatest satisfaction. In any event, as the study drew to a close it appeared that despite the real satisfaction which she gave, neither Heather nor her parents were wholly happy, and the vicissitudes of life extracted their inexorable toll.

SUMMARY

A. EXPECTATIONS

1. Maternal Expectations. Mrs. Harris had some anxiety about the experience of motherhood and concern about her adequacy. She seemed to need reassurance that "someone would be around to show her how to care for the baby" but did not anticipate need for help at home. Although she did not openly express her satisfaction, there was a general air of happiness about her pregnancy and there was no doubt that she was happy to have a child. Much of her anxiety was centered about religious reconciliations in terms of the baby's baptism and rearing. She was not unduly apprehensive about motherhood and declared her intention to be a "modern mother." There was no interest in outside employment even when difficult economic circumstances might have warranted it.

2. Specificity of Expectations. Mrs. Harris had many specific expectations that took the form of opinions rather than questions about what would be the course of events. She was committed to breast feeding, an ad lib feeding schedule, and a permissive mode of child-rearing. Despite inability to assert herself on many matters, Mrs. Harris tenaciously pursued the matter of an early baptism for the baby. Questions of how to deal with child-care problems were largely practical, related to the child's actual environment and her response to it.

3. Motivational Orientation. Both Mr. and Mrs. Harris were predominantly child-centered throughout the period. In the adoption of permissive child-rearing policies and in the enjoyment of their daughter, the Harrises were in complete accord. Sometimes they were permissive to the point of inconvenience to themselves. Heather's advanced development brought them great satisfaction, which seemed to "feed in" to a continuing warm relationship between child and parents.

In terms of child-care routines, Mrs. Harris was primarily concerned with the well-being and comfort of Heather. Even the child's sleeping difficulties, which greatly interfered with their rest, were tolerated and handled to best suit Heather. There was flexibility towards the child's food likes and dislikes and a gradualness in shaping her behavior.

During the second year Mrs. Harris put greater stress on values of social behavior, health and performance. But she maintained the same permissiveness and lenience she had shown earlier in matters of discipline. With the second pregnancy and concern about marital difficulties there was some shift in orientation, but it was not of a nature to indicate any basic change.

4. Role of Child in Fulfilling Mother's Expectations. Heather was indeed the center of her parents' world. Responding to criticisms that they were "spoiling her," the Harrises proudly pointed to her advanced development as proof of their parental accomplishments. On her part, Heather fulfilled every possible expectation in her behavior, charm, development, and response. Actually, Mrs. Harris's demands for achievement and conformity were somewhat more lenient than those of other mothers with high social and intellectual standards. Her motivations in the process of socialization were more unequivocally child-centered than those mothers, and consequently Heather happily fulfilled the maternal expectations under no pressure.

5. Paternal Expectations. Despite having had two children by a former marriage, Mr. Harris behaved like a "new father" and was immensely pleased at the prospect of a child. He anticipated the future in terms of both the child's needs and his own responsibility for satisfying them. He saw the child as an individual who would require loving care and a good environment in which to grow, which he as a father should provide. Thus paternal expectations were related to the child's well-being rather than to demands for conformity or achievement. This attitude persisted through Heather's first two years. His attitudes were mostly permissive, and he also showed consideration for the limitations of the child to conform and to go at her own pace.

B. BEHAVIOR

1. Communication. From the beginning Mrs. Harris was a "talker" to her baby for the purpose of expressing feelings rather than achieving specific goals. The talking was accompanied by a good deal of physical contact, holding, and comforting. As Heather grew older, her own soft continuous chatter was almost a replica of her mother's, and it served to maintain constant contact between them.

Mrs. Harris was astute in understanding the clues of her child and seemed able to interpret and respond to them unerringly. Communication between Mrs. Harris and Heather was so well attuned that she seemed able to explain each of Heather's actions and development in the greatest detail and to know intuitively the timing of her functioning, her general preferences, and when she was ready to give up breast feeding or naps. Mrs. Harris adjusted her own behavior to those needs. On her part, Heather was a baby who gave clear clues and responses, which facilitated her mother's handling.

2. Regularity and Flexibility of Scheduling. Emphasis was on the child's "demand" schedule, and from the beginning Heather had no great regularity. Her feeding in the early months seemed erratic and not scheduled, while her sleeping patterns were highly irregular. Although her appetite was never large, feeding did not become a problem either in terms of intake or habits. Mrs. Harris acceded to Heather's eating preferences by frequent variation in both the timing and selection of food. A serious weaning problem was anticipated by her, but the actual process occurred without a struggle. Elimination was never a problem because Mrs. Harris was flexible and unconcerned. Discipline similarly was not made an issue because of the family's general tendency towards permissiveness and Heather's usual cheerful compliance with the few restrictions put upon her. Mrs. Harris coped with Heather's severely irregular sleeping patterns in various ways but generally accepted the situation. It could be said that in the Harris family any irregularities of Heather did not produce undue problems.

3. Techniques of Management. There was little recorded non-permissive behavior, and Mrs. Harris lived up to her belief that "you can't spoil a child by giving it love and attention." She seldom used pre-arrangement of environment; rather she was accommodative in terms of the particular situation. At the worst of Heather's sleeplessness her mother only called her "pesty" and would not even consider the use of a temporary mild sedative. In her unsuccessful and sporadic attempts at toilet training she tolerated Heather's refusals and at the most rebuked her for soiling after disdaining the toilet.

In the second year of Heather's life there was an increase in reported non-permissive behavior, attributable to Mrs. Harris's pregnancy, marital difficulties, and shared living conditions. When the second baby was born, Mrs. Harris complained of Heather's willfulness, tears, and demandingness, which sometimes resulted in a spanking. But this slight change toward non-permissive behavior was also consistent with the pattern of a growing child whose activities required more social control. Of all the mothers, Mrs. Harris alone showed no great difference between permissive and non-permissive behavior during each of the two years.

4. Relation of Expectations to Behavior. Of the group who had many specific expectations concerning their children, Mrs. Harris was the most consistent in suiting her activity with the child to the fulfillment of her expectations. These expectations were largely of a permissive kind: one should be lenient in rearing a child; one should show attention and love without worry about "spoiling"; the child should not be pushed or hurried into achievement. Within the limits of available data Mrs. Harris's child-centered behavior carried out these expectations.

She set no unusually high standards and did not push Heather towards greater excellence.

Whatever reservations Mrs. Harris had concerning her own adequacy, she functioned smoothly in motherhood. Those who saw her remarked on the easy confidence with which she managed child and home.

5. Paternal Behavior. Mr. Harris's participation in child care was somewhat limited because of his working hours and carpentry tasks at home. His pleasure in Heather was enormous, however. He played with her at every possible moment and was most indulgent. His pride in Heather's achievements and advanced development was exceptionally great. For him, as for his wife, Heather was the bonding cement of the marital relationship.

During Mrs. Harris's confinement when Heather was nearly two years old, Mr. Harris briefly took over her management and apparently did it well. When living conditions became chaotic after Mrs. Harris's return with the new baby, Mr. Harris took Heather back to their old home, where he cared for her until routines became more established. The father-daughter relationship was loving and well developed.

C. SOCIO-CULTURAL INFLUENCES

1. Socio-economic Status and Values. Although neither of the Harrises was dominated by intense feelings for social and economic achievement, they did find satisfaction in the middle-class values of good housekeeping, neatness, and respectability. Yet throughout the study they were frustrated by financial insecurity, neighborhood unpleasantness, and social isolation, which mounted as the months passed. These difficulties weighed progressively on each of them.

When Mrs. Harris married her husband she felt secure in his economic position and abilities. But she was alternately gratified and thwarted by her husband's fluctuating work history and the consequent instability of their home. When he found it necessary to take a factory job Mrs. Harris found his semiskilled status an affront to her aspirations. Towards the end of the study she became discouraged by her husband's repeated vocational rebuffs and came to be skeptical of his ability.

Mr. Harris keenly felt his financial responsibilities and struggled to keep his head above water. He changed jobs no less than five times during the first two years of Heather's life. It was humiliating and bitter for him to move in with his wife's family and sell the house upon which he had lavished so much attention. He became increasingly taciturn and morose, a further factor in their deteriorating relationship.

Exclusion from their respective churches also contributed a sense of status loss but affected each of them differently. Mrs. Harris felt a deep personal loss and had a great desire to be accepted back into the fold, but her husband reacted with resentment and hostility.

Mrs. Harris's social inclinations were not shared by her husband. Her desires for strong family ties and contact were at odds with his disinclination for involvement with extended families. Thus, in terms of family, neighbors, friends, and an active social life there was lack of fulfillment for Mrs. Harris and a dichotomy between husband and wife. The Harrises were characterized as a family with equivocal mobility aspirations.

2. *Extended Family.* Because of the rivalry with her sister-in-law, Mrs. Harris felt alienated from the brother to whom she had been so attached in earlier years. Despite the strong attachment to her mother, Mrs. Harris had always felt a sense of emotional deprivation. Both Mr. and Mrs. Harris were annoyed and resentful at implications by family members that they were spoiling Heather. Nevertheless, Mrs. Harris remained quite attached to her family and longed for close ties with them.

Mr. Harris was quite the opposite. His family isolation had begun early, when he left a turbulent home situation to "go it alone." His insistence on independence not only applied to his own family but to his wife's as well, at least during the early period. As his economic position deteriorated, they called more on Mrs. Harris's parents for help. The combination of financial need and psychological isolation made for an unrealistic pattern of moving in and out of the maternal grandparents' home toward the end of Heather's second year. The sharing of the grandparental home further contributed to the disruption of the already unstable husband-wife relationship.

3. Spatial Arrangements and Values. In her parents' home Heather was allowed freedom of the house, with no evidence of restrictions. She had a fair share of toys despite straitened family circumstances, and her comfort came first with both her parents. However, as the living arrangements shifted back and forth to the maternal grandparents' home, Heather received an inconsistent and uncertain experience in terms of opportunities for exploring, freedom of movement, and sleeping arrangements. Under extremely crowded conditions she had little space in which to crawl, or later, to walk. The severity of her sleeping problem during these troublesome times led to further disruption of the family's patterns.

D. FAMILY RELATIONSHIPS

1. Marital. Of all the families in the study the Harrises came closest to disintegration. There was a basic lack of sharing and agreement on life values and goals, as well as extremely sharp conflicts between personalities. From childhood Mrs. Harris had felt deprived and excluded, unable to assert herself on matters of importance to her. She had many fears, some almost approaching phobic proportions. Various dependency needs had been inadequately met by her mother and even less so by the father who scarcely played any role in family life. In her first marriage she had had many disappointments, and she counted heavily on her second marriage. But many of her expectations in the marriage did not materialize, and she was faced with disillusionment.

Mr. Harris had grown up with strong feelings of loneliness, deprivation, and separation from others. He tended to isolate himself to avoid establishing relationships with other people, which he found difficult. His perspective of women was somewhat distorted, and he viewed them as a threat to his independence. Furthermore, he needed to be always in the right as a way of self-assertion.

The feelings of Mr. and Mrs. Harris were also affected by the disapprobation of the Church and possibly by the fact that their first child was conceived before their marriage. Mr. Harris's financial obligations to his first family and minimal success in business created an economic problem that added fuel to the fire of marital discord. The marriage was also characterized by inability to adequately express their feelings to each other and intermittent periods in which there was no communication between husband and wife.

The major factor in the disharmony, however, was basic personality conflict. This, plus difficulties in the socialization process for each marriage partner, combined to make the marital relationship unstable.

2. *Mother-Child.* The infant was the mother's chief source of emotional satisfaction. With her child Mrs. Harris found the satisfaction, warmth, and belongingness which she had failed to find in other relationships. Heather's attractiveness and advanced development provided her mother with self-confidence that she lacked in other areas. Communication between mother and daughter was on a high level of rapport and understanding. In the crescendo of marital discord the mother-child relationship continued to be greatly satisfying for both.

3. *Father-Child.* Mr. Harris's pleasure and satisfaction in Heather made it possible to establish an empathy with her that was lacking in his adult relationships. While he had small part in child-care routines, he shared experiences with the child in play, outdoor activity, and interchange of teaching and learning. Mr. Harris established this relationship early, and it continued during the two years. His pride in her accomplishments was great, and he was concerned that she should not be deprived of any advantages in child-rearing. Heather became the unifying force in the marital crisis because the threat of losing her made divorce intolerable. The child had much affection for her father and enjoyed activities with him.

E. PERSONALITY CHARACTERISTICS

1. *Handling of Anxiety and Hostility.* Because she was fearful and passive, Mrs. Harris was unable to express either negative or ag-

gressive feelings. In some respects these inhibitions resulted from the forced independence and self-reliance of her early childhood. Her self-described nervousness was expressed in a number of fears and fantasies associated with loneliness and the possible exposure of her inner feelings.

There was considerable ambivalence toward her husband throughout most of the two-year period. She deferred to his wishes in a number of things but harbored resentment at doing so. She resorted to subterfuge and "hiding" things from him, but the need for subterfuge distressed her. She was even uncertain whether to reveal her earlier tuberculosis. In general, she felt that it was better not to tell her husband how she really felt about things.

Infrequently she would express her hostility verbally, with sarcasm and double-edged bickering. Sometimes, when she felt the deepest despair, she screamed at him. But characteristically the most common defense against anxiety was silence and the concealment of her deepest feelings. The security which she had expected from her husband did not materialize, and she was especially disillusioned with his role as economic provider.

However, these anxieties did not affect her handling of Heather, and she was able to cope with all elements of child care in a reasonable way. Hence, while the handling of tension and anxiety became a divisive force in the marital relationship, it did not affect the mother-child relationship.

2. *Dependency and the Sense of Security.* Although Irene Harris had a number of dependency needs which had not been adequately met in childhood or in either of her marriages, these did not seem to be the major source of her difficulties. There was no marked dependency in relation to her family of origin, even though the maternal grandmother helped the Harrises at various times. The help was supportive in a practical rather than emotional sense. In the stress and strain of her difficult marital relationship, her mother provided support. While there appeared to be a strong relationship between them, there was some reason to believe that there was a fair amount of ambivalent hostility on Mrs. Harris's part. She was often embarrassed by her mother's forwardness and manners as well as critical of her mother's failure to provide proper parental control during her own youth.

Severe dependency needs were also not part of the marital difficulties. In the early period of marriage Mrs. Harris found her husband someone she could idealize and in whose life she could enjoy participation. Since she valued his apparent financial stability and secure middle-class status, she accepted his undisputed lordship in the household and bowed to his decisions. With the advent of Heather, however, and the beginning of Mr. Harris's financial and vocational stresses, the situation changed. As her sense of security in her husband diminished, Mrs. Harris became more self-assertive and less inclined to accept his domination.

3. *Feelings of Adequacy or Inadequacy.* Mrs. Harris presented an attractive, smiling, composed appearance, which served as superficial protection against revealing her self-critical feelings of inadequacy. She had always experienced difficulty in meeting people and later in making friends. She looked upon herself as having no special ability or talent, and she felt there was little about her which would be attractive to others.

Her feelings of inferiority and lack of acceptance continued for the duration of the study. She was very hesitant about describing her experiences with the child unless she could feel certain of having her comments favorably received. Because the new process of child-rearing proceeded smoothly enough, these inadequacy feelings did not seem to interfere with her care of the child. Mrs. Harris's six months of successful breast feeding made her extremely proud. At the same time she wondered if she were too unintelligent to give any intelligence to Heather. Hence, Heather's advanced development brought enormous satisfaction to her mother.

4. *Planning and Impulsiveness.* This did not seem to be an area of significance for the Harris family. Mrs. Harris appeared neither to be a compulsive planner nor impulsive in handling her life situations. Although she gave thought to her many problems and reflected on possible solutions, she was not driven to impulsive decisions.

5. *Self-Assertion.* Difficulties in self-assertion characterized the adult relationships of Irene Harris but did not significantly influence the mother-child relationship. Mrs. Harris had always found it

difficult to assert herself and tended to hide her feelings in a cloak of silence and hurt. Often she did not assert herself with her husband on matters that were very important to her. However, with the advent of Heather, she became able to act more assertively. She had Heather baptized, and she maintained close ties with her family. During the study it seemed that as Mr. Harris's economic stability decreased, his wife became more self-assertive, which also contributed to the marital discord.

6. Recapitulation of Past Experiences. Irene Harris perceived considerable deprivation in her early years from tangible hardships and emotional insecurities. She felt that her mother was a controlling parental force who had not provided the necessary elements of intimacy, education, and understanding. Remembering her own circumstances, she was determined that Heather should have every advantage of comfort, emotional security, and good rearing. The prominence that this assumed in child-care routines was not delineated, but it was clear that Mrs. Harris and Heather had an exceedingly close, warm, and mutually perceptive relationship.

F. EMERGENCE OF FAMILY INTEGRATION PATTERNS

1. Family Structure. In a family tending toward segmental and divisive organization Heather Harris seemed to constitute the chief unifying force in the midst of more marital discord than was found in any other family in the study. Despite the effective and satisfying relationships between Heather and each of her parents, the sharp marital conflict could not be overcome. All that can be said is that in the absence of Heather, this marriage might well have ended in the divorce court.

In terms of Heather, there appeared the semblance of a triadically integrated family, but the marital dissatisfactions of the parents were such that only strong separate dyadic mother-child and father-child relationships emerged. Unquestionably there was not a genuine pattern of three-person sharing, a cornerstone of unitary family structure.

2. Division of Labor and Balance of Power. In their own home the Harrises followed the customary pattern of the father being responsible for management of home repair and the grounds outside the home and the mother for the inside of the house. Herb Harris was a skillful craftsman who enjoyed building and improving things for the house. He also assumed, especially in the early period of marriage, a dominant role in decision-making concerning the home. He seemed also to make the financial decisions and to control what they should or should not purchase. Generally Mr. Harris played the dominant role in the family, and there was less sharing in decision-making than in unitary families.

3. Development, Achievement, and Social Behavior of Child. Heather showed above-age adequacy in the developmental landmarks. Her performance in almost every task at a given age level was higher than her actual age. These achievements were matched by her social behavior, which was winning and attractive from the beginning. She exuded happiness and was a pleasure for all concerned, especially for her parents. Even though Mrs. Harris did not pose unusually high goals for her child's achievement, she recognized that Heather had advanced quickly, and she compared her favorably with her peers.

4. Prospect of Siblings. During Heather's first year Mrs. Harris spoke of wanting another child, and she couldn't understand why her husband was opposed to it. She strongly felt that another child would be a companion for Heather and that there "would be someone left" when Heather grew up and left home. However, when she did indeed become pregnant by "accident," her response was ambivalent. This pregnancy was physically more difficult for her, and Mrs. Harris only wished that it would be over. The new baby had no problems, but Mrs. Harris's dissatisfaction was accentuated by Heather's demandingness and difficult behavior. There was evidence before the study ended of forthcoming sibling rivalry between Heather and her brother.

5. Status of Family in Community. The Harris family had tendencies toward relative isolation from community influences and pressure. Contacts with the study staff literally provided Mrs. Harris with her only extended contacts beyond the boundaries of her family group. Because of conflicts that developed with neighbors, Mrs. Harris was excluded from the usual area friendships. Although she longed for a social life, her husband was antisocial and preferred solitude. They were involuntarily isolated from their respective churches. Mr. Harris's general attitude towards families, plus his wife's conflict with her sister-in-law, further limited extended family relationships.

6. Types of Parent-Child Adaptation. The Harrises' severe marital disorientation and conflict inevitably led to a pattern of segmental family operation. The positive relationship that each parent had with Heather could not overcome the unsatisfactory husband-wife interaction. Both parents were consistently highly involved in the child's life and essentially child-centered, despite difficulties in family life. Their management of Heather was largely permissive, although Mrs. Harris's stressful situation in the second year produced some minor conflict with the child. The Harris family was characterized as segmental in structure, child-centered in orientation, and permissive in management.

POSTSCRIPT

Living arrangements were resolved by the purchase of a rundown house with considerable land in an outlying area. Although it seemed that Mrs. Harris concurred with her husband on its purchase, sharp dissent immediately appeared. In terms of comfort, the house was extremely inadequate. It was decrepit, and the structural defects were almost irremediable. For heat and hot water they had to depend on an old stove. Despite Mr. Harris's intention to "fix up the home," the job was so vast, tedious, and expensive that it became a discouraging process. Furthermore, its isolation accentuated Mrs. Harris's fear of loneliness and solitude. Although she had learned to drive, the very old car which she had at her disposal was mostly inoperable.

Mr. Harris applied himself to those repair jobs which he thought necessary. Often they were not the ones which had the highest priority for his wife. She resented the time he gave to outside gardening while living conditions inside the house remained intolerable for her. The economic problems and handling of family expenditures remained a prominent difficulty, especially since there was little joint planning. Mr. Harris acted unilaterally, and Mrs. Harris nursed her grievances in cold silence until their accumulation erupted in angry outbursts which set off violent explosions.

Strife mounted to the point where Mr. Harris lost self-control and physically assaulted his wife on several occasions. Relationships with Mrs. Harris's family were, as ever, part of the conflict. The turbulence of marital strife on at least two occasions led to seeking of legal advice. However, no actual steps for separation and divorce were taken. Mr. Harris could not tolerate the thought of being deprived of his children, and Mrs. Harris "could never do that to him." Feeling helpless and trapped "with two small children," she resigned herself "to do nothing until the children were grown." During reconciliations, attempts were made to understand each other and work out problems and the situation would temporarily improve. Then complaints and dissatisfactions would again accumulate, whereupon a minor incident would serve as the incendiary spark for a full-blown family crisis.

The children and Mrs. Harris herself had frequent episodes of illness from upper respiratory or gastrointestinal infections. It was felt that the inadequate heating possibly contributed to this situation. The infant Jimmy was more trying for his mother than Heather had been reported to be. He nursed frequently, yet had unexplainable severe crying spells which made her "frantic." Mrs. Harris continued to breast feed for a long period because Jimmy disliked the bottle. It seemed, however, that her own desire to breast feed was also involved.

As with Heather, the infant's sleeping patterns were highly erratic. Night-time sleeping was especially precarious. In fact, sleep problems remained a perennial difficulty with both children. The chore of comforting and attending the children at night in order for her husband to get his rest was most exhausting to Mrs. Harris. Nevertheless, she handled it with her characteristic devotion and without hostility. As she said, "It's not their fault. They didn't ask to be born."

Jimmy was an attractive, responsive, large, and moderately obese infant, who functioned in almost all areas at somewhat advanced development similar to Heather's early performances.

Heather took to her brother with affection, pride, and helpfulness, even though there was some reaction to the fact that she was no longer the sole focus of her mother's attention.

The relationship between Heather and her father remained very warm, and she continued to be "the apple of his eye." There appeared to be considerable competition between the parents for Heather's affection. As a matter of fact, Mr. Harris was extremely devoted to both his children, seeming to hold their interests above all else. This was not entirely well tolerated by his wife. Frequently marital disturbances were focused on the children. Mr. Harris had high standards for their good behavior and conduct. Despite Mrs. Harris's consistent, devoted, and perceptive care of the children, he blamed her for any transgressions and was critical of her ability "to raise them properly."

In nursery school Heather initially had some separation difficulty. But her unease gradually vanished, and she showed "balanced judgment and a thoughtful approach to objects and humans." She was assessed as a gentle but determined child who knew what she wanted, could wait for it, and could follow through to obtain it. One comment was that she "was the least disturbed of the study group children."

Nevertheless, Heather was not immune to the stressful family atmosphere. With other children she held herself somewhat aloof. Although she did not initiate contact, she was responsive when included. At times, coinciding with the greatest family tension, Heather was depressed, fearful, and subdued. There were days in nursery school when she closely attached herself to an adult and participated little.

Her sleeping continued to be erratic, and her eating was now described as minimal. At home it was reported that she had periods of willfulness, silliness, demanding or provocative behavior. These seemed more noticeable during or after special family crises. In play therapy sessions Heather was characterized as a very pleasant, somewhat inhibited and constricted child. Developmental evaluations continued to assess her as somewhat advanced for her age, although the outstanding charm and individuality of her earlier years had diminished.

When she entered school Heather had no adjustment difficulty. Later reports indicated that she did not perform scholastically as well as might have been expected. Nevertheless, she maintained a moderate B and C record, while Jimmy performed as an A and B student.

A third child (male) was born to the Harrises when Heather was about 12 years old. The family had sold their house and had purchased a more modern and desirable one in a nice suburban area. Mr. Harris's financial status appeared improved. He was conscientious in his efforts to improve the family economically, although it did not always turn out that way.

He remained rather exacting about the children's upbringing and was especially careful to restrict Heather from early socialization with boys. Otherwise, Heather had friends and was engaged in a wide variety of group activities. She was well groomed and highly interested in her appearance. When last seen at 14½, she was an attractive, nicely rounded young girl with quiet charm. She seemed "very well put together," poised, friendly, and cooperative but with certain constriction and conventionality. There was a sense of disappointment that "the remnants of superior function seen from years ago were no longer evident."

As for the marital relationship, it seemed to have settled down to a status quo, or "the same as ever." It would be easy to assume that the intactness of the family rested solely on the satisfactions and devotion of parenthood. But one cannot ignore other possible emotional satisfactions which kept the bond from being severed as well as the memory of a former broken marriage for each. Perhaps the fabric of family continuity for the Harrises was made of sterner stuff than met the eye.

The Neville Family

MOTHERHOOD IN CONFLICT

The emotional legacies of her mother's unhappiness and dissatisfaction had made a deep impression on Maria Neville long before she herself became a mother. For the woman who was "tortured by the ghost of her frustrated mother" there was little promise that motherhood would moderate the hunger for security, achievement, and satisfaction. "I'm not one of these women who just have to have children around for the sake of having children. . . ."

Maria's mother was widowed in World War I and was left with a six-year-old son. Some time later she met an attractive man and "it was love at first sight." After a six week courtship they were married and lived in Hungary, where Maria was born. Although they were "terrifically in love," they were not a "companionable couple," and her mother was very unhappy throughout the marriage.

Her new husband was adamant that she give up her small business lest "the townspeople think that he could not support her adequately." They lived on a large estate, with servants to do the housework. Maria's mother had little to do. "She brooded and became desperately unhappy." Maria was ashamed of her father in little ways, "because he was so different from all the other fathers." He was "much too dapper and flashy for his own good or the happiness of his family. And he really seemed out of place in our simple community."

In any event, family life was of short duration since both parents died when Maria was about twelve or thirteen years old. She went to live with her brother, who was ten years older and already married. Soon they moved to England. Maria remembered this part of her life as a happy period, although her brother was much stricter than her parents had been. She stressed that both he and his wife were "very responsible people," well able to take care of her from the time her parents died.

Maria studied advertising and began to work in that field. When her brother and his family emigrated to America she remained in England, where she shared an apartment with a girl friend. Soon she met English-born Paul Neville, a promising young architect. He was tall and "not slender but plain skinny." Six months later, while they were riding in the noisy subway, he proposed. "It was hardly a romantic scene," Mrs. Neville said, laughing, "but within half a year we were married." The next two and a half years "were the most fun I'd ever had."

They saved their money for special holiday trips to France and to Italy. Paul Neville shared his wife's interest in art, which made their travels especially exciting. Then they decided to emigrate to America. For one thing, Mrs. Neville wanted to be closer to her brother, and for another, it seemed auspicious for her husband's career. Mr. Neville secured a position as junior architect in a New England firm. It was fairly close to the town where Mrs. Neville's brother lived and taught in a college.

The Nevilles rented a third-floor apartment on a broad shaded avenue in an old but quiet and respectable section of the city. They tastefully decorated the modest apartment with sophisticated art and a décor that demonstrated how much could be done in homemaking even with limited resources. Mr. Neville was engrossed in his work, and his wife resumed her advertising career, which had progressed so well in England. They were beginning to make friends, especially in connection with Mr. Neville's job, and life seemed exciting and full of promise.

Then the unexpected occurred. Mrs. Neville found out that she was pregnant. Suddenly it seemed that life was inexorably changed. Now there was no hope of continuing to enjoy the freedom they had known in England. Now travel, which had been one of their greatest joys, was impossible. And the creativity of an advertising career would be replaced by the drudgery of housework and diapers.

It was no wonder that Maria Neville often spoke nostalgically to staff members of the carefree London evenings and the satisfactions of engaging in rewarding work. Cast as she now was in a maternal role that she did not cherish, she remembered the unhappiness of her mother, and her father's wish that she had been a boy. She dwelt also upon her parents' early death and her own subsequent emigration to England.

As a patient in the obstetrical clinic of the Grace-New Haven Hospital, Mrs. Neville was introduced to the study. She was immediately eager to join the group, no matter what was entailed. The first interview took place in the fifth month of her pregnancy. Mrs. Neville was described by the interviewer as short, dark-haired, and quite chubby. Her face was not particularly pretty, but she gave a neat and well-groomed appearance. Her speech had a soft English accent, and she was lively and smiling. Candidly she said, "I don't know what having the baby will do to us. I know it's going to be different." To many mothers, pregnancy seemed almost endless in the light of their eagerness to have their babies. But for Mrs. Neville it was otherwise. "I'm not in a hurry," she explained. "It doesn't have to come so quickly. I don't want to see what it's like all that much."

Mrs. Neville had no particular worries but admitted that she was "a little scared." She hoped to be helped by the study "not to be so afraid" and said, "I'm a terrible sissy about physical pain. When I go to the dentist, I'm ready to shriek and jump out of the chair the moment he touches me." However, she had read a story on natural childbirth in *Life* magazine which interested her a great deal, and she was very enthusiastic about natural childbirth.

Physically, she reported, she had been slightly nauseated during the whole first month but had never actually vomited and "it wasn't too bad." Pregnancy had made her sleepier than usual, and it was irritating to her that she needed more rest. She had always craved sweet things because "I guess I never grew up," but now her desire for sweets had diminished and she craved fruit. When specifically asked, she said that her breasts had enlarged considerably. She said that she had gained only one pound. She did not look pregnant but merely plump.

Mrs. Neville expressed enthusiasm for rooming-in with the baby and intended to breast feed as she had been breast-fed by her own mother. When asked if she would be disappointed if she couldn't breast feed, she replied, "Oh, I would be very disappointed. I am really quite keen on breast feeding the baby." Although they had certainly not planned to have a baby at this time, Mrs. Neville said she felt that she wanted it. She definitely wanted a boy, she said, "because that's the way it had been in my family and I was ever so happy with my brother." Her husband, however, "didn't care one way or another." A boy's name had already been selected. At this time Mrs. Neville was looking for some part-time advertising work to do at home since she would be happier "doing some kind of work."

The second interview took place after Mrs. Neville had come from the exercise class. She said that some of the exercises hurt when she squatted and that the front of her leg was quite strained. She reported a five pound gain in the past four weeks and was certain that the obstetrician would "scold" her for this because she was "already too fat" when she became pregnant.

Mrs. Neville asked the interviewer what was the best spacing between children. She commented that her husband wanted three or four because there were three in his family and they had had a very happy time. However, she felt, "After he's taken care of the first one, maybe I'll be able to get him down to two." Her husband also thought that children should be spaced about eighteen months apart, again because it had been that way in his family. She imagined that it was more of an upheaval to have children in the late twenties and early thirties than when one was very young, "and we're already twenty-eight years old." Also, she said that "a mother can't really get back to work until the children are at least four or five." She was pleased to report that she had gotten a couple of small ad copy jobs to do at home.

Concerning preparation for the baby, Mrs. Neville said that she was going to "leave all of that to the last two months." She planned to get a crib from a friend and would buy a few new things for the baby, but she hoped most of the baby's things would come second-hand from this friend.

Mrs. Neville was next interviewed after she had been seen by the obstetrician. She said that the doctor had praised her for her small weight gain, although the previous week "he had wiped the floor" with her because she had gained four pounds. She found that if she stuck to her diet, she didn't gain, but when she went visiting or ate with friends it was impossible for her to keep on the diet. "If you ate only what the hospital told you to eat, there just would be nothing at all."

As usual, Mrs. Neville was talkative, enthusiastic, and gay. The night before, they had been to a Horowitz concert, and she commented that he was a brilliant pianist. Although the day was rather gray, Mrs. Neville commented on the nice weather in an effort to be friendly and sociable. She said that they had received a letter from a relative in England to the effect that her baby had been strangled by the umbilical cord during delivery. This frightened Mrs. Neville into switching from Ward to Resident service in order to assure completely satisfactory care during her delivery. "Even though we can't afford this extra outlay of money, it seems the best thing to do."

Then Mrs. Neville reported that she had been told she was Rh negative. Although the doctor had explained that it didn't matter with a first baby, Mrs. Neville wondered about subsequent ones. It was suggested that this be discussed with the pediatrician, who could be helpful in advising about the care of the baby and the kind of things one might expect from newborns. Mrs. Neville said that it was "all quite frightening because once the baby is born, everything will be different, and it is a very final kind of change because we'll always be responsible for this youngster and we'll never be free again."

She believed that some of her apprehensions came from unfamiliarity with babies. She was the baby in her own family, and all her cousins were considerably older. She was sure her husband would be better with the baby than she because she herself had "a terribly quick temper which flares up suddenly and then it's past." Also, she was "extremely impatient" and often felt "like sticking a pin in people to make them hurry up."

Mrs. Neville discussed her fear of how the baby would change her life, but she did not state specifically what she was afraid of losing, other than her "freedom." It was suggested that she meet with the pediatrician a number of times before delivery and perhaps gain more confidence about caring for an infant. She was also invited to observe the children in the nursery school and seemed eager for the opportunity to do so.

Mrs. Neville asked whether it would be all right to spend some time at her brother's home right after the baby's birth, since her sister-in-law could help during the first few weeks. The interviewer approved, and then Mrs. Neville said, "Well, we'll go there and stay long enough to thoroughly disrupt everything and then we'll return home."

Just before the next interview the obstetrician performed a version procedure to turn the baby around from a breech position. When Mrs. Neville came from the examination she did not seem particularly upset by the experience, although her hair was a bit mussed and her face flushed as though she had been perspiring. She said that the doctor had performed this same procedure two weeks earlier. It seemed that the baby "won't stay in the right place; it keeps moving around." Also, she had the idea that fatty tissue was pressing on the uterus, which caused the baby's movement. Up to now she had gained seventeen pounds, and the obstetrician wanted her to start losing weight because her hands and legs were puffed. She didn't seem confident of success in this because weight had always been a problem with her. He had also put her on a salt-free diet.

Mrs. Neville asked the purpose of the psychological testing program and then inquired if her husband could also have these same tests "if it wouldn't be any trouble." The interviewer said this could be arranged. It made her feel much better, she said, "because then I won't be the only one subjected to this kind of thing. . . . After all, the baby's going to get its brains from both sides of the family." Laughingly she commented, "If it's a little girl and looks like him, it's going to be a pretty sad baby." They hoped that if it were a girl, she would inherit her mother's looks and not her father's.

To questions about her husband's family, Mrs. Neville responded that his father had died when he was six. His mother had raised the three children and worked in a gift shop. After being a widow for twenty years she had recently married and now lived in Arizona. Her husband was retired from business and was quite a bit older than she. Mr. Neville's brother and sister both lived in England. Mrs. Neville said her mother-in-law was quite excited about the coming baby because it would be her first grandchild.

At the next session Mrs. Neville asked the interviewer about the results of the psychological test. She felt that she had been "so very stupid," that there had been so much of it that she could not do. When asked to which things she referred, she said, "Well, mainly it was the numbers." The interviewer asked Mrs. Neville whether she believed her husband was brighter than she in most things. Mrs. Neville said, "No, it's just in science and the kinds of things I've never been able to do."

The interviewer commented that it must be nice to be back near her brother after the four year separation. Mrs. Neville replied that it certainly was, but that the separation had really been quite good because now he no longer treated her as a young child but accepted her as a grown-up equal.

The pediatrician met with Maria Neville and described her as very neat in her navy blue dress, quick and sure in her movements. Mrs. Neville's interest in the rooming-in plan seemed not so much a matter of wanting the baby with her as wanting to be instructed in the baby's care. She expressed some fright at the prospect of caring for a little baby since she had never been around young children and knew little about them. She said she "might be too hard on the baby" and that maybe her husband would help her because "he's calmer and seems to have more common sense." The thought of being a mother still seemed quite unreal to her since she had no way to imagine herself as a mother.

She told how shocked she was to learn that she was Rh negative, and since then she had heard stories from various people which made her quite anxious. She told about an Rh negative woman who had had one baby but decided not to have another for fear it might have erythroblastosis fetalis. The pediatrician felt that Mrs. Neville possibly was implying that "one is enough." She seemed to be reassured by the pediatrician's explanation of the Rh factor.

Mrs. Neville's health was pretty good on the whole, although lately there were some episodes of dizziness, which disturbed her. The doctor said that everything was fine. The exercise class was discussed, and Mrs. Neville said she did some of the exercises at home but didn't have time for all of them. She said that if they were terribly important, she would make it her business to do them.

In a discussion about natural childbirth and the need to relax between contractions, Mrs. Neville spoke of how difficult it is to relax in the way she was told to do. "How can you just lie there and think of nothing when your mind's going a mile a minute? How does one go about thinking of nothing?"

As for feeding the baby, she said, "I plan to do it myself." Then she asked if it was all right to give the baby a bottle occasionally. She seemed relieved to learn that the pediatrician felt the baby should occasionally have a bottle for the sake of both the baby and the mother. Mrs. Neville commented that she and her husband cherished their freedom to move about and didn't know what they would think about being "tied down by a baby." Then she added, "But of course I'll be the one tied down most of the time because I will have no one with whom to leave the baby."

Mrs. Neville mentioned the fact that she had her "heart set on a little boy," although her husband didn't really care. "I don't know why I want a boy, but I just do."

The interviewer next met with Mrs. Neville after she had seen the delivery room. She was not upset by the instruments but by "the straps for your hands." The interviewer explained that these were not always used and that actually they were for the mother's protection. Mrs. Neville replied, "Probably the nurses and doctors are afraid that we will grab at them." She described the nurse who took them through the delivery room as "a bit too sweet" and said that she "romanticized the whole experience too much." She would have preferred someone who had had children herself and would therefore be able to give a more realistic view of what might happen.

Mrs. Neville then volunteered that she thought her husband was trying to "squirm out of being tested" and that she "wasn't going to let him do that." She said this with great seriousness, adding that she had been careful not to tell him any of the answers because it wouldn't be fair. She had an air of victory, as though she were going to make him prove how intelligent he was.

In the seventh interview Mrs. Neville as usual was enthusiastic about being part of the study. Throughout, she seemed most anxious to please and to describe as frankly as she could her views and attitudes on certain issues. She reported that the baby was remaining in the right place after the obstetrical procedure and that she felt fine. Because of slight varicose veins she had been wearing a rather heavy maternity girdle and rubber stockings, which were uncomfortable in the warm weather. Except for that, she had no complaints.

When asked if things were ready for the baby, she said, "Absolutely everything is ready for him." Then she added that they always referred to the baby as a boy and that they "would be a bit surprised if it turns out to be a girl." They had decided on a boy's name but had no selection as yet for a girl. They had "played around with several girls' names" but were not really pleased with any of them.

Mrs. Neville's tone of voice became quite serious and low as she apologetically asked if her husband could take his test at a later date because he was exploring the possibility of taking courses for a higher degree in his field. The interviewer asked whether Mr. Neville brought much of his work home. Mrs. Neville answered, "Yes, he does a lot of it at home, but it doesn't mean a thing to me." She felt that "one ought to either know a lot about the husband's work and really work with him, or know nothing at all." Her view was that a little knowledge could be a dangerous thing. As it was, she didn't bother him in any way and just kept completely detached from his work.

She agreed, however, that he should get a higher degree before he became too much older since the lack of it would handicap his future. Finances would be a problem if he had to relinquish his job in order to study, because with a very small child she could not make any contribution financially to their family.

In the next visit Mrs. Neville complained that she really had felt quite bad the past two weeks and had been "more uncomfortable than in all of the pregnancy put together." A week ago Sunday she had felt so wound up and jittery inside that she could hardly sit quietly at all. When the doctor saw her, he became quite concerned about the increased blood pressure and gave her various medications, including phenobarbital. She had to take thirty-five pills a day, which she found quite an ordeal. For four or five days she took the phenobarbital and felt so "dopey" that about the only thing she could do was sleep. The obstetrician advised her "to just vegetate," but she knew she couldn't possibly do this without the help of phenobarbital. Mrs. Neville characterized herself as feeling "just like a dead body" the past week.

The interviewer asked if Mr. Neville was particularly perturbed about the forthcoming birth. Mrs. Neville answered, "If he is, he certainly doesn't show it. . . . He reads his book, and I moan to him about this and that, and he sort of hears me but is not particularly demonstrative." He had also told her that she was strong and it wouldn't be much trouble. Mrs. Neville thought he had got that idea because she had been so completely well until the last two weeks. She added, "It might be nice to be a bit weaker so that you get more sympathy and consideration." Mrs. Neville had lost four pounds in the last week because of the medication to decrease her blood pressure.

The interviewer asked if they had finally decided on a girl's name, but the answer was "no." Mrs. Neville said that she had spoken to a woman in the waiting room, who told her a child need not be named immediately in the hospital, and that they wanted to wait a week or so after the baby's birth. Throughout the interview Mrs. Neville giggled quite a bit and spoke gaily. She did not seem depressed by the past week's illness and was pleased by the fact that there were only two more weeks to go. When asked if she felt the time had gone quickly or slowly, she noted her surprise at how fast it had gone, except for the past two weeks, which had seemed longer than any other time of her pregnancy.

In the following interview Mrs. Neville said that she had gained six pounds within the past two weeks and knew that she would be "scolded" for this by the obstetrician. She said that she was getting more panicky and couldn't do anything because she tired so quickly. She wondered, "How much will it hurt?" and added that she hated the sight of blood or pain. The interviewer asked Mrs. Neville if she had ever given thought to how the baby would come out. She answered, "That's just it. I don't see how it will do it." She said that no matter how much she had heard in the exercise class concerning birth she felt that "no one can really tell you about this kind of thing." When asked if it seemed more mysterious than other kinds of important things, she commented, "You can sort of plan anything else but in giving birth you're not really in control of the situation." She felt that she was powerless and at the mercy of pregnancy, that "it is mostly God's will which decides these things."

The interviewer asked if religion meant quite a bit to her. Mrs. Neville said that she had not had a religious background but during pregnancy she felt very definitely that a strong faith would help. She said she planned to give her baby a solid religious education. Laughing a bit, she observed, "You always want the opposite for your children from what you had as a child." She added, "It's impossible for a child to develop religious attitudes and beliefs if the family does not have them and really live them." The Nevilles had not gone to church since coming to this country but planned to go to some Protestant church as the baby grew up.

The interviewer asked why she did not have as much religious experience in childhood as she seemed to want. Mrs. Neville said that her mother had been religious but her father had been "pretty much of a heretic"; "a child senses it and cannot build up a strong faith."

Mrs. Neville was very enthusiastic about what she had seen of child-rearing in America as compared to England. She felt that in England they kept their children babies for too long, sent them off to school, and did not permit them to take their fair share of responsibility in the family. "Everything is decided for them and when they grow up they find it quite hard to be independent, assertive, easy-going people." She added, "If you raise a child to be independent, you have to be willing to take a little bit of rudeness and talking back as a youngster grows older."

Mrs. Neville reported that she had seen a disturbing film the week before. It stated that a child with cerebral palsy was born every fifty minutes, and she wondered "if you would know right away whether or not the baby is really all right." Also, she had seen a Mongoloid child in the clinic a few weeks ago and "would hate to be pitied by other mothers for having such a child." Mrs. Neville commented that her own fears about the baby were most likely just part of every pregnancy and not too unusual.

At the last ante-partum interview Mrs. Neville was asked if she felt any differently the past day or so, since the baby might be born in a few days. She said that she didn't think the baby would be born very soon because it had not dropped as yet.

Mrs. Neville was very pleased to have lost four pounds in the last week and attributed it completely to the pills. Her diet had also changed a bit because she was not quite as hungry. She expected that the baby would be rather late because her irregular menstrual periods made it difficult to estimate accurately her last period. Menstruation was usually painful and the flow lasted about seven days. Since marriage, however, the periods had been less painful. She characterized herself as feeling "irrational" the week before she menstruated and said her husband used to know by the way she acted that she was going to have a period. She did not specify except to say that she just "flew off the handle, was very sensitive, and picked a fight for no good reason at all."

She questioned whether it was better to "fly off the handle and get it out of your system or to hold it back." The interviewer asked how Mrs. Neville thought she would manage the baby when she was angry. Mrs. Neville said quite simply, "I'll spank him," and made the gesture of a neat little pat on the buttocks. Then she changed the subject and asked the interviewer if she liked the name Rita, which they had selected from the name book.

Two days later Rita was born. Mrs. Neville came to the hospital because she had passed a rather large blood clot the night before. She did not appear particularly upset by the experience and was very pleased that labor was beginning. She commented that she had had the first really good night's sleep in a long time.

The obstetrician examined her to determine whether there was a placenta praevia and if a Cesarean was warranted. This frightened her a bit, but she said that whatever was best for the child she wanted done. She also commented that she hated to be examined vaginally but knew it had to be done. Two or three hours after the examination it was decided that labor and delivery should go along normally. Mrs. Neville's face was flushed, and she looked as though she had been crying, but she was relieved to know that she would have the baby in the normal way.

During the afternoon and evening little happened. But somewhere around 3 A.M. she was having frequent, very forceful, and vigorous contractions. She complained of considerable leg cramping and seemed very tired. Upon examination the obstetrician found her almost completely dilated and decided to move her to the delivery room. He felt there was plenty of time to get her there for preparation and draping in the usual way. However, she suddenly said, "I believe I'm about to have this baby." When the doctor looked under the sheet he beheld the crown of the baby's head. The baby was delivered right there in the room, with Mr. Neville looking on and cheering from the bedside. Despite the doctor's embarrassment that a primipara had precipitated in the bed, he felt that it had been a fairly nice experience for both the Nevilles. After the delivery Mrs. Neville was removed to the delivery room for repair of a small tear in the perineum.

The obstetrician recorded several comments about Mrs. Neville. He had not anticipated that she would do well during labor, delivery, or the post-partum period and was therefore quite surprised at the way she conducted herself during labor, particularly during the second and third stages. He felt her attitude in general was better than it had been during the pregnancy period.

When the interviewer saw Mrs. Neville the morning after delivery she looked well and not particularly worn after the day's experience. She seemed enormously pleased at having done such a speedy job in giving birth, and commented, "Having the baby in the room was something like having it at home and yet you had the security and protection of the hospital." She said that "the baby was just a bit over five and one-half pounds, but she tore me apart." Although the baby was a "Rita" and not a "Stuart," she said it was beautiful and she didn't care.

The psychologist's evaluation of newborn Rita outdid itself in superlatives. "I have seen many young babies but never one so enchanting and ravishing as Rita. She is perfection in miniature. Her head is round and well-shaped, the lips soft, full and beautifully curved. Her skin is immaculate, her cheeks rosy, her whole appearance full of health but wonderfully dainty and feminine."

In addition to her physical beauty there was an unbelievable peace of expression, a calmness untouched by all the rush and disturbance of the world. During ten newborn observations Rita cried less than any other child, and her crying was of short duration. It gave the impression that for a newborn she was unusually free from discomfort and that "she was in control of suffering." Of the seven crying episodes, two were from hunger, three from sudden change of position, and one from noise. But she succeeded in comforting herself quickly and lastingly by motor discharge or by mouthing.

Rita could relax in many different ways: by startling, by moving a number of parts or only one part of her body, by squealing or crying. But she almost always relaxed completely, her body at ease and her position looking comfortable. Her responses did not seem as unpredictable or unreliable as other newborns. She responded to most outside stimulations by becoming more active and matched her response to the intensity of the stimulation. The startle occurred only in reponse to acoustic stimulations. In one instance she responded to a very sharp and sudden noise by crying. At touch, she became red, or withdrew. There was the vague impression that touch was unpleasant to her, and there was no further experimentation with tactile stimulation.

At change of position Rita cried briefly and then "adjusted" to her position. It seemed that she had to "add a last touch" to find her own position before settling down. With amazing regularity she became restless when the blanket was removed but quieted when it was restored. While this involved touch, it was of a different nature from the localized sudden touching which seemed objectionable to her. During one observation, when many noises accidentally took place, Rita showed herself able to adapt to the environment by decreasing her response to them consistently and regularly. It seemed as if her organism was quite capable of always using its potentialities in an optimal way.

Her hands frequently touched her head, cheek, or ear and reached her mouth fairly frequently. The hand-mouth contacts were mostly with the right hand and occurred when she was moving. These contacts did not last for any length of time and she sucked only once. Nevertheless, the contact with her mouth seemed to contribute greatly to her peace and quiet. Rita was not a baby who slept all the time, but it was fairly easy to distinguish sleeping from waking. She moved three times as much when awake and reacted to twice as many stimulations. There was also a difference in the nature of her behavior when sleep or awake. When awake, only eighteen percent of her movements were startles, but in sleep, forty-three percent of her movements were of a jerky variety. This permitted the speculation that in sleep Rita did not achieve maximum peacefulness but that in waking she was better prepared for meeting and responding to the outside world.

Her reaction to hunger was always an increase of movements, and sometimes crying, with hand-mouth contact or motor discharge. This suggested that it would not be difficult to determine when she was hungry and that she could rather easily be put on a self-demand schedule. Furthermore, hunger did not overwhelm her, at least if it did not go beyond a certain stage. She reacted to it more or less as to outside stimulation. Her position was mostly supine and turned to the right. When in prone she moved more, but in supine she was more at rest. Her pattern of movement consisted of two distinguishable acts. In the first, the whole body seemed to tense, and in the second, the whole body seemed to relax. Rita's general activity level seemed to top the list of the study children.

Summarizing the newborn picture, Rita showed a high level of organization and seemed to be an unusually well-endowed child with optimal potentialities which were heightened by superior charm and attractiveness. But two considerations kept the staff from being too optimistic. Her mother did not seem captivated by her charm, and her independence might reduce the adult's desire to serve a "helpless" infant. It was strange that such a perfect picture of a newborn tempted such dreary speculations. Perhaps it was just superstition about the "too glamorous" and the "too perfect."

After examining the baby the pediatrician visited Mrs. Neville, who asked if breast feeding would start right away. Later in the day the pediatrician returned and found the baby established at Mrs. Neville's side. She had been put to breast once, and Mrs. Neville reported that things had gone pretty well. But the next day she told the pediatrician that she really was not managing very well. She said, "The breasts are so large and heavy that I'm afraid they will smother the baby." The pediatrician suggested ways to support the breast during feeding and recommended a proper brassiere.

The baby awakened and cried a bit. Mrs. Neville said, "She looks so funny when she cries." The pediatrician reported a feeling that Mrs. Neville exhibited real detachment and separation from the baby, as if she were not concerned whether the baby was crying from discomfort or anything else.

One of the obstetricians reported that he was impressed with the enormous number of questions Mrs. Neville had about her own physical condition. It seemed to him that each day she reported a pain in her neck, back, or legs. He had the definite feeling that she had rather little interest in the baby and was primarily interested in herself.

One day when the interviewer commented how pretty Rita looked, Mrs. Neville said that she didn't think she was pretty but imagined that she would be all right in time. She commented that the baby looked like her husband. It was a marked change from her characterization of the baby immediately after birth as "beautiful." She complained how very uncomfortable she was feeling, that she was dizzy and her stitches hurt. Also, she mentioned that feeding wasn't going well and that Rita was a "bad girl" and wouldn't take her food.

To the pediatrician Mrs. Neville said that feeding was difficult because her breasts were so heavy. She added, "I can do it here with help, but I'm sure I won't be able to breast feed at home." The pediatrician then told her it might be more satisfactory to bottle feed, which would be perfectly reasonable. Mrs. Neville seemed quite relieved but said, "I don't want anyone to think I'm trying to get out of anything, but I can't see how breast feeding would be good if I can't do it well."

For a few days Mrs. Neville ran a fever, complained of headache and dizziness. She was given penicillin and aspirin. After she had expelled a bit of membrane that was left in the uterus, she began to feel better. During another visit the interviewer again commented on Rita's prettiness. Mrs. Neville asked, "Do you think so? I'm proud when people say she's pretty because I did have a hand in it." She said that her husband thought the baby was the most beautiful thing in the world, but she didn't think Rita was particularly pretty. Mrs. Neville was pleased with the change to bottle feeding because she was "learning how to do it before going home."

From the hospital Mrs. Neville went directly to her brother's home and remained there for three weeks. In a letter to the pediatrician she said that Rita was getting along well; "her main achievement has been to raise and hold her head fairly steadily when I burp her. . . . She has just started to suck her thumb but has not made a habit of it yet."

At home Rita's feeding became marked by irregularity in frequency and amount. By the beginning of her second month the day feedings became better regulated and lasted only from twenty to thirty minutes, but at night she would spend up to an hour and a half taking the bottle. To the Nevilles, as to so many parents, it seemed that the baby had stolen their sleep. The long night feedings continued for several weeks. Solids were introduced near the end of the second month, and Mrs. Neville thought this accounted for the variations in milk intake. But she was willing to try almost anything to prolong Rita's sleep, and thus she wanted to include solids in every feeding. Often in the middle of the night she took the baby to bed with her to keep her quiet. Rita was reported to be intolerant of waiting for her bottle and punctured the silent night with her screaming, which prompted Mrs. Neville to "scream back at her." At least once in the early months Rita screamed for an hour. Her distracted mother tried everything, including spanking. And then she was swept up in guilt over what she had done.

It was thus with relief that the parents left her with Mrs. Neville's brother at the age of seven weeks while they took a week's trip. The Nevilles found it refreshing once more to indulge in the carefree joy of travel together, and the week seemed much too short. Rita did very well in the sister-in-law's home and her mother commented, "Everyone tells me I should be glad that I can get rid of my daughter so easily." To her surprise she found that she had missed Rita.

The Nevilles' attractive apartment was reached by going up the building's back steps. The living room was warm and friendly, dominated by hundreds of paperback books and three original watercolors. In a middle-sized bedroom next to the living room the baby slept in a small crib at the foot of the Nevilles' bed. At the end of a very long hall was another room, now used as Mr. Neville's study, which they planned for a nursery when Rita was older.

At nine weeks of age Rita was brought by her mother for the first well-baby clinic visit. The feeding irregularities were discussed, but it could not be determined how disturbing they were to Mrs. Neville. She said that she didn't have anything else to do all day so she didn't worry whether or not Rita was regular. It was observed that she fed Rita by holding the baby at quite a distance, supported on her knees, with no cuddling at all. Although it appeared awkward, she seemed to have good control of the situation and handled the baby's body without difficulty.

On the whole, Mrs. Neville seemed pleased with her daughter and noted that Rita liked best of all to be talked to in her crib without being handled. Spontaneously she said she didn't pick Rita up much as she didn't want to spoil her. The pediatrician suggested that Rita might enjoy more attention and social stimulation. Mrs. Neville agreed that it would probably help her to develop faster but did not comment on the idea that it might be enjoyable as well. On the physical exam Rita was found to be well nourished, well developed, and in good condition. Her development as rated on the tests was normal, with perception and social responses exceeding gross motor development and body mastery. She seemed content to lie in the crib, looking at the adult and responding to facial expressions and voice of the adult. She apparently had less need to be handled physically than some other babies.

Mrs. Neville reported being able to do her housework in the mornings, leaving the afternoons free for other things. The fact that Rita required little time pleased her. Although she did not plan to return to full-time work, she thought she might take a part-time job or two if it were presented.

It was apparent that Mrs. Neville was anxious for her daughter to perform well. Several times she said, "Since she won't be beautiful, she had better be clever." Somehow Mrs. Neville thought that babies should be chubby to be attractive, and Rita did not conform in that respect. She displayed old pictures of herself as a baby, which she considered the model of a beautiful child.

In a home visit Mrs. Neville characterized the baby "as no trouble at all and very easy to take care of." In order to show the interviewer around the apartment, she left the baby strapped to the bathinette. At that time Rita was fussing and crying a little, but Mrs. Neville did not look back to see whether or not she was going to cry more vigorously. She gave Rita part of her bottle as she prepared lunch, but it did not seem to comfort her. When the baby continued to fuss during lunch Mrs. Neville arose with considerable determination, picked Rita up, blankets, pads, and all, and swooped out of the room, saying, "We must be excused." She put the baby on the large bed in the bedroom, where Rita continued to cry for possibly five or ten minutes. Mrs. Neville said that she would quiet in a matter of minutes if left alone and "the crying does her no harm."

Mrs. Neville was rather proud that she found it so simple to care for the baby and spontaneously said that if it were possible, she would like to be pregnant right now except that her husband had to complete his advanced study first. The interviewer asked how she planned to limit her family, and Mrs. Neville said, "Frankly, we have not had intercourse since the birth of the baby." They had used contraceptives in England, but she found them difficult to obtain here and wondered how one went about it. A nearby clinic was suggested.

The interviewer asked if she had missed sexual intercourse and

Mrs. Neville said that "It doesn't mean very much to me and it really is not important." Her husband had an orgasm in about ten minutes and she wouldn't have one for another half hour so there really wasn't much point in even trying. She said, also, that she imagined sex might be more important for other people because it was the only thing they had, but she and her husband were so close to one another and had so many common interests that it wasn't important.

Through most of these first months Mrs. Neville was subject to one or another physical disorder. Chief among these was her inability to lose weight, and she was as heavy as in late pregnancy. She found it difficult to limit her food intake because of her "sweet tooth." Beyond this difficulty she also was liable to severe menstrual distress and irregularity, as well as varicosities of her right leg.

Rita was free of serious illness during this period, although on several occasions a slight facial rash was reported. When Rita was two months old, her mother said the baby had episodes of "abdominal cramps," which disappeared as soon as cereal was discontinued. In the third month Mrs. Neville telephoned the pediatrician with much excitement over the fact that she had left Rita in the carriage and the sun had inadvertently shined directly on her head and face. Rita was hot and sunburned, and Mrs. Neville was quite distressed. Her worry was "that the heat might have done damage to the brain."

The irregularity which characterized feeding was also true for Rita's sleep pattern until about the middle of her third month, when Mrs. Neville discovered that the baby would sleep soundly through the night if put down in prone. Rita was reported to have four bowel movements a day during her fourth month, usually just after feeding. Mrs. Neville asked about toilet-training procedures, but added that she did not think much of using rewards in training. "The child should want to do this for its own sake."

In her third week Rita had started regular thumb-sucking and by three months would lie quietly in bed after awakening, sucking her thumb for as much as an hour. Sometimes she would put herself back to sleep with thumb-sucking. As early as three and a half months she was observed to respond differentially to her mother and another person, smiling at Mrs. Neville and crying at the pediatrician.

In clinic when Rita was three and one-half months old, Mrs. Neville asked if Rita's weight was satisfactory "because she doesn't eat as much as some babies." She described Rita's impatience at waiting for the bottle and how upset she became with the intensity of Rita's crying. She couldn't understand why Rita became so unhappy "when I'm trying to warm the bottle as fast as I can."

Throughout the examination Mrs. Neville constantly asked if the baby was "doing it right." When the baby began to cry she made an effort to calm her. When the baby continued to cry Mrs. Neville approached the crib, put her face quite close to Rita, and said, "Now you be a good girl." The baby looked at her mother and stopped crying. Each time Mrs. Neville held the baby she immediately quieted and looked around the room. Her mother reported that Rita smiled at everybody, but during the examinaton it was apparent that she smiled only at her mother and that crying was her uniform response to the examiner. Mrs. Neville seemed disappointed that Rita was not smiling, friendly, and performing the tasks set before her. She tried to do everything she could to improve Rita's mood to cooperate, but it was of little avail.

When Rita was four and a half months old, the psychological examiner who had seen her as a newborn declared, "The picture definitely contradicts my memory of Rita's earliest months." She felt that the pediatrician and the mother's interviewer were reluctant to reveal unpleasant feelings about developments or to clearly voice their disappointment. And the psychological examiner was equally reluctant to admit that "misery" had started much sooner than the staff had realized.

Rita screamed almost without provocation and for a longer duration than one would expect from a child of that age who had company and toys. It was difficult to decide whether the sound was pain, rage, or both. Her position was tense most of the time. Just once, when she was held and patted by her mother, did she look relaxed and at ease. But in no case did Rita smile.

In contrast to the baby's sad or angry mood, her mother seemed predominantly cheerful, with many smiles and numerous instances of laughing. But this mood did not transfer itself to Rita.

Upon second thought, it seemed that the mother's "cheerful mood" was artificial and that her laughter covered anxiety and a keen awareness that she was being observed behind the screen. This led to the hypothesis that Rita was quite sensitive to her mother's moods and was reacting to her mother's tension. It was also noted that Mrs. Neville showed no surface response or sympathy for Rita's misery.

She held the child with her left hand in a stiff unrelaxed way while the other arm was held empty and unused. The mother's body did not meet the child's. When she undressed the baby, she moved very quickly, and as the baby cried, her movements became even quicker. As the mother's movements gained rapidity, Rita's own movements became more hectic and accelerated. It became apparent that she diapered the baby as if she were "a thing" and was quite unaware of the baby's unhappiness.

Considering this, it was somewhat surprising that Rita was comforted when picked up by her mother. Although she neither cuddled nor really relaxed, she never cried in her mother's arms. Perhaps the warmth of the mother's body provided a promise of contentment to come, as contrasted with the absence of hope if she were not held.

When the rattle was put only three inches away from Rita's hands, she only approached it, and when it was placed in her hand, she did not manipulate it. There was no response to either the presence or absence of a toy. For a child close to her fifth month she showed unusually little investment in the things around her. In body mastery it was hard to evaluate Rita's potential. She was capable of turning from prone to supine but she never supported herself by the hands, and her head quite frequently "dropped" down altogether. Another feature of her motor behavior was that her movements were either very quick or strikingly slow. When lying in her crib kicking, the movements were quite rapid. When approaching an object they were hesitant and slow. It seemed that in her movements she expressed anger or anxiety more readily than by her facial expression.

The psychological examiner had the impression that "something had gone wrong with Rita's development" and that her response to the surrounding world had become negative and unrelated, that she lived unhappily in a void. Her wonderful independence as a newborn had transformed itself into a dreary and drab withdrawal. It was hypothetically postulated that perhaps the mother-child contact may not have developed satisfactorily, that Rita's initial self-reliance may have decreased the mother's motivation to comfort. Thus, the child was deprived of the warmth and human contact which it needed in order to grow. However that may be, it was obvious that Rita was at odds with her world. Despite these disturbing signs, however, Rita was still described as attractive and alert by staff members.

For the pediatric examination at the third well-baby clinic Mrs. Neville had prepared a number of written questions because she felt "her memory was so poor." One of the questions was whether Rita's hair would fall out before it began to grow in again. Another was whether to wake Rita at 11 P.M. for a late feeding in the hope that she would sleep longer during the night. She said that Rita had only recently been moved to a full-sized crib, and she wanted to know if the delay may have retarded her ability to turn over or move about. Now she felt guilty that they had not put up the crib sooner. There was an urgency in the manner in which she asked questions, as though she could not wait.

She related that the paternal grandmother had come East for a month's visit. Rita "was just perfect" throughout the visit, she said, and had not disturbed her grandmother's sleep at all. During the visit, however, Rita seemed to have a slight wheeze. Since the paternal grandfather had died of tuberculosis, the grandmother wanted to make certain that the wheeze was not associated with lung disease. The grandmother had also suggested that Rita should be started on a toilet pot, and Mrs. Neville wanted to know if "this was too early." She had read an article about toilet training and did not quite agree with the emphasis on praise and rewards. In her opinion, a child should "want to cooperate with toilet training for its own sake" and not just because the mother wanted it.

In a telephone conversation with the pediatrician when Rita was about five months old Mrs. Neville reported that she required feedings every two or three hours, and she asked about giving more solids with each feeding in the hope that this might lengthen the time between.

A week later she reported that Rita was sleeping from twelve to thirteen hours at night without any late feeding. Then she raised the question of moving the baby out of their bedroom to the far bedroom, which was quite isolated and rather cold. Instead the pediatrician suggested that Rita needed social contact and perhaps the playpen should be placed close to the mother's activity area. Mrs. Neville said that Rita vocalized a great deal and made noises described as "rather shrill, high-pitched screams like a cat on the back fence"; "but you can't do anything about this, like you can with a cat."

In the fifth month visit the interviewer described the apartment "as a lived-in home with quiet artistic color, clean but not scrupulously neat." Rita was in her crib in the bedroom, cooing and playing happily by herself. She smiled at the interviewer, who was again struck by her prettiness and delicacy. Mrs. Neville said that Rita was undressed because she had just had her bath and was waiting to be fed. She usually dressed her after the feeding so she wouldn't get her fresh clothes dirty. The interviewer picked up Rita and carried her to the kitchen. Rita looked at herself in the mirror, cooed, gurgled, and seemed quite happy.

Mrs. Neville placed Rita on a blanket on the floor and asked the interviewer if the baby didn't seem pale. On her back Rita bicycled, played with her hands, and picked up the rattle her mother had brought. Mrs. Neville reported that Rita sometimes cried and screamed and "nothing would stop her, even spanking." She said that when she heard Rita cry that way she "felt wild."

With considerable pleasure Mrs. Neville told the interviewer that she had lost seven pounds by dieting. Her mother-in-law provided the motivation, as she had really "given it" to her for becoming so heavy. As she talked, Mrs. Neville started to give Rita her bottle. Rita did not try to hold the bottle but extended her left arm and looked at her hand as she drank. Her mother said that Rita now waited patiently for her bottle and no longer screamed before the bottle arrived. She showed some recent pictures of Rita and remarked in her daughter's direction, "You will get on with your charm and not with your looks." She characterized her daughter's looks as "mousey, completely colorless."

The question was again raised about moving Rita to the far bedroom, which was close to a staircase that led down to an outside door. There was no way of locking that door, and Mrs. Neville said, "I'm nervous and quite afraid of being in an unlocked apartment."

She was also worried about fire hazards, and when she left the house she checked the burners and the heat two or three times to be sure they were off.

At the fourth well-baby clinic, when Rita was six months, Mrs. Neville again looked quite matronly and heavy-set, as if she had gained rather than lost weight. Rita's mood was better than at previous visits. She smiled broadly and vigorously kicked both feet against the bed. Mrs. Neville remarked that Rita did this so frequently that they had taken to calling her "thumper." She reported that the baby's feeding was rather stable at this time, but that the major feeding difficulty was that "she won't concentrate on eating." Rita was so distracted by sights and sounds that her mother "couldn't read" when she fed the baby because Rita looked up at each turning of a page.

Rita slept through the night from 6 or 7 P.M. until 7 A.M. and during the day had three brief naps following her meals. There was a persistent rash on Rita's cheeks, which disturbed her mother. She explained that Rita drooled a great deal and then rubbed her face so that it was constantly wet. She reportedly sucked her thumb only just before falling asleep, with no noticeable hand preference.

Mrs. Neville asked if it was all right to make a scheduled visit to her brother's home, since her niece had been exposed to chicken pox. Mr. Neville felt that it was too much of a risk. It seemed to the pediatrician that Mrs. Neville was reluctant to give up her pleasure, although she was concerned about possible scarring from chicken pox lesions.

The physical examination showed Rita to be rather frail in appearance, with a small skeletal frame. On the growth chart her weight appeared at the 3rd percentile level, and in length she was between the 10th and 25th percentiles. Her sitting was poor, showing a rounding in the lumbar region. At 26 weeks her performance was at the 24-week level. The impression was that she did not have much interest in inanimate objects. Mouthing of hands and objects was marked. There was a fine papular rash across both cheeks and a linear area of redness on both thighs, which corresponded to the area rubbed by the diaper edge or the edge of waterproof pants. No teeth were present.

When Rita was 7 months and 25 days she came for the fifth well-baby clinic. Mrs. Neville looked tired, not very well groomed, and as if she had continued to gain weight. She reported that she had given the liver and beef mixtures which had been suggested at the previous examination but that Rita took no more than three or four teaspoons at a feeding. Also, she had been unsuccessful in getting Rita to take egg in any form. She said that Rita was using her left hand a great deal and she had consciously tried to move objects from the left to the right hand in an effort to change her. Now she felt that this was wrong and had guilt feelings about having done it.

Mrs. Neville had been to a party where a baby three weeks younger than Rita already sat alone and pulled to stand. Since Rita was behind this child in development, Mrs. Neville asked the staff if she was "delayed in any way" and would the pediatrician tell her "if there was something wrong." She looked relieved when told that progress was along normal lines.

Mrs. Neville then reported that Rita recently had screaming and crying spells fairly often. These came at times when Mrs. Neville was sure she was not hungry, wet, or physically uncomfortable. It made her angry at Rita because "there was nothing to cry about." These episodes happened most frequently on Monday, a day in which she herself generally felt very depressed and unable to do her work. She wondered if the baby could sense her moods. She mentioned that her husband was engrossed in his work and studied from twelve to fourteen hours a day, and that it was quite lonely for her in the apartment. She said she would very much like to have some kind of a job because it would give her a feeling of being able to do something again. Being a housewife and mother were not sufficient. But her husband thought her job was to stay home and take care of Rita.

Upon examination the pediatrician found that Rita now appeared to be at least two months younger than her actual age. Her weight was now below the lowest 3rd percentile and her length remained between the low 10th and 25th percentiles. She was unable to pull herself into sitting position, and when assisted, she sat only briefly erect and then fell to one or another side. Her body contour except for her face was thin, and muscle tone was poor. Her skin was clear, head was symmetrically rounded, and one lower central incisor was present in the mouth. Chest, heart, abdomen, genitalia, and extremities were all within normal range.

At 34 weeks of age Rita gave a fairly solid performance in all four areas on the Gesell test at the 28-week level. Her performance on the Viennese test showed a depression below her age in all areas. She was two months below in body mastery, one month below in social response, one and one-half months below in learning, and two months below in material usage.

Generally the child gave a test profile which was typical of an institutionalized child. She was retarded in weight as well as in her developmental performance. Since the extent of retardation was not known, it was not discussed. The pediatrician planned to make a home visit as soon as possible to attempt to find out more about the handling of the child and to suggest ways in which Mrs. Neville might extend her areas of contact and stimulation.

For the first time the pediatrician recognized that Mrs. Neville had used most of their contact time to talk about herself and only superficially about Rita. Now the pediatrician clearly felt that by keeping herself in the foreground Mrs. Neville had possibly kept the pediatrician from knowing about the child and had obscured the quality of her inadequate relationship with Rita.

The psychological evaluation at this well-baby clinic emphasized these impressions in more concrete detail. The report noted that the usual eight-month stranger anxiety was reversed with Rita. With the mother's approach her whimpering became definite crying or screaming, but it was just the opposite in reaction to the examiner's approach. In fact, in one instance the baby smiled when the examiner talked to her. It appeared that Rita exhibited an intense and unique emotional reaction to her mother.

In grasping objects Rita still raked them in rather than firmly grasping them. When she finally reached an object she pushed it away from herself instead of bringing it towards herself and handling it. Except for the bell, she did not keep any object for more than a few seconds. This was consistent with the observation four months earlier that inanimate objects had no emotionally positive quality for her but reflected instead the negative reaction to her mother.

For the short periods that Rita held an object she held it at the wrong end. Not even by accident did she ever grasp any of the rattles by their handles. The same applied to the cup. However, when the bell was offered and softly rung, she smiled slightly and grasped first at the bell part then quickly and skillfully shifted to the handle, manipulating it quite expertly. It became apparent that her grasping and handling difficulties were not due to neuromuscular immaturity or deviation but more plausibly to lack of investment or to negative emotional investment. It looked as if she deliberately "tried" not to hold or to keep objects.

She hardly mouthed at all, did not suck her fingers, and did little contacting of any part of the body with any other part of the body. When set in front of the mirror, Rita started to cry. It was not clear whether crying was due to displeasure at seeing her mirror image or to discomfort created by the sitting position. In sitting she was only at the four to five month level, with an amazing limpness of the shoulders that gave the physiognomical impression of not enough "resistance" in this body to keep it erect.

There were very few active leg movements. Creeping in prone, as far as it was observed, was mostly produced by hand movements with the legs dragging rather than pushing. When lying quietly in prone, she did not support herself by her hands only. Nor was she able to remain resting on one elbow when grasping a toy with the other. Then she lay almost flat or tumbled to one side.

The psychological observer commented that "this child looked like four or five months at best." But even for a child that age she showed some peculiarities. She was not thin in the usual constitutional sense of some skinny and bony babies, but with the limp unmuscular thinness that is seen in very sick or institutionalized children. Her face was prevalently sad. Even if she was not crying, and she cried most of the time, the corners of her mouth drooped and her eyes were wide open in a pained and painful stare.

The dismay of the staff was matched by Mrs. Neville's own discouragement. It seemed that every conference with pediatrician or child psychologist was an occasion for tears and screaming by Rita. Mrs. Neville had never seen any beauty in her baby, but she had set great store on her being charming and intelligent. And now her daughter perversely embarrassed her efforts to calm her and steadfastly refused to perform. Mrs. Neville's spirits were at a very low level.

On their part, the pediatrician and child psychologist saw an undernourished and desperately unhappy child whose behavior seemed reminiscent of the effects of "hospitalism" and maternal deprivation. The psychologist declared, "If attempts to improve Rita's emotional environment failed and the next test showed a further decrease of general developmental level, serious preventive measures would have to be taken, as such disturbances tend to become irreversible."

It was decided to make specific recommendations for systematic body massage of the child, systematic play periods to introduce toys and social stimulus, and increased food intake if possible by improved mother-child contact during meals. It was also agreed to make more frequent home visits during this critical period.

The interviewer was invited to supper on the same evening of the above distressing clinic examination. She described Mrs. Neville "as very fat now, with her face, hair, and whole appearance depressed and unattractive." Mr. Neville was described as moderately tall, slender, rather shy, and in need of a haircut. Rita was in her crib for the night, but the interviewer was told that she might see her. The baby greeted the interviewer with a smile and played with her bracelet when she offered it. Mr. Neville knelt beside the crib and tapped the slats on the side, saying that each slat made a different noise and one could play a song on it. He laughed with Rita and played peek-a-boo with her. When they left, Rita whimpered and cried for possibly a half hour. But her mother made no effort to have her join in any way in the social event.

At dinner Mr. Neville discussed the taxing demands of his work and studies. Mrs. Neville added that he was often away from home until late at night and that she was so lonely "she could scream." She said she was looking forward to spring: that it could not possibly be as bad as the winter has been. Mr. Neville listened rather stoically but sympathetically and did not try to minimize her trouble.

Mrs. Neville then asked the interviewer if she would be told if something were going wrong with Rita "not only physically but mentally." She was concerned, because at a party she had noticed a younger baby who was much more advanced than Rita. She said it made her miserable because she wanted Rita to be "the best person in the room." Her husband commented that he just wanted his daughter to be a genuine person and would like her just as she was, no matter what she was. Mrs. Neville interrupted to say, "He wouldn't like her if she were a genuine half-wit." He answered that obviously she wasn't and he still believed that people should only be expected to be themselves. He added that though he disagreed with his wife, he knew she was a good mother and loved Rita. Mrs. Neville said she knew she was a good mother. She was strict, and she "would hit Rita and hit her hard, but also love her and love her hard."

Mr. Neville commented that the way his wife talked about Rita to outsiders and friends, it appeared as if she "didn't like Rita and was always pointing out her weak points." His wife answered, "Maybe so, but there's no point in wearing your heart on your sleeve." She thought it was ridiculous to go around pretending your child was absolutely perfect when you knew she was not. She could not understand why her husband never saw any of Rita's faults and added quite bitterly, "How can love be so blind?"

She said that she worried terribly when Rita did not perform well at the Child Study Center, and she had cried all afternoon after the last test. She spoke of a baby who was not developing properly but who improved after being given some kind of injection and she wondered whether Rita should have such treatment. The interviewer said that the staff would watch Rita's development very carefully to determine what if anything might be the trouble at this point. She also pointed out that some babies needed a little more stimulation than others and suggested that Mrs. Neville play and talk with Rita more.

Mrs. Neville immediately stated that she played very little with Rita and didn't do much with her because being with her was "really a bore." She had never liked babies even before Rita, and it was all new to her. Then she asked, "How do you play with a baby?" She felt that her "blue moods" were transmitted to Rita, especially on "blue Mondays," and then Rita screamed so long that in the end Mrs. Neville found herself spanking her hard. As she reported this, Mrs. Neville became disturbed to the point of tears. She said that some days she felt so bad she just sat around and read a novel, giving Rita little or no attention. She said she had anticipated this trouble before having the baby and that was why she had hoped to find part-time work.

Mr. Neville praised his wife's creative activity in London and hoped that she would continue her ad copy work at home. But she said that it was not the specific work she needed but "just to get out and have a job which would make her feel better because she was respected for her work." She stated that having a baby was definitely not enough for her; that maybe if she had another baby she would feel better because then she "would really be fed up with the diapers" and would have more than she could do. Mrs. Neville said she knew she made everyone miserable but that she was driven into those patterns by "the ghost of her frustrated mother."

A few days later the pediatrician visited and reported to Mrs. Neville that the tests showed that Rita's development was not satisfactory and she seemed in need of more stimulation and contact. Mrs. Neville said she had tried to point out to her husband and mother-in-law that Rita had problems, but they just thought she was an overly concerned mother. Her husband could see no fault with Rita and did not like continued discussion over and over on the same thing. She felt she had nobody to talk things over with, especially since she could not freely discuss things with her brother as before.

The pediatrician outlined in detail how to play with a baby, to massage the body, flex the extremities, and stimulate the skin with some kind of oil. She prescribed propping the baby in a sitting position on pillows for a ten-to-fifteen minute daily play period with three toys: a rattle, a soft cuddly animal and soft bells. She also suggested music records, particularly containing a human voice, which Mrs. Neville and Rita could enjoy together.

The pediatrician further discussed the area of feeding and suggested that solids could be taken better in a sitting position. She urged that Mrs. Neville keep a simple diary and record what Rita ate, what she liked and disliked. Above all, the pediatrician stressed the hope that Mrs. Neville would get some pleasure from playing with and caring for the baby. Another suggestion was that she should eat at the same time with Rita and thus make eating more of a pleasure through the "sharing" process.

At a subsequent visit Mrs. Neville demonstrated how she gave Rita the massage. In one brief motion she rubbed some drops of oil on both legs and the lower part of the baby's back and rubbed briskly for a few strokes. The whole procedure took aproximately five to ten seconds and appeared as if she were applying polish to furniture. Mrs. Neville then mentioned that she had noticed a slightly discolored area over the lower sacrum (Mongolian spot) and wondered whether this had anything to do with Rita "being slow." It surprised the interviewer that after having cared for the baby this many months it had just come to Mrs. Neville's attention.

Mrs. Neville pointed out that Rita had cut another lower incisor and it looked as if her teeth "were coming in crooked." She seemed quite concerned because her own teeth had been crooked as a child and several had had to be extracted before they straightened themselves out. It had made her quite self-conscious and unhappy.

She showed the interviewer pictures she had taken of a squirrel that came to sit on the window sill of the living room. The squirrel was rather repulsive to her because it reminded her of a rat and she had always feared dogs, cats, rats, etc. She told how her father tried to overcome this fear by making her get close to a dog. He wanted her to be "a big brave girl" while all she wanted was to be "a little girl behind her mother's skirts."

In school it had been important for her to "excel with distinction," and if she brought home a poor report card, her father wouldn't speak to her for two days. She said she "hated school and had no mind for facts," that her "mind is like a sieve, things stay a while and then are gone." She often had tutors and finally came through "with distinction."

When the pediatrician visited two weeks later Mrs. Neville said that she had been "working on a fifteen-minute play period a day" as suggested, plus the massages, but that it was a rather "boring" period for herself. She demonstrated the "play period" by placing Rita on the floor in prone and surrounding her with three toys. Then she turned away from her and made no further contact with the baby during the visit. Soon Mr. Neville arrived and greeted Rita in a soft voice. He took her in his arms and seated himself in a chair. She began to whimper and he held her close against his body and face as if to comfort her, saying, "I don't see her very much but we get a chance to get acquainted on weekends." The crying was brief but Rita continued to look at him soberly and intently.

At the well-baby clinic in Rita's ninth month her mother reported with great pleasure and excitement that she had pulled herself into a standing position the night before by holding onto the side of the crib. She said that now Rita reacted to strangers with strong crying. During a carriage ride one day Rita "screamed for a solid half hour until she exhausted herself and fell asleep." The pediatrician said that Rita needed to be held and reassured during this period, and to "spoil her as much as possible at this stage." Mrs. Neville said if she held her for five minutes then it would soon be ten, and it would become "an unending cycle." When she commented that Rita provoked her to the point of slapping, the pediatrician explained that it was inappropriate to spank Rita as she had no way of understanding but instead needed to be reassured of Mrs. Neville's presence. Mrs. Neville retorted, "I always hit the people I have close relationships with; that's just the way I am."

She discussed her "blue spells" and said she did not know what caused them. The pediatrician suggested that Mrs. Neville might be helped by professionally trained people to understand and manage her feelings. She immediately answered that she "didn't believe in psychology, no one was really well adjusted, and psychologists were cold persons who did not have any liking for people as individuals." She felt that "as long as an individual got along all right, that's the important thing; people do have problems and difficulties, but that's life." She said that her own mother had not known what to do in bringing her up, and didn't have anybody to tell her, but she had turned out all right after all.

The pediatrician's examination disclosed that Rita's weight still fell well below the 3rd percentile and height was maintained between the 10th and 25th percentile. Body contour was thin and muscle tone poor. Skin was clear except for a slight diaper rash. At 39 weeks of age on the Gesell tests her only age adequate performance was in the fine motor coordination. In all other areas she was from two to seven weeks below age. On the Viennese tests her developmental age was rated at 6 months, 27 days, with a developmental quotient of 76.

The impression was that this child continued to be retarded in weight as well as in her developmental performance, and there was little indication that the program which had been instituted had made any real or significant change. It seemed that Mrs. Neville tried to deny her lack of progress and had strong feelings against seeking help for herself. It was evident that circumstances had produced an almost complete breakdown of the mother-child relationship and that Mrs. Neville's own unhappiness clearly threatened her mental health. She felt imprisoned in her house and the cold gloom of the winter fed her depressed feelings. She felt that her husband did not understand her problem and was immersed in his own world. As the winter progressed, tension within her rose to such a point that on some days she was almost incapable of functioning at all.

The effect of these moods on Rita was clearly obvious. Physical contact between mother and child had always been minimal, now it was reduced to the briefest possible duration. She did not hold the child lest she be involved in an unending cycle, and she shied away from close physical or social contact with the baby.

Signs also appeared that she had become indifferent to her hitherto expressed concern about Rita's appearance and behavior. Sometimes she didn't appear to notice that Rita's clothing was twisted and out of place. Mainly she was angry that the child screamed and cried inconsolably. Her attempts at soothing were sporadic, awkward, and ineffective. It was discovered that Rita often wakened several times a night and fought sleep for up to an hour, yet Mrs. Neville said that her daughter presented "no particular sleeping difficulties."

Rita's response to these experiences only intensified the problem. Her appetite was poor and became poorer; physically she appeared younger than her age; mentally her development showed an alarming lag. Always irritable, she now began to have days when she seemed to scream constantly. Frequent upsets complicated the problem.

It was climaxed by an episode of illness, which started when Rita vomited throughout the day and had a fever. In panic Mrs. Neville brought Rita to the emergency clinic when she couldn't reach the pediatrician. It was diagnosed as a slight throat infection. The ailment receded in a few days under an injection of penicillin and modifications in Rita's diet. Two days later Mrs. Neville herself had a temperature of 104 degrees and was seen by her doctor. Mr. Neville stayed home and took care of both of them. He moved Rita out of the bedroom so as not to disturb his wife, and from his reports of Rita's progress it appeared that he was managing quite adequately.

In the meantime, a meeting of the research staff was held to evaluate the situation. The staff felt that if there was no appreciable change very soon, severe measures should be proposed because the child was in jeopardy. The situation was complicated by the fact that Mrs. Neville denied that anything was wrong and refused help for herself. Yet she realized that something was seriously wrong with Rita by her question, "Can physically weak children develop intellectually?" Methods of bringing Mrs. Neville to accept psychotherapy were outlined, including telling her directly that the baby was not developing properly and that "mothers are not always the best thing for babies." It was also noted that the study group had not missed clues that this mother's attitude would create difficulties but that they had not acted on this insight. Also emphasized were the particular kind of clues that could be regarded as serious danger signals in a mother-child relationship.

A visit was made by Mrs. Neville to her brother's home after the birth of his second child. This apparently helped to break the cycle of her depression. She was pleasantly surprised that care of her three-year-old niece was easier than she had expected. The comings and goings of many friends and neighbors provided companionship and conversation which she had sorely missed in the drab dreary confinement of winter. During her stay she lost five pounds without any effort. She also felt that Rita had improved during the sojourn as she had very much enjoyed being with her three-year-old cousin.

Since her holiday Mrs. Neville felt that "things were all right now between Rita and me." A further cause for her elevated spirits was that the Nevilles had received an unexpected income tax refund and were planning to rent a cottage at the shore for the month of June. Mr. Neville would have a two-week holiday, and the other two weeks he would commute by bus. Mrs. Neville recalled the dreadful winter and vowed that she "would never go through that again." To prevent it, they were trying to find living quarters closer to Mr. Neville's office so that he could be home more often.

The subsequent pediatric examination in Rita's tenth month disclosed that there was some improvement in her general development. Her weight continued to be retarded, but the retardation had not increased in the last six weeks. Her age-adequate behavior with the pellet seemed to exclude the possibility that there was neurological involvement. For the first time there was some definite upward trend in the development quotient. At 10 months,

12 days on the Gesell test she rated a development quotient of 94.2, and on the Viennese test her developmental age was 8 months, 24 days, with a developmental quotient of 84.6.

Mrs. Neville showed a decrease in anxiety and seemed less tense in her relationship with Rita. While her response to the child's unhappiness was still different from other mothers, it appeared that she was at least better able to meet needs than before, that it might be sufficient to permit continuing progress and growth.

On this same date the psychological observer noted, "It is difficult to get in contact with Rita or sustain her interest." She still showed little interest in toys, grasping and letting them go without much investment. The greatest interest and even possibly pleasure was provoked by the bell, but when it was taken from her and covered with a diaper, she made no attempt to reach it but cried and moaned in a heart-breaking way. When the diaper was removed and the bell returned to her, she went on moaning for quite a time and up to the end of the examination showed no further pleasure or interest in the bell.

A facial tic had developed, with one eye squinted and the corner of her mouth drawn up on the same side. This occurred mostly when she was faced with a more intense stimulation than she had expected. The same grimace also appeared when a person started to talk to her. Although she was now able to sit without support, her equilibrium was precarious. If any unevenness was created on the surface where she was sitting, Rita could not compensate by any positional change of hips, pelvis, or shoulders and therefore tended to tumble to the side.

Despite the poor body integration it seemed highly improbable that the developmental picture was due to neurological damage because the fine motor coordination of her hands was excellent. And it also seemed unlikely that mental retardation on a congenital basis was responsible for Rita's condition.

Three days later a new interviewer from the research group visited the Nevilles at home. She found Mrs. Neville sociable and chatty. Mrs. Neville told her how difficult it was to change her occupation and way of life to that of a housekeeper and mother. She thought it was hard for a person "who had a place in the world" to be spending all her time doing housework and taking care of a baby.

The interviewer's impression of Rita was that she was even more subdued, passive, and deprived at home than was obvious at clinic visits. Her face had a kind of blank staring expression, and the interviewer was struck by the silence of the child and her isolation. On a couple of occasions Rita rocked violently in her chair, but there was no smile or pleased expression, only intensity. Her mother said she rocked like that frequently "and likes it." It seemed to the interviewer that Mrs. Neville wanted to do the right thing but didn't know how. At the same time, her heart went out to Rita for the unsympathetic, unresponsive, and even forbidding climate in which she lived.

A few days later the pediatrician was called about Rita's "screeching" for the past several nights. It seemed that the nighttime awakenings and crying had been taking place for some time. There was also "screeching" during the daytime as well. The pediatrician made a house call to see if Rita were physically well. Her appetite had further decreased, according to Mrs. Neville, and she ate little during the day. During the night disturbances she occasionally took some milk, which seemed to satisfy and return her to sleep. The pediatrician found no evidence of physical illness.

The well-baby clinic visit when Rita was almost a year of age was an ordeal for all concerned. Mrs. Neville and Rita had come by bus from the summer cottage at the beach. Whether the baby was tired from lack of a nap or other causes, she cried from the moment of arrival. It did not seem possible to reach her in any way or to comfort her. The psychological observer said, "I have never heard a crying quite like this in all my experience with children. One could not help feeling that Rita revealed utter despair relating to a terrible past, to an unbearable present, and to a future which she did not want to experience."

At the examiner's suggestion, the mother gave her the bottle. She sucked eagerly for a very short period, then let the bottle go and started to cry again. The examiner made numerous attempts to comfort her in a soft and tender voice, with smiles and delicate patting. Nothing helped. At the examining table Rita tentatively began to approach the objects, and her eyes lost their empty stare. Finally the crying stopped while she played with the toys. She looked neither at her mother or the examiner but only at the toys and nothing else. One had the impression that this small inanimate world around her was all she could bear.

She grasped the objects without really closing her fingers around them. The main aspect of her play was an approaching of the objects on the table in front of her and pushing them away afterwards, repeating the game over and over again. When the mother tried to put Rita down in the crib, she became so stiff that one could not sit her down. The whole body, and especially the legs, formed a slight arc. Her screaming and behavior began to look like a temper tantrum full of frustration and pain. Mrs. Neville's anxiety and frustration added to the tension.

The pediatrician noted that Rita was a very attractive but utterly miserable little girl with a small, thin, but well-proportioned body. There was a fine papular rash over the face and shoulders. All physical findings were negative, genitalia and extremities were normal. But her anxiety and inconsolable reactions were unique for a child of this age. The inability of the mother to provide comfort was startling. It was a miserable experience for everyone, including the staff, and the examination ended quite early under the circumstances.

While waiting for Mr. Neville to pick them up, Mrs. Neville made many apologies for Rita's behavior. The interviewer commented that Rita's crying must be hard on her, but Mrs. Neville said it didn't bother her at all. She knew there was nothing she could do about it and so she just let her cry. She further commented that she was bothered only when Rita "screamed," especially when she was supposed to go to sleep. Apparently, she differentiated between the extreme crying that the staff had heard and what she called screaming. Rita had fallen asleep on Mrs. Neville's lap, and the interviewer was struck by the changed appearance of her little face, which was puckered up in a worn out, ravished, and anxious expression.

Rita's first birthday was celebrated with a party in the beach house. At this time she impressed those who saw her as a most attractive little girl. Superficially it seemed that her life had been tranquil. Mrs. Neville had worked out a child-care regime which seemed to satisfy Rita's basic needs but still involved minimal physical contact. As the child's powers grew, however, her mother enjoyed being with her more and more. Like her husband, Mrs.

Neville loved to teach Rita the names of colors, of objects in her baby book or in the room.

As Rita began to walk, outsiders marveled at the way knick-knacks and other breakable items were left unscathed within the child's reach. Mrs. Neville saw no need to put a protective gate at the end of the long hall to guard Rita from falling down the staircase. Instead she felt that she could teach Rita to avoid it. In deportment, some thought Rita could be called a "model child." But this was not wholly true. She still had a marked and prolonged fear of strangers and could but poorly tolerate changes of place or routine. She continued to have tantrums of screaming, and there developed a pattern of the child hitting the mother in anger — and receiving payment in kind.

Mrs. Neville had given up hopes of finding a new and more conveniently located apartment. As her husband's studies demanded more and more time, she was left pretty much to her own resources. She rejected the thought of getting a job because she could not leave Rita unless she found the proper person to care for her, and that was an insurmountable difficulty. She thought about evening teaching, but her lack of citizenship prevented it. She compromised by becoming more interested in other mothers and their children.

At fourteen and one-half months Rita had a fever, lost her appetite, and had diarrhea. These symptoms, together with a blotchy rash on face and body, continued for several days and were diagnosed as roseola infantum. From that time, and throughout her second year, Rita's appetite for both solids and milk went down. She could not "manage" thick or lumpy foods and had a tendency to gag and retch on them. She was chronically reported as "a poor eater." She shared meals with her parents but was likely to play with her food. Mrs. Neville tried to prohibit this messing.

Sleep continued to be interrupted several times during the night. Mrs. Neville took to leaving the bottle in the crib, and Rita no longer cried but drank her bottle and continued to suck on the nipple until she went back to sleep. During and after her bout with roseola the child tired easily and took longer daytime naps. Her mother was concerned about her general fatigue and asked if a "tonic" was indicated.

Soon after Rita's first birthday Mrs. Neville started to put her on a seat which fit on the toilet. Because the baby's first bowel movement of the day was quite regular, just after breakfast, she managed to catch it quite easily. But after the roseola, toileting did not go well because Rita's bowel movements became quite irregular. Although her mother reported that Rita "mouthed everything," rarely was any mouthing seen during home or clinic visits. If Rita even ventured to put something close to her mouth, Mrs. Neville immediately said "no, no."

At this time Rita could walk if her hands were held, and she crawled with a crab-like gait on hands and feet. Clearly she enjoyed the locomotion and had evolved a chasing game with her mother. She was not particularly interested in toys or books but preferred moving from room to room or playing with water. Her speech, too, was limited, confined mainly to specialized sounds. Rita was more manageable outside, where she was interested in everything. Mrs. Neville remarked, "She is unbearable if she doesn't get out." Rita's fear of strangers was still remarkably strong. Some of this sensitivity was seen at the clinic, where Rita was so fearful and uneasy, even on her mother's lap, that she was distracted by the slightest noise.

But as Rita began to improve her capabilities, her mother was more able to relax her insatiable demands for perfection. There was greater interchange between mother and child, and Mrs. Neville said, "She's a sweet human being now." She looked forward to teaching Rita things and playing with her. Mrs. Neville's fears of spoiling her daughter were also tempered. Although she felt strongly that it was bad manners, she allowed the child to wander away from her place at the table and sometimes to finish a meal on her daddy's lap.

It was in the routines of child care that this greater flexibility on Mrs. Neville's part was most marked during Rita's second year. Perhaps there was a correlation between Rita's continued poor appetite and her mother's willingness to allow latitude in behavior at meals. Or perhaps the child's alternate attacks of diarrhea and constipation which followed the roseola caused her not to enforce strict toilet training. In any event, Mrs. Neville did not make it an area of struggle. Throughout the whole second year Rita's sleep was again irregular, but Mrs. Neville did not react to this in any marked way and was willing to let Rita fall off to sleep with a bottle.

In home visits the pediatrician found Rita less frightened of the stranger and able to tolerate women better than men. She responded to the pediatrician amiably and even initiated some contact with her. The pediatrician's impression was that Rita's increased activity and better behavior, and development had improved the relationship between mother and child. Mrs. Neville found it easier to fulfill the role of teacher and guide than to give emotionally of herself to a helpless infant.

At the well-baby clinic in Rita's fifteenth month the psychological observer noted that her face had lost its childish softness and appeared hard, bitter, and hostile. She still cried much more easily than other children did, but the character of the crying was completely changed. It was no longer a cry of despair but the screaming and yelling of rage. Its main quality was protest, directed against the adults around her. The staff was struck by the terrifying amount of hostility, by the grotesqueness of her expression.

Even in laughter, or what was defined as laughter, the eyes did not laugh but remained wide open and anxiously staring. Her face reminded one of a mask which did not know whether to laugh or scream with pain. If the sounds which accompanied this facial expression had not sounded like laughter, it would not have been understood as such.

In her reaction toward inanimate objects, however, she no longer showed the same hostility as she did toward people. She seemed interested in the toys offered to her and functioned quite adequately with them. Observed while playing, she did not differ considerably from any other child of her age. If any toy was taken from her, however, she clung to it so desperately that the examiner had difficulties in going through the routines of the examination. The emotional quality of her reaction was so great that the adult was apprehensive of taking anything away from a child who seemed to need it so desperately.

It seemed that in her experience of deep disappointment with the human object she had given up mourning for it and had turned toward the world of inanimate objects, which she "could hold on to." This turning away from the human being, however, could only be done by reversing the emotions, by hating instead of loving, and the staff wondered how such a transfer to inanimate objects would influence later development. The research group speculated whether this was a "deviant" child, whose structure had become manifest in the second year whereas in the first year it could only be spotted as retarded development, or whether the development was totally the result of the environmental picture. It was felt that the course of further development might support either the environmental or the constitutional hypothesis.

At the evaluative observation when Rita was 16½ months old, she looked rosy and less frail than before. For the first time in over a year she had made a significant weight gain, and the developmental tests showed her to be performing not only age adequately but above the norms in all sectors.

On the Gesell test she was given a general maturity level at 17 months and a developmental quotient of 103. On the Viennese test she was given a developmental age of 21 months and a developmental quotient of 132.5.

Rita was matter-of-fact and busy at her tasks, at times even concentrated. She spent more than five minutes filling the cup with cubes and taking them out. Throughout this activity she left one cube on the table and one cube in the cup. She never emptied either the table or the cup completely.

With the spinning top, Rita touched it once, then startled, shook her head, but touched it again. The second time she backed off without losing sight of the top until she reached the wall but returned and touched the top again, and then again. After the fourth attempt she picked a dry leaf from the table and used it as an intermediary to touch the top. Her favorite object was the ball, which she threw with a gesture that other children would use to catch or grasp it. When the ball was gone, she giggled, squealed, laughed, and screeched with excitement. Her eyes gleamed and glowed radiantly. Her whole body became tense. But she did not get up to get the ball. Instead she waited until it was given to her and then she repeated the game.

She fed the teddy bear adequately with the little milk bottle. She did not hold him but placed him on the table and fed the bottle with her left hand. It seemed that Rita was basically left-handed but used her right occasionally because of her mother's instructions. When she finished feeding, she hit the teddy bear's head with increased speed and vigor, then suddenly interrupted this "spanking" to give the bear to the examiner. She shook her head and said "no." She did not stop the head-shaking "no" gesture until the examiner took the bear away. When the rubber cat with the protruding tongue was shown to her she reacted with an immediate "no" and withdrew. Although she did not whimper, cry, or scream, her facial expression was unmistakably anxious, and she could not be induced to touch the rubber cat.

Rita's reluctance to be touched by the examiner did not mean that she was not in contact with her. On the contrary, she remained in constant contact but on her own terms. She gave objects to the examiner or pointed at her to provide objects. Except in the ball play Rita hardly looked at her mother. Most of the time Rita remained in her chair and left it only when her mother invited her to do so, such as to play ball. When she walked, she walked slowly and hesitantly as if to find out whether it was safe to walk. No impulse or pleasure in locomotion was observed.

Rita no longer appeared like a retarded child. The formerly observed bizarreness of facial expression had disappeared. But some action patterns had developed to indicate that her recovery had been made at a rather high cost and that some personality problems had developed. These showed in terms of separation (the trauma when an object was removed from her grasp, the lack of impulse to get it back); the reluctance to be touched and the reports of hitting herself; the outside compulsion to be active versus the inhibition in locomotion; and the need to avoid (as in refusal to touch the rubber cat).

In Rita's seventeenth month the paternal grandmother and her husband visited the Nevilles a number of times. The grandmother was critical of Mrs. Neville's handling and urged that she be stricter with Rita "because she has a terrible temper and needs breaking." This made Mrs. Neville uncomfortable, and she kept her contacts with the mother-in-law brief and superficial.

Mr. Neville continued to carry a heavy work load, which left little time for his wife and child. He discussed his choice of a profession at length with the interviewer during a home visit and impressed her as a talkative, friendly but serious man. On the subject of Rita he was an enthusiastic and spontaneous reporter.

During the period when Rita was cutting her pre-molars she was quite irritable and refused a number of foods for a while. Other than this, her eating went quite well and she was almost exclusively on table foods, insisting on feeding herself. She still preferred her bottle to the glass, and Mrs. Neville was slightly embarrassed that "such a big girl still takes a bottle." Her sleep at night was still interrupted with episodes of crying, but a bottle usually helped to pacify her. Mrs. Neville reported that upon her mother-in-law's insistence she tried to let Rita "cry it out" but on one occasion after fifteen or twenty minutes "the baby was near hysteria." Rita seemed to remain dry for two or three hours at a time, and Mrs. Neville habitually put her on the toilet after meals. On this she reported that "we are coming along nicely."

Mrs. Neville reported that Rita would hit her own body "whenever she doesn't get her way." She discussed possible ways of stopping it for fear that Rita would "begin to have temper tantrums." By the time Rita was eighteen months old this pattern had been supplanted by episodes of hostile staring in which mother and daughter engaged in silent and controlled struggle, sometimes for minutes at a time. It seemed to the staff that in these recurrent struggles early feelings of rejection and hatred, now mostly controlled, would flare briefly.

Rita delighted in walking and walked quite well by now. She followed her mother around the house and imitated her in household chores. On outdoor walks she kicked leaves and ran about. Also she began to develop friends of her own, particularly two little boys with whom she loved to play.

Mrs. Neville giggled at the "romance" she fancied was being enacted before her eyes. She said that Rita "held her own" with other children, "growled like a tiger" when she wanted something, and revealed fighter qualities. But she noted that Rita never hit any of her playmates because "I've never spanked Rita, so she doesn't know about hitting."

As Rita's second year progressed, the Nevilles' social world expanded. For the first time Mrs. Neville was willing to leave her daughter with a baby sitter, which enabled them to make several trips to New York. And Mrs. Neville began to cooperate with other mothers in arrangements whereby each would take the others' children on specific days. Mrs. Neville became much more attractive and lively than in former months, with more attention to dress and grooming. She had lost ten pounds without having to diet. Nevertheless, she reported that she had not been feeling well and suffered from pains in the back of her head and dizzy spells.

During a home visit Mrs. Neville discussed at some length her criticism of psychologists and psychiatrists. She cited in detail the case of a friend who was made worse by going to a psychiatrist, and commented that "even if you start out with only a little wrong, by the time you're through you have a real complex." She expressed relief that the study psychologists "only observe Rita and don't do anything to her."

Rita had three attacks of diarrhea and vomiting between her sixteenth and eighteenth months but no specific pathology could be detected. Restriction of food intake, prescription of boiled milk, and some medication on the last occasion resulted in a recession of the symptoms. The rash on elbows, knees, and buttocks persisted, however, as it had for several months. Food intake was quite selective, and Rita's appetite was only fair. Milk intake was between 24 and 32 ounces per day, almost all by bottle. Mrs. Neville had solved the problem of night-time interruption by leaving a bottle of milk in Rita's crib after she was asleep. The bottle was usually empty in the morning.

Mr. Neville still spent long hours in the office or at study and came home after Rita was in bed. He insisted on getting her up to play despite Mrs. Neville's objections that "he lets her get away with murder." However, Rita had no difficulty returning to sleep after such arousals.

After a fairly long period of cooperation Rita began to refuse being placed on the toilet. She would run away and say "no." The Nevilles bought a potty chair, which she seemed to like, but then Mrs. Neville reported that Rita "became agitated" at seeing the bowel movement or detecting the odor and "seemed for a few moments to be about to vomit."

At well-baby clinic visits Rita appeared to be an unsmiling, sober child who performed adequately in most situations but showed a low level of social responsiveness. At home she was observed to have a special way of showing anger towards her mother and strangers by suddenly becoming tense, her body rigid, her arms raised and an expression of great intensity upon her face. Mrs. Neville called it "looking daggers." Rita also continued trying to stare her mother down, and Mrs. Neville's own attempts to outstare Rita were unsuccessful. She remarked that "the princess is hard to live with some of the time" and felt that the glaring may have become a substitute for Rita's hitting behavior.

Rita was quite willing to cuddle up with her father and display affection toward him, but Mrs. Neville could make affectionate advances to Rita only by making a game of it. Rita was also reported to glower at any display of affection between her parents. Most of the observed interplay between Rita and the parents was of an educational nature consisting of naming pictures and colors in very precise terms.

At the twelfth well-baby clinic the pediatrician reported that Rita was an apparently normal and healthy child, although poorly nourished. She found no consistent abnormality in gait to which Mrs. Neville had called her attention, and the lower extremities appeared normal. The "no" stage reported by Mrs. Neville also seemed to the pediatrician not a true negativism but rather a selective rejection of the mother. For the first time it seemed there was a definite turning towards the father, with resultant feelings of jealousy by Mrs. Neville.

The pediatrician felt that there was a feeding problem which would probably increase in severity, a mild constipation, and a non-specific dermatitis. Mrs. Neville made some extremely contemptuous and scathing remarks about Rita's failures in the testing but said nothing about her successes. The pediatrician explained that Rita could not be expected to accomplish all the tasks as they covered a wide span going beyond her age, but Mrs. Neville remained anxious in this connection.

To the psychological observer at the thirteenth well-baby clinic, when Rita was almost twenty-one months, she appeared more filled out and healthy-looking. Her ribs were less prominent, and she was well dressed and groomed although still sober-faced. Everything she did seemed quite deliberate, well planned, and outstandingly cautious. The world around her, according to the observer, was still an extremely dangerous world.

Rita did not seem overtly afraid of the examiner but kept a watchful eye on her and tended to remain as near as possible to her mother. This is a typical development at Rita's age, but in view of the existing relationship between mother and child it was somewhat surprising. It suggested that some new bond may have developed between them. There were a few brief episodes in which Rita smiled. The smiles and delight with which she viewed herself undressed in the mirror resembled those of a happy, little girl, and the observer felt they demonstrated more pleasure and self-acceptance, a positive development in this child.

Rita's responses and actions in the structured play contact were at a minimum. She took what was given but hardly did anything with it, as if she could not respond to the invitation for reciprocal human interplay. Instead she took the object and offered it to her mother or somebody else. One had the feeling that it was easier for her to "share objects" than to "share contact." Even when she wanted to play with an object she first had to go through the procedure of "getting rid of it." This contrasted with the unstructured play situation, where she pulled out what she wanted from the toy chest and immediately interested herself in it.

This same impression applied to language: Rita did not share her experiences verbally with others but used language only to share objects intellectually, by naming them or colors correctly. This may be the initiation of intellectualization as a defense mechanism for human contact on a less threatening level. The speculation for the future was whether Rita's intellect would dry out in withdrawal from human contact or whether it would succeed in giving life to her human relations. The hypothesis was that it depended on the fate of her bond to her mother, and the continued improvement of that relationship.

In the latter part of Rita's second year there were few changes in the structure of living. But the home interviewer noted that a barrier had finally been placed at the head of the stairs to protect Rita from falling. At first Mrs. Neville put the playpen there to prevent a visiting friend's little boy from falling down. Then Rita had several falls during this period, including one down this same staircase. After this fall Mrs. Neville called the pediatrician in some alarm, fearing that Rita may have injured her head.

To the interviewer Rita seemed much more lively than before

and apparently had a superficially smoother relationship with her mother. Rita's vocalization at times seemed compulsive and quite repetitive, as did her compulsion to have her hands cleaned immediately if they were soiled in the least way. Also, there seemed fewer overt expressions of hostility by Mrs. Neville and more sociable interaction between them, even some real satisfaction in Rita's achievements. Although the observer detected no particular warmth towards Rita, it seemed there was more for the child to hang on to in terms of her mother's acceptance of her. And Rita seemed to the observer a quite delightful and charming little girl.

The observer noted that Mrs. Neville was somewhat derogatory towards her husband's progress with his studies. There was some fear that he would not attain the advanced degree without an additional year's work. This seemed to threaten Mrs. Neville's confidence in his ability to provide support and security for the family. Her attitude toward her husband possibly also reflected a change of family alliances. As Mrs. Neville's attitude towards Rita became more positive, her husband became more of a focus for disappointment. Another factor may have been defense against the father-daughter axis, of which she had shown disapproval in the past. Mrs. Neville spoke of desire for another child, and it appeared that career ambitions had finally been shelved.

There was a return to the gastrointestinal upset in Rita's twenty-second month and also a chronic mild constipation, for which a laxative had been prescribed. Otherwise Rita was free of illness except the recurrent rash, which was now on the scalp, back, shoulders, and buttocks. She ate well but remained highly selective, refusing almost all vegetables except potato. She fed herself with fingers and spoon. Almost all her milk was taken by bottle, most of this in bed at night. Her sleep again showed an increased tendency toward night wakefulness and some crying, despite the bottle. She finally would return to sleep with Mrs. Neville's firm admonition of "not another peep out of you."

Rita's "agitation" on defecating was accompanied by a spell of retaining both feces and urine and partial refusal of the potty. After discussion with the pediatrician, Mrs. Neville was able to relax her toilet training. From that point on, elimination problems were less frequent. By the end of the twenty-first month she was "fairly consistently trained" for bowel movements and urine during the day but consistently wet at night.

While being bathed Rita was observed to examine her nipples closely and pinch them. Also, she stared intently at her genitals, pointing towards them and saying "wee-wee," which was her name for the genital area. Although Rita was more lively and active, she remained sober and solemn in her approach to the world. Even her activity had a restless, compelled quality that led her mother to describe her as "nervous and high-strung." This was seen in Rita's response to her rashes, at which she clawed repetitiously and "nervously."

In general, she was "a very good child" and not too demanding. Mrs. Neville looked forward to nursery school as a chance for Rita to learn to share with others, as "she has the earmarks of an only child." During this period Rita became increasingly jealous of affectionate signs between her parents and was reported to insist that her father care for her when he was at home.

Rita was able to make a remarkable number of discriminations and verbal identifications of pictures in books. She was also well able to differentiate subtle shadings of color. But little of this linguistic equipment was used for communication or experiencing the human give-and-take. It was invariably tied to her books, which she carried about clutched to her in a most insistent way. Or else, her speech was used for demonstration in drill sessions with one parent or the other.

At the final psychological evaluation towards the end of Rita's twenty-third month one could not believe that Rita had been an outstandingly pretty child. It was hard to decide whether this was because of her expression, which seemed to be one of deep hostility, or because of the odd quality of her movements. Her smile had all the ambiguity and tragedy that a clown might display, along with a depersonalized quality. This same depersonalized quality was also present in her movements, which seemed divorced from any communicative purpose. The impression of unrest in Rita was aggravated by her constant scratching of herself and conveyed a sense of physical discomfort to the observers.

Despite all this, Rita could not justifiedly be called a child for whom gross motor outlet provided any adequate pleasure. Although she seemed to hurry, she hurried in a "driven" way, as if she were driven from the outside and not from within. It was an excited stumbling that one associates with accident proneness. The clumsiness of quick motion was accentuated by a tenseness of her whole body, which moved as "one piece" without a separateness of limb movement. In the end, her hurried quick movements covered little space, and she mainly remained in the center of the room. She refused to climb on the chair and told herself continuously, "Sit down."

In contrast to her gross motor activity Rita's verbal behavior was extremely advanced, and she was capable of naming almost everything in her surrounding with apparent ease. She spoke well and quite a bit, but did not give the feeling that she addressed herself to a social partner in so doing. She addressed herself in the second person or spoke of herself in the third.

Consistent with this, she showed little interest in objects. Her behavior with the formboard puzzle was on the fifteen-month level because she did not try to achieve any correct solution through trial and error, having no real interest in it. Even when she was interested and wanted something, she did not exert herself to overcome obstacles and reach it. She did not retrieve the ball from the Gesell problem box nor did she use the chair or stick to get the cherished milk bottle. She did not even open a drawer to get the toy telephone, which she obviously liked very much. This was not ascribed to lack of discriminatory perception but was partly determined by her negative relationship to adults.

In addition to taking an interest only in those objects which she handled, Rita had a strong perception for those which produced alarm. At a prior examination she had been scared of the rubber cat with the tongue but now she reacted with panic. She screeched in a quite inhuman way, her movements became uncoordinated, and she seemed to move blindly in the direction of her mother. It reminded the pediatrician of her disintegrated despair of about one year ago. Only after she had been on the mother's lap for some time did Rita's tension subside and she say "all gone." Later in the examination, when she approached the chest of drawers in which the rubber cats were stored, she showed the same expression of anxiety on her face. It showed that her memory could function intensely and well under very specific circumstances.

Her relationships with people were the hardest to describe. At no point did she give the impression of listening to what the adults were saying. Rarely did she look at what they were doing, yet she imitated the examiner easily and efficiently. In fact, she performed better than adequately in all imitative items. Although she imitated the examiner, this did not impress one as a game of social sharing but only as a series of imitative acts. Her advanced language also had an imitative aspect, as she spontaneously repeated a number of the sentences which the examiner said to her or in front of her.

Both the Gesell and the Viennese tests were given. At 23 months and 21 days Rita based at the 18-month level on the Gesell test and was given a general maturity level of 23 months and a developmental quotient of 96.8. On the Viennese test she based at the 15- to 18-month level and was given a developmental age of 26 months and 12 days with a developmental quotient of 111.39.

As the two-year study came to a close it seemed that the heavy skies showed lighter patches. Mrs. Neville felt better about her relationship with Rita, was more able to relax her standards and to find some pleasure in her role. And on her part Rita had come to better terms with her environment. While Paul Neville's professional progress was slow and his hours of work were long, nevertheless his family relationships seemed to be of a healthy and stabilizing character.

Though circumstance and the emotional legacies of the past made the first two years of Rita Neville's life stormy, they also made possible the development of adjustment patterns that gave hope for the future. While these patterns seemed to involve no fundamental change in orientation on the part of any of the Nevilles, they at least seemed to become more accommodative. During those dark days of Rita's first winter Mrs. Neville remarked that she was "tortured by the ghost of her frustrated mother," that inexorably she walked in those footsteps of unhappiness and discontent. One could wonder how long this ghost would continue to haunt the Nevilles.

The Neville Family

SUMMARY

A. EXPECTATIONS

1. Maternal Expectations. Mrs. Neville was clearly reluctant to assume the maternal role. Her anticipations were negative and focused on the disruption of her own and her husband's lives by the coming of a child. This situation was met with a high degree of intellectualization. She held that home and motherhood were insufficient for a modern intelligent woman who has "a place in the world," and she was ambitious for an outside career. The fears expressed during pregnancy that the child would "change everything" and she would be irrevocably "tied down" became a reality. Yet by the time Rita was two years old, her mother found herself reconciled to the situation and had given up expectations of a career. She was now ready to "settle down and raise a family."

It appeared that an important factor in this decision was the prospect that her husband would eventually establish himself in a position of status sufficient to satisfy his wife. Another factor was Rita's growing ability to achieve in intellectual areas, which were highly valued by her mother. Thus, Mrs. Neville found some satisfaction in the child, even if only to a limited extent.

2. Specificity of Expectations. Mrs. Neville emphasized the importance of intellectual achievement and had many expectations for her daughter's development. She had very specific ideas of what children should do, how they should be reared, and how they should behave, though she repeatedly asserted that she had never been with children and knew nothing about them. In the first six months of Rita's life, Mrs. Neville's expectations dealt largely with such matters as eating, sleeping, and holding, and Rita's behavior in response to these activities. Expectations in the earliest period were also based on not "spoiling" the child and ensuring that she would be unobtrusive, rather than being related to her own activities in carrying out maternal duties.

By the time Rita was six months old Mrs. Neville expected her to give up infantile ways. During the first year she hoped to establish very specific ideas about what could be expected of a child at any given age. She had recourse to Dr. Gesell's books in order to check up on how well Rita was doing. Her expectations of Rita from the age of six months on, and throughout the two years, were increasingly in terms of the child's developing in a superior fashion, performing well, and being independent; that is, they were directed toward Rita's functioning according to her mother's conception of what the child should be.

3. Motivational Orientation. Mrs. Neville was clearly and consistently mother-centered in terms of her goals. She felt a child would intrude on her activities and make demands for time, energy, and attention which she was unwilling to give. Her ambitions also conflicted with the maternal role. She preferred a baby that would lie quietly in her crib and not bother her mother.

She wanted the kind of response from her child which could more reasonably be expected from older children. She had little tolerance for Rita's impatience and thought the baby should have the sense to wait quietly until the bottle was ready. Her values were consistently in terms of her own satisfactions, and it was to the degree that Rita conformed to them that she was accepted by her mother. By the end of the two years, when Mrs. Neville found qualities in Rita which could satisfy and please her, there was some shift and moderation towards the child.

4. Role of Child in Fulfilling Mother's Expectations. Rita demonstrated a type of adaptation characterized by a capacity to respond to demands for achievement and social behavior. Although there was a contest of wills a good part of the time, Rita was quick to understand what her mother required of her and capable of satisfying these demands. She used this kind of conformity to win approval and affection. In the second year it appeared that Rita's success in winning some approbation from her mother was due not only to her high level of achievement in learning but also to her skill in adapting to her mother's expectations even when no specified clear requirement was expressed. Mrs. Neville commented that Rita "had learned what was expected of her."

5. Paternal Expectations. Not much is known about Mr. Neville's expectations. During his wife's pregnancy he expressed a desire for a family of three or four children, like the one in which he grew up. He showed rather permissive attitudes during the two years, more so than his wife, as well as consideration for the limitations of the child's ability to conform. He did not believe in pushing children "too fast." Like his wife, he put high value on Rita's intellectual achievement, but he was far less insistent about it and had none of his wife's intense determination that Rita should "be the best." He nevertheless encouraged her to learn to do things, and his gifts were often books, from which he taught her to recognize and name objects.

B. BEHAVIOR

1. Communication. From the beginning Mrs. Neville used verbal communication to direct and control rather than to express pleasurable maternal feelings. In Rita's first year Mrs. Neville talked to her frequently as a substitute for picking her up or holding her. When the mother reached her limit of tolerance for Rita's crying, she would scream back at her. Scolding and yelling were more frequent than the soft words she sometimes used to console her. In the second year Rita's excellent comprehension and use of words provided a greatly welcomed opportunity for Mrs. Neville to concentrate on teaching her and directing her activities. Through these means she derived some satisfaction from her daughter, and Rita won a measure of approval and esteem. It is clear that a minimum of physical communication was achieved in routine child-care activities and play. Mrs. Neville kept as much physical and psychological distance as possible between herself and Rita.

Mrs. Neville was at the far end of non-responsiveness to her child's clues. Much of the time the child was restless, fretful, and unhappy; she cried a good deal. Her mother recognized these states but was annoyed and frustrated by them. She saw no reason for the crying. She made unsuccessful efforts to appease the child only after the limits of her own tolerance for crying were reached. She might, in succession, pick up the child, put her down, hit her, or give her a bottle, trying various ways to make her stop crying.

Rita, on the other hand, seemed more responsive to her mother's clues. During the crisis of the second half year of Rita's life, when Mrs. Neville fell into periods of depression, Rita was reported to respond to her mother's feelings with manifestations of deep unhappiness. It is likely that the child was reacting to the withdrawal of even the minimal attention her mother usually gave her.

2. Regularity and Flexibility of Scheduling. Regularity of the child's eating and sleeping schedules did not appear to be a matter of major concern, although it was not always achieved. Throughout the first two years of Rita's life there was irregularity in both going to sleep and in night sleeping. This was reported primarily as an inconvenience to Mrs. Neville, and no systematic effort was made to deal with it.

In feeding there was irregularity in both timing and amount. Mrs. Neville responded with considerable flexibility to Rita's apparent preferences regarding types and amount of food. Shifts in both the amount of food and the timing of meals were influenced in part by gastro-intestinal disturbances which Rita experienced during the first year, in part by the irregularity of her sleeping, and in part by the child's frequent crying spells.

In toilet training, which was begun during the second year, considerably more regularity was established by Mrs. Neville. But from time to time she gave up attempts to toilet train because she felt unable to fight over this issue. However, she did convey to the child the necessity of conforming, and by the end of the second year successful training was accomplished.

3. Techniques of Management. The paucity of physical contact between mother and child was marked. The poverty of their relationship was such that Mrs. Neville held Rita at arm's length for feeding, or strapped her to the bathinette, or laid her supinely on the floor — anything rather than hold her closely. Substitution was used a great deal. When Rita started to pull books out of the low bookshelves Mrs. Neville brought out a set of beads which she could string. Prearrangement was used by placing a bottle in the crib at night so that Rita could have it without waking her parents. An example of avoidance technique was also seen in Mrs. Neville's delay in preparing and offering Rita the bottle.

Non-permissive behavior by Mrs. Neville was the general pattern. However, during the second year there was a noticeable increase in permissive behavior, attributed to the impact of experience on expectations and to greater acceptance of the maternal role.

4. Relation of Expectations to Behavior. Mrs. Neville's behavior was consistent with her clear reluctance to assume the maternal role and its responsibilities. She saw her responsibilities as the provision of physical care for the child, and the child's obligation as being orderly, regular, and compliant with her mother's requirements. Mrs. Neville fulfilled what she considered her own obligations and insisted that Rita do the same. This concept was obviously ineffective, and the first year was marked by overt and unhappy struggle.

Mrs. Neville's major shift in expectations for her daughter was from requiring non-interfering passivity on the part of the infant to demanding active achievement and performance. With the shift of expectations to the child's performance and achievement, Mrs. Neville became more actively engaged with Rita during the second year, especially in the last six months. Finally, she was able to adjust her values to be more accepting of her own role and to find satisfactions in her intellectually successful child. However, both expectations and behavior were based on mother-centered values throughout the two years.

5. Paternal Behavior. Mr. Neville, despite long hours at work, tried to spend some little time with Rita. From the beginning he found her "beautiful" and approved of her. He could not understand why his wife "downgraded" Rita. The child responded to her father warmly, which occasioned some ambivalence on Mrs. Neville's part. Clearly, Mr. Neville provided a balance to the demands made by his wife and was more demonstrative, affectionate, and warm with the child than was his wife.

C. SOCIO-CULTURAL INFLUENCES

1. Socio-economic Status and Values. This family clearly held upward mobility aspirations and appeared to be maritally compatible.

They agreed upon upwardly striving occupational and social class values and shared cultural and artistic interests. Mrs. Neville found intellectual achievement and a professional career most rewarding to her as she grew to adulthood. Consequently, she experienced a great deal of satisfaction and prestige in her husband's professional status even though it meant long hours and extensive blocks of time away from home.

This embryonic professional family had an unplanned and unwanted baby who interfered with her mother's career. The baby's coming seemed to pose a special problem to the Nevilles. Children were not part of the goals defining the things in life worthwhile to them. It is likely that Mrs. Neville would feel that if children were at all desirable, they should not come until her husband was professionally established. As it was, she experienced much dissatisfaction with her role as homemaker and preferred a professional career, almost until the study's end.

2. *Extended Family.* For the Nevilles, conflict occurred in contacts with Mrs. Neville's mother-in-law. Her visits were occasions for criticism of Mrs. Neville's way of bringing up Rita. The criticism touched on one of the aspects of child care with which Mrs. Neville was most concerned — the question of strictness of discipline and "spoiling" the child. In this, her mother-in-law thought her to be lax, and she was blamed for not achieving the very value she held most highly. Her resentment and uneasiness were further intensified by the fact that they were under financial obligation to Mr. Neville's mother, a fact of which the mother-in-law often reminded them.

In contrast, Mrs. Neville derived strength and support from her own family, namely her brother and sister-in-law, with whom she had frequent and close contacts. Advice and help were forthcoming from them at times of crisis, and more than once they helped Mrs. Neville and Rita through critical periods by their understanding, sympathy, constructive advice, and practical help.

3. *Spatial Arrangements and Values.* There were three points where physical arrangements and space in the home appeared to affect the child-care practices in the Neville household. One was the delay in moving Rita from her parents' bedroom to a separate

one at the end of a rather long corridor. This move did not occur until Mrs. Neville thought Rita was able to cry loud enough to be heard. The second involved the steep stairway at the end of the hall, with no physical safeguard for so small a child. From the first, Mrs. Neville made Rita responsible for staying away from it. In the course of her learning, there were several falls before a barrier was set up. Mrs. Neville expected that Rita would not damage her prized possessions and made no changes to guard them from the child's explorations. Surprisingly, Rita conformed to what was expected of her.

The one situation in which space was used constructively and pleasurably by Mrs. Neville in relation to Rita was the practice of outdoor walks. These offered the mother more contact with others and gave the child expanded opportunities for physical exploration. It was one of the few areas of unequivocal mutual enjoyment.

D. FAMILY RELATIONSHIPS

1. Marital. As has already been said, the Nevilles were predominantly compatible. Mrs. Neville's emphasis upon neatness, orderliness, and social striving was quite consistent with her husband's status as a junior professional who was just beginning to climb the rungs of a successful career. She derived a great deal of satisfaction through vicariously participating in his progress as well as through working on her own career outside the home. Prior to the arrival of the child their marriage had been carefree and happy.

However, there was periodic evidence that Mrs. Neville found it hard to take the immediate frustrations of their struggle towards achieving status. Her husband's absorption in work and lack of time for shared activities fostered periods of depression, with feelings of loneliness and isolation. Mrs. Neville's denial at times of the importance of their sexual relations suggested the existence of some marital incompatibilities. But deeper levels of their relationship were not uncovered, and they appeared to be a harmonious, sympathetic couple.

2. Mother-Child. For a long time Mrs. Neville failed to find any emotional or psychological satisfaction in her child. In fact, Rita was a chief source of emotional dissatisfaction, which Mrs. Neville clearly made known by word and act. Until Rita began to meet her mother's demands for high performance, Mrs. Neville was unable to respond to her daughter. Even so, Mrs. Neville very slowly relinquished her personal ambitions and reconciled herself to the maternal role. It appeared likely that Mrs. Neville's demands on her daughter grew out of her feelings of failure in her own childhood, her use of intellectualization as a defense, and her expectation that Rita should somehow help "make it up" to her.

Although Mrs. Neville expressed some resentment at the growing attachment between father and child, she also found his presence and the attention he gave to Rita something of a relief for herself. Even more remarkable than her second-year shift to a greater child-accepting (though not child-oriented) attitude was Rita's capacity to adapt to the demands made on her.

3. Father-Child. Mr. Neville had small part in child-care routines but shared experiences with the child in play and in the interchange of teaching and learning. When necessary during his wife's occasional illness he took over Rita's care quite adequately. He was responsive to his child from the beginning, although his absorption in work limited his time with her. Partly because of the difficulties of mother-child interaction there resulted a close alignment of father and child, with marked evidence of the child's preference for the father

E. PERSONALITY CHARACTERISTICS

1. Handling of Anxiety and Hostility. We have seen that Maria Neville had an intellectual way of relating to the world as a means of getting approval and affection from her father during her childhood. The use of intellectualism as a way of achieving satisfactions carried into her adult life. It also provided a cover for her many anxieties, which included forebodings about Rita's development, normality, and potentials. Through this intellectual detachment Mrs. Neville found a way of handling her own anxieties, but in the maternal role it proved inadequate by promoting a separateness from her child that left little room for the satisfaction of Rita's emotional needs.

At times, the veneer of intellectualism was no defense against Mrs. Neville's anxiety. Her feelings exploded in uncontrollable outbursts of anger and hostility. Thus, her predominantly negative feelings toward Rita would occasionally erupt in screaming at the child, spanking her, ignoring her, or sometimes denying the existence of such feelings.

2. Dependency and the Sense of Security. Mr. Neville's long hours away from home accentuated his wife's sense of loneliness and isolation. In many ways she needed more companionship and more sharing in life from her husband. Her feeling of isolation was most acute in the winter months, when she was seldom able to be with friends and felt unable to discuss her difficulties.

Her early dependence upon her brother, who served a parental role for her, changed somewhat to a relationship of more equality after her marriage. For the most part, her deep-seated dependency needs were concealed by the detached appearance which she presented to those around her. She tended to reject those neighborly contacts which were available and could accept social support only on her own terms.

3. Feelings of Adequacy or Inadequacy. Mrs. Neville did not appear to be either concerned with or troubled by feelings of inadequacy and demonstrated a minimum of problems in this connection.

4. Planning and Impulsiveness. Planning did not seem to be too significant for Mrs. Neville. She managed her household tasks without great emphasis on planning. There was no evidence of impulsiveness. Her inability to schedule effectively body massages and play periods with Rita was due to the absence of gratification from care of the baby rather than to inability to schedule.

5. Self-Assertion. The question of self-assertiveness did not, by itself, appear to be a source of difficulty.

6. Recapitulation of Past Experiences. Mrs. Neville dwelt on the trauma of parental loss at an early age. Memories of her mother were mainly of severe brooding discontent and unhappiness. Her parents had wanted a boy when she was born, and she felt a similar disappointment that she had had a girl instead of a boy. She stated that in "making everyone miserable" she was following her mother's pattern. Her routines with Rita demonstrated remoteness, separation, and general discontent, perhaps reflecting her own experiences of the mother-child relationship. It was apparent that the recapitulation of past experience did not develop gratification for the sustained nurturing role of motherhood and provided no positive model of mother-child relationship.

F. EMERGENCE OF FAMILY INTEGRATION PATTERNS

1. Family Structure. Rita did not become a part of a triadic relationship because she did not easily fit in with the mother's psychological and social needs or values. Her father's brief and sporadic participation was not sufficient to offset the weak mother-child relationship. While the husband-wife dyadic relationship was compatible, the child's dyadic relationship with either parent was not strong, and the family emerged along segmental lines. Although Mr. Neville was generally more permissive and protective of the child, the general character of family development was toward a parent-centered adaptation.

2. Division of Labor and Balance of Power. There was sharing between Mr. and Mrs. Neville of professional and intellectual interests but minimally in household and child management. Mrs. Neville was the dominant one in family management and was mainly responsible for Rita's care because of her husband's heavy work schedule. There was little evidence of incompatibility or stress over household affairs.

3. Development, Achievement, and Social Behavior of Child. Despite Rita's outstanding picture and prognosis as a newborn, an alarming retrogression took place and she was barely age-adequate in developmental tests for a year and a half, notwithstanding her mother's unusually high standards for growth and development. However, Rita did begin to show a great capacity to respond to her mother's demands for achievement and social behavior in an effort to win approval and affection. By the end of the study she performed appropriately at age-adequate developmental levels.

4. *Prospect of Siblings.* On a few occasions Mrs. Neville spoke of her desire for a second child. At one time it seemed that she hoped another child would provide satisfactions that Rita failed to give. This was during the period when the relationship between mother and child was at its worst and Mrs. Neville feared that Rita was "retarded." On another occasion she said disparagingly that Rita "had the earmarks of an only child." As Mrs. Neville became more reconciled to her maternal role and shelved career aspirations, she spoke of her desire for a larger family.

5. *Status of Family in Community.* Mrs. Neville was characterized as being active in social life outside of the nuclear family, although her social activity was much more prominent in the spring and summer months than during the winter isolation. Also, she longed for a social life of status and professional prestige and felt that motherhood basically interfered with the development of such a life.

6. *Types of Parent-Child Adaptation.* The relationships in this family, particularly between mother and child, were such as to preclude unity. The orientation was basically towards parent-centered goals, and child management was essentially non-permissive. While there was a significant shift toward greater permissiveness and child-acceptance during the two-year period, this did not vitally alter the overall quality of the relationship. The Nevilles emerged as a segmental, parent-centered, non-permissive family.

POSTSCRIPT

The relationship between mother and daughter consistently improved, although it was not indicative of fundamental changes in interaction. As Rita developed intellectual skills, Mrs. Neville began to praise her achievements and to show greater warmth and affection for the child. While she was aware and troubled that her demands might have been "too strict," it was difficult for her to alter completely the patterns of her nature.

In the contest to make Rita conform to her exacting standards, overt struggles continued to erupt from time to time to jar the relationship. The hostility of her mother was poorly tolerated by the child, for whom maternal security had ever been tenuous. The toll it took of Rita was evident in a continuation of nervous scratching, some ritualistic body movements, exceedingly poor eating, a solemn and "lowering" expression and strong resistance to bottle-weaning.

Rita gave the impression of anxiety and tension, like a coiled spring which would move in an unpredictable direction when released. Although spontaneous childish enjoyment was infrequent, Rita developed rapidly in areas which gave her mother the most satisfaction. Her speech was on a high level of precision and clarity, she was attached to books and learning, she adapted to social situations along standards established by her mother. Thus, she earned genuine commendation, warmth, and approval, which resulted in a more gratifying relationship to both.

Rita was found well able to function in nursery school. Surprisingly, normal separation anxiety did not appear at the beginning. Only later, after Rita had settled down in nursery school, did she undergo a separation problem with respect to her mother. The staff assessed this as a positive development in that the child abandoned her artificial adjustment and worked out the normal separation process Mrs. Neville began to report that Rita was now more affectionate with her and permitted Mrs. Neville to "touch" her. The school experience was gratifying to both mother and daughter. Mrs. Neville felt that it helped Rita to become more adult and self-reliant. Rita held her own with other children and derived pleasure from the group, although she kept herself somewhat on the periphery of interaction.

As Mr. Neville struggled for his advanced degree, his wife became more critical and concerned about their future. In the preoccupation with this, some of the pressure was transferred from

Rita. The child began to eat better and seemed more carefree. With the evaporation of Mrs. Neville's own career ambitions, she was eager to enlarge her family. Despite concern about an existing Rh factor, she became pregnant.

To prepare for the new baby the family rented a desirable private home with spacious yard and extra space. The pregnancy was not difficult, and Mrs. Neville enjoyed good health and spirits. A normal male child was delivered when Rita was just past three years of age. Mrs. Neville was delighted with her male offspring and admitted that she had been quite disappointed with Rita's sex. However, she said that she now enjoyed having a daughter.

The baby was started on breast feeding, but this was found too demanding, as he seemed to require very frequent feedings. Mrs. Neville demonstrated more appreciation and satisfaction with the infant than she had had for Rita. However, her pattern of mothering remained unchanged. The same awkwardness of handling was seen, with a lack of fondling, cuddling, or demonstrable affection. In contrast, Mr. Neville's warm approach to the infant had more maternal quality than that demonstrated by his wife.

Rita accepted her sibling with tenderness and affection. Mrs. Neville considered her attitude as "very good." The baby asserted himself with lusty crying when hungry or uncomfortable. He required a good deal of holding, and Mrs. Neville wondered about "spoiling him." Although much of her behavior was similar to that with Rita as an infant, she surprised the staff with many detailed and perceptive observations of the baby's clues. As she said, "I'm learning all the time."

When Mr. Neville completed his studies, the family settled in the Midwest, where he had accepted a position which promised to be rewarding in terms of his career Upon a brief return visit to the area Rita was again seen. She was slightly over four years of age. At that time she demonstrated an insatiable drive to achieve through intellectual power, and her capacities in this direction were rated high. Her outstanding way of relating to others was through performance with material objects rather than by direct personal interaction. She appeared attractive, poised, friendly, and competent.

A subsequent letter from Mrs. Neville indicated that Rita was progressing well but that the contest of wills still existed. However, as Rita was reported to say, "Even if I want to do so and so, we can still like each other, can't we?" And indeed these words may be prophetic of what the future holds for the dynamics of the relationship between mother and child.

The Callini Family

TAKING LIFE AS IT COMES

Familiar cultural patterns and a stable communal life were substance enough for Mary and Tony Callini. For some, the teeming streets and dilapidated buildings of the crowded Italian neighborhood might appear to be a slum. But beauty is in the eye of the beholder, and the area was eulogized in Mary Callini's statements. "I don't want to leave this place. I've lived here all my life and I'm sure there isn't a better place to live anywhere."

The patterns of life were well defined for the Callinis amid the bustle and the laughter of large Italian families. But childhood was sometimes hard. There were days when there wasn't quite enough food and their mothers were too busy to cater to them. Instead, older siblings acted as auxiliary parents. Sickness and death, deprivation and sorrows, were not unknown. But the impact of these was cushioned by the security of their large family groups, where each member had his accustomed duty and his assured place. So when the children grew up it seemed only natural that they would marry and settle down in their parental neighborhood. And so it was with Mary and Tony Callini.

Although they grew up but five blocks apart, they did not meet until after they were both out of school. Tony first spied Mary at a neighborhood wedding, but it took him almost a month to find courage to ask her for a date. She was nineteen and he was twenty-two. Tony had served three years in World War II and had had some trouble finding work afterwards. In the first flush of their romance, they had wanted to get married right away, but there were obstacles to overcome. Mary was the last daughter at home, which meant that her mother depended on her for cleaning, sewing, and companionship. Despite her own impatience, Mary "understood how her mother felt about it."

And then there was the matter of finances. Although Tony had finally landed a job, there "was not even a shoestring" on which to begin married life. The courtship continued until Mary was twenty-one. Then Tony said, "You're twenty-one and can do as you please." "A nice family wedding" took place, and even Mary's mother was very pleased with her new son-in-law.

The couple was welcomed into the Callini homestead, where they shared the ground-floor apartment with Tony Callini's parents and an unmarried brother. Mary Callini was certain that if they both worked, they could get a home of their own in about a year. Although the five-room apartment was large, it was cluttered with so much heavy overstuffed furniture and so many knickknacks that it appeared small. Italian and religious pictures, plus two large statues of Christ and the Virgin, testified to the family's religious values, while an elaborate cocktail shaker outfit and a gleaming new television set were prized symbols of newer ways.

As the months passed, Mrs. Callini's hopes for an apartment of her own grew dimmer. But it did not seem to matter too much. The couple was happy in their wedded life, their filial roles, and their work. They did not plan to have babies until they had their own home. Although Mrs. Callini had douched and "counted on the safe period," the pregnancy "just happened" after all.

In the fourth month of her pregnancy she had the first interview in connection with the study and was described as a short, slender, black-haired young woman of twenty-three with a slight but definite lisp and several missing back teeth. She was quite shy and seemed to feel that there was little to talk about which would be of interest to anyone. She leaned forward, listened intently to everything, and was most eager to cooperate with the interviewer.

Mrs. Callini was still working as a press operator in the same factory where she had worked for almost five years. She planned to leave the job shortly and did not intend to return after the baby was born. With some pride, she reported that they had enough money to get by, now that her husband had a good steady job, and she did not have to worry about the Army because he had served for three years in the last war. It was also pleasing to her that her husband's job was "right around the corner from home" and she could see him for lunch and coffee during the day.

The fact of her pregnancy was almost unbelievable to Mrs. Callini. Time and again she said, "I don't feel I'm a mother at all." It surprised her that she felt so well and had no trouble. She had thought that pregnancy would be as bad as the severe menstrual cramps which used to incapacitate her. But other than a small weight gain and enlarged breasts, there was scarcely any difference. She had been hungry and more thirsty, but her weight had not changed much. She added, "I hope I'll stay this way forever. I know I'll get bigger, but I hope I'll stay healthy this way." Only when she felt the baby move did Mrs. Callini finally believe that she was pregnant.

With some embarrassment she asked the interviewer about several puzzling things that "the girls at the factory talked about." They had said that "the husband gets sick and has symptoms when the wife is pregnant" and also that "the husband gets labor pains." Mrs. Callini said, "I don't see how that can be."

At the following interview Mrs. Callini was still quite shy and hesitant but remained eager to please. Piece by piece, some details were learned about her background and family. Her mother had married at seventeen and had quickly started to raise a family, consisting of three boys and nine girls. Mary was the eleventh child and the youngest daughter. The oldest son was already forty-five and had a twenty-one-year-old son of his own. There were now nine grandchildren. Mrs. Callini's father "definitely wanted his twelve children and liked all of them."

About her mother, Mrs. Callini said that "none of the children were close to her because there were so many of them." Mrs. Callini couldn't remember whether her mother had breast fed her or the child that followed her. When asked how she got along with her brothers and sisters, she answered "fine." The interviewer pressed to find out her favorite sibling and learned that she was closest to her sister Dorothy, nine years older. Mrs. Callini had "baptized" this sister's children and expected that Dorothy in turn would "baptize" her babies. "I'll do anything for my sister and my sister will do anything for me," she added.

The interviewer asked if she had any special hobbies. Mrs. Callini seemed to find this difficult to answer and finally stated that she had always liked sewing class in school and had been good at it. She still did the sewing for her mother. Her reserve was evident in the interview, and she did not speak readily. She seemed more eager to please the interviewer than to discuss life situations. She gave specific answers to direct questions without elaborating on her feelings or introducing any new elements.

At the next interview Mrs. Callini looked very well. Her hair was attractively curled, and she wore a pretty green sweater with a simple black skirt. Although she appeared heavier, she did not look at all pregnant. She reported happily that she had not dieted and had eaten anything she felt like but had only gained two and one-half pounds in the last month. She felt very well and was constantly surprised at this. Later in the discussion she wondered whether the two and one-half pound gain might be a little too much. The repetitiveness of astonishment at feeling so well suggested some hidden fears about child-bearing and body changes. She asked the interviewer why "some women have it so difficult during pregnancy and childbirth." Two of her sisters had had rather difficult deliveries. She said she knew what to expect and imagined "it will hurt to have a baby."

During this interview Mrs. Callini gave the impression of more intelligence than at earlier meetings. Her poise was greater, and she sat more quietly as she talked. She had regard for the people at the hospital and expected them to answer her questions intelligently, clearly, and without ambiguities. At each interview she asked some specific factual question concerning pregnancy and childbirth. She wanted enough of an answer to help her learn about the physiological basis of changes that were taking place within her.

At the fourth interview Mrs. Callini still seemed to feel that there was nothing in her life that would interest the study staff. As in all interviews, she answered questions to the best of her ability but rarely did she start a topic of conversation or offer information except when she asked a specific question. At this interview she asked, "Why do other women say time drags in pregnancy?" To her it seemed as though time were passing terribly quickly and before she knew it, "the whole pregnancy would be over."

When she asked this question her face became alert. One felt that she wanted to learn from us but was not particularly interested in communicating her own family experience.

Again Mrs. Callini mentioned that she hoped she would "keep small" and not gain any more weight. She reported that she had attended all but the last of the exercise classes and had learned a lot from the nurse. She expressed desire to "meet with the doctor who will take care of the baby." Time and again she said, "Everything is going fine." There was no doubt that she seemed happy and that living arrangements at home did not present problems for this happy couple.

Only two minor problems were noted. Mrs. Callini was sometimes frustrated by the tendency of all the Callini family, including her husband, to lapse into Italian. Mary had never developed confidence in using the language, since her own parents rarely spoke it. Also, her own family, though they liked Tony Callini, always felt a little uncomfortable in the Callini home. So for the first time in her life Mrs. Callini found she had to leave home to see her parents. This made even five blocks sometimes seem like a long distance.

No names had yet been chosen for the baby, and Mrs. Callini said this seemed "like a mistake" but there was nothing she could do about it. As far as she was concerned, she didn't care if it was a boy or girl "just so it's healthy," and her husband felt the same way about it. To the question of how many children she planned on having, she said, "That would depend on whether or not we get our own home, but I don't plan on having as many babies as my mother." She said that she had knit a sweater for the baby and that all other things were ready. She had not decided whether she would breast feed.

At her meeting with the pediatrician Mrs. Callini said she had no complaints whatsoever and felt fine. Though pleasant and smiling, she seemed slightly ill at ease during the early part of the interview. Later she relaxed and asked specific questions such as, "How do you know how to make formula for babies?" Mrs. Callini listened with great interest to the pediatrician's explanation. Then she commented that she was glad to hear about it because she had "always wondered how much milk and sugar to put into the formula for little babies at different ages." She then declared her intention to breast feed "because it's better for the baby."

The methods of the study group in observing the babies were discussed, and the pediatrician had the impression that Mrs. Callini was somehow pleased by the idea that her baby would be one of those observed. She asked about the details of rooming-in and listened carefully to the explanation. She said her reason for choosing rooming-in was, "It will be awfully nice to have the baby with me," and also "If I have help from the nurses during that period I'll feel much more comfortable about going home."

A question or two was asked about "how babies are bathed" and "Do the nurses show you how before you have to do it yourself?" The interview was rather brief because Mrs. Callini seemed to have little she wanted to talk about. "I'm sure," she told the pediatrician, "that there'll be questions after the baby arrives, but I can't think now what they'll be."

At the next meeting with the interviewer Mrs. Callini mentioned that she had seen a play at the mental hygiene session about how different mothers handled the same problem. It impressed her that "everyone has their own way of doing things." She did not spontaneously discuss any personal matters at length but commented briefly, "Apartments are so very expensive that I don't think we'll find a place very soon." In speaking of the coming baby, she smiled and commented that her husband wanted the baby very much and she imagined he would spoil it.

The next interview proved to be the last before the baby's birth. During this session Mrs. Callini was considerably more talkative. She still felt "perfectly fine" and remained surprised at her state of good health. She had gained just fifteen pounds, carried the baby attractively, and was quite small. With some impatience, she commented, "I'd like to get out of maternity clothes."

There was some discussion about her family. Mrs. Callini said that her mother had "never had anything to do" with her father's barbering business. With some gaiety, she commented on how well her father handled little children's fear of haircuts. If his grandchildren "sat quietly in the barber chair and let him do a good job, he gave them a quarter." She reported that her mother was taking care of her sister's four-year-old child, as both parents worked. She said that this child "was developing very slowly," and she had spoken about it during her interview with the pediatrician of the study group. However, the pediatrician had not given any specific reason for the slow development but had said that the youngster might "catch up as time went on." Mrs. Callini said matter-of-factly "After all, a four-year-old ought to be talking a little bit," and that she was slow in everything.

Her preparations for the baby had all been made. She had also sewn a few kimonos and knitted a sweater. She asked why it would be necessary to take the baby to the Child Study Center for well-baby checkups. This was explained, and Mrs. Callini listened intently. Then she said, "You are most likely interested in how babies differ and develop." In a roundabout way she questioned the interviewer to learn whether the pediatrician had reported anything of their interview. She asked whether the pediatrician had said she was "all right and everything."

Mrs. Callini had been given a pill at the clinic and had wondered what it was for. When told that it was vitamin K and for what purpose it had been given, she appeared relieved that it had no other significance. She mentioned that at the last exercise class they had been taken on a tour of the operating room. She said it frightened her because she had never seen one before. The table looked "scary" and she "didn't like the stirrups" but imagined that these things wouldn't worry her when she was having the baby.

Two weeks later Johnny was born. The nurses' notes described Mrs. Callini as calm and in good spirits during labor, which lasted six hours and twenty-four minutes. The delivery was uneventful, and Mrs Callini was reported "quiet, smiling, radiant, content, and pleased with everything." She said the delivery was "just wonderful" and everything about the baby was "absolutely perfect." She said she wanted to have another baby very soon. Mr. Callini was also joyously excited.

The staff failed to share Mrs. Callini's enthusiasm over her "beautiful baby." Johnny's face was yellowish grey and puffed up under the eyes. Long straight black hair covered his pin-shaped head, his mouth and nose were large and poorly shaped, and nobody ever saw his eyes. His body was fat and flabby, with thin black hair on arms and legs. The observers described his appearance as "porcine" and "very unattractive."

But he was an easy baby to observe, as his movements were so few and he maintained approximately the same position in all observations. His head was turned left but snuggled into his body in what seemed a far from comfortable position. Yet Johnny appeared quite relaxed and slept through eight of the ten observations. Once he was observed forty-five minutes after circumcision. Neither hunger nor other discomfort interrupted his sleep for longer than a few moments. He responded to continuous noise only with some startles, then returned to his deep and peaceful sleep as soon as the startle was over. When stimulations accumulated, he woke up crying, but soon his peace was restored. When he was uncovered "to the bone" he responded with some fussing, but a few soft strokes on his stomach quieted him immediately.

Johnny's sleep was surprisingly well defined for a newborn because his movement production was reduced almost to nil, and his breathing was slow and regular. From observations during his infrequent wakings it appeared that sounds increased Johnny's activity whereas touch decreased it; that cold had an exciting effect and warmth a quieting one. If these indications were reliable, they implied that Johnny would be a rather responsive child when awake and that his behavior could be influenced in either direction — stimulating him into action or by helping him to relax.

A marked difference in pattern was created by changing his position. If he was placed in supine, he became more active and less at ease, but if placed on his stomach, there was a quick and short period of tensing followed by a long and slow period of relaxing. Johnny's demands were well defined. On three different occasions his crying was comforted only by changing his diapers. When he fussed because of hunger he could only be comforted by food. His crying never sounded too despairing or unhappy but was more like a signal of protest or demand. He neither lost his breath nor did his movements become disorganized. Altogether he cried very little.

One of the factors that may have contributed to Johnny's relaxation was the nature of his hand-mouth contact. Both hands were successful in reaching his mouth, although the right established the contact slightly more easily. He rarely established a perfect hand-mouth contact, but whether the contact was casual or definite, it was sufficient to quiet Johnny. Johnny was put to breast within an hour after his birth. Even though Mrs. Callini's milk did not come in for several days, she was pleased at how well the nursing was going. He "held on well to the breast," and his sucking was vigorous and regular though slow. Altogether he functioned surprisingly well and maturely for a newborn.

Johnny and his mother returned to the rickety wooden house, unbelievably crammed with furniture and with people. In the bedroom were several wardrobes, a bassinet, stroller, knick-knacks, two large religious statues, and a large double bed. Aside from the five adults who lived in the apartment the dwelling often contained other Callini children and grandchildren, who visited constantly. Everyone in the household became involved with the baby, and someone was always ready to play with Johnny or take him up. During coffee breaks his father dashed home from his nearby factory job to play with his son. And Johnny's mother had eyes for no one else. It soon became obvious to her that Johnny was going to be "spoiled" but it didn't bother her. She thought her infant son "would grow up to be smart because so many people talk to him."

Mrs. Callini was observed to be competent and warm in all her activity with Johnny. Most of the time she seemed content and free of anxiety. On the rare occasions when she did express some concern, about his eating so much or being fretful at a clinic visit, she accepted the staff's reassurance readily. Under the eyes of doting parents and relatives Johnny grew rapidly. He was solely breast-fed for a month, then some supplementary formula was added. Two weeks later he went on formula exclusively, although the termination of breast feeding was never raised or discussed with the pediatrician.

Solid food was first given at one month, and by the third month Johnny was eating cereal, vegetables, meat soups, orange juice, and fruit in addition to eight or nine ounces of milk four times a day. This large amount of food was taken easily. By his fifth month Johnny was close to a three-meal-a-day schedule. In his fourth month Johnny started to awake at night and take a bottle of milk. Upon pediatric advice the formula was manipulated until it was found that giving him whole milk rather than formula during the day ended the night wakening.

Shortly after his homecoming Johnny started to sleep through the night so deeply and quietly that his mother used to get up "to see if he's okay." He slept in prone in his little crib, and it was characteristic that his head and shoulders remained hunched until just before he went off to sleep when they flopped down. He was transferred to a larger crib in the fourth month, and Mrs. Callini reported that he crowded against the bumpers so that "he has the feeling of being up against something."

Johnny continued to fuss when he was wet or dirty, just as he had in the hospital, and complained bitterly until he was changed. He usually had four or five bowel movements a day, during or just after feeding. He would stop feeding, strain, and get red. His mother was natural and efficient in changing and cleaning him. She showed neither distaste nor embarrassment. Johnny played frequently with his hands and occasionally took them to his mouth. This play continued to the fifth month, when he was reported to "talk and talk" to his hands. He was observed once or twice to suck and chew on his thumb.

His development, on the whole, was quite even through the first five months, and there was no doubt that his performance in prone was markedly better than in supine. He showed more interest in retaining objects than in getting them, and there was some indication that there was more active response to visual than auditory stimulation. Despite the fact that Johnny's wants were fulfilled by many adults, an instinctive close rapport soon developed between mother and child, each seeming to adjust almost instantly to the clues of the other.

At the well-baby clinic observation at 4 months and 7 days Johnny was seen as tall, big, and husky, with his fat so well distributed that he did not appear either flabby or chubby. His face was still far from handsome, although his coloring had somewhat improved. But his "double chin," broad nose, and slightly protruding eyes were not pretty in themselves, and his expression was sober. He was serious and behaved purposefully. Contact and interrelation with his mother or any adult, for that matter, seemed rather meager in this observation, and Johnny was far from active. Except for repeated crawling movements made in the prone position there was heightened activity only twice. He looked at any toy that was offered and followed it with his glance. He smiled at the sound of the bell and at his own image in the mirror. The smiling response was comparatively rare, however, and as a rule, his observation of objects was serious and concentrated.

For a child as well developed as Johnny, his grasping attempts were minimal. Although his hands were on the diaper that was placed on his face he did not pull it off. When the rattle was shown, he lifted his left hand but lowered it without touching the rattle. However, when the rattle was actually placed in his hand he became quite interested and fingered and "talked to it." When the examiner tried to remove the rattle he held on to it and showed unmistakable signs of displeasure. It appeared that "having" was more important for Johnny than "getting."

On the Viennese test he was at the 6-month level in body mastery, learning, and the handling of inanimate objects, and at the 5-month level in perception and social response. Both on this test and the Gesell there was a consistently good developmental picture.

He could support himself on hands and arms in the prone position, and his crawling movements were purposeful and well coordinated. But this mastery did not hold when he was pulled up to sitting position. He showed a definite head lag and tumbled twice when placed in the supportive chair. There was no clear picture as to the beginning of hand dominance. He used the right hand in fifteen instances, the left in twelve, both hands in seven. The picture was even more ambiguous as far as handling of toys. He used his left hand with the rattle but was expert at manipulating the dangling ring with his right hand.

Johnny vocalized repeatedly in a way that related to the object with which he was involved. This early communicative function may have had something to do with the constant noise, music, sound, and speech which prevailed in the Callini household. Or it might have been related to the fact that his mother frequently interfered with his mouthing attempts and the vocalizing might have been a substitute function of the mouth. Although Johnny appeared purposeful, mature, and well balanced in this observation, his developmental picture was not altogether clear.

In the next well-baby observation Johnny was far more active than before and was characterized as "rolling, crawling, and twisting out of the hands of the examiner." Still his picture was not too clear. Possession seemed more important to him than acquisition, but this did not prevent him from approaching the world around him and accepting what it offered.

Johnny continued to thrive in the busy communal home that served as a clearing house for the large Callini family. There were always enough relatives present to insure that he was never alone and rarely in need of anything. His parents were proud of their little boy and enthusiastically reported his latest accomplishments. At home the interplay between mother or father and son was zestful, warm, and genuine. There was no doubt about Mrs. Callini's competence and control in almost all situations. She even managed to help with the arrangement of testing equipment at the clinic and to persuade the home visitor to eat larger portions of cake than she cared to have.

At this time Mr. Callini left his nearby factory job to take a more lucrative one in a city not far away. The commuting was long, and he worked the swing shift from 3 P.M. to 12 P.M. Johnny's sleeping hours were rearranged so his father could see more of him. Nevertheless, Mr. and Mrs. Callini missed the informal coffee breaks and the pleasant evenings they had shared. Evidences of restiveness and dissatisfaction began to appear within the family, accumulating as time went on.

In his sixth month Johnny had a somewhat heavy cold, from which he made a smooth recovery. But it showed a discrepancy in Mrs. Callini's sure handling of him. She was quite distressed that she could not easily comfort the boy and felt so unable to give Johnny his medicine that she was markedly relieved when the pediatrician offered to do it. He was scarcely over his fever before she asked how soon she could take him out-of-doors. The pediatrician observed, "She seems to have a need to skip the period of convalescence." Similarly, there was a sharp decrease in her customary skill with Johnny when he was given an immunization injection at the clinic.

Johnny's intake of food dropped both in quantity and variety in his sixth and seventh months. Although Mrs. Callini expressed no overt concern about his eating, she communicated a sense of uneasiness. She reported that he made a "great sport of razzing his food," blowing it all over and messing with it. He slept through the night from 8 or 10 P.M. until 8:30 or 9 in the morning. Once in a while he awoke when his father came in after midnight, but he returned to sleep without difficulty. His naps during the day went better when he was outside in his carriage because "there's so much going on inside," his mother said. She didn't like him to miss the afternoon nap because then he became overtired and resisted his night sleep.

By the middle of Johnny's sixth month his mother seemed to know when to "catch him" for bowel movements because of clear facial signs. She would place him on the toilet seat, where he defecated unless somebody else was around. Her primary concern did not seem to be regularizing Johnny's toileting but rather diaper washing. At the end of his sixth month she reported some success at getting him to urinate in the potty. She thought he was "beginning to get the idea."

It was clear at the next well-baby clinic evaluation that Johnny preferred the prone position, from which he could more fully creep, grasp, and move. When he was put on his back he rolled over to prone in one quick movement. However, if his mother placed Johnny in supine and kept her hand quite lightly on his arm he remained in supine. Her touch served as a prohibiting factor. While on his mother's lap, Johnny was vocal in more variety and quantity than when he was away from her. In none of the observations did Johnny react to the stranger with anxiety, fear, or discrimination. But he did distinguish between his mother and other people in his visual contact. With others, the visual contact was a separate act in itself. But with his mother it was an inherent part of his every action.

His imitative behavior showed incredible progress and also seemed emotionally important to him. He imitated knocking in rhythm and at the same place where it was carried out by the examiner. When he fell and hurt his head his cries were calmed by being induced to imitate the examiner. It suggested that Johnny had begun to recognize the difference between his own and other people's actions and that the recognition was successful and pleasurable.

Johnny resorted to mouthing relatively infrequently compared to other study children of the same age. He had a greater interest in manipulating toys than in mouthing them. He mouthed a spoon very briefly and then began to bang it. His whole body and face participated in the banging. It demonstrated that his emotional preoccupation with motor behavior was so strong that it left little room for anything else. It may also have been related to his mother's prohibition of mouthing by words, gestures, and facial expression.

Johnny was quite skillful in using his own body as a helping tool. He played with parts of his body, actively moving one part with the help of the other. He could grasp his foot without looking at it. His extreme tendency to move to desired objects interfered with his faculty for perception. Thus, when an object was attached to a string so that he could get it only by using the string he made breathless efforts to reach the object directly and did not notice the string at all.

At the age of 6 months and 29 days (30 weeks) Johnny remained amazingly high in development. On the Viennese test he had a developmental age of 9 months and 9 days, which was almost 2½ months above his chronological age. While Johnny obtained a high test score, this was not necessarily predictive of high intellectual performance because the test focus was mainly on body mastery, which was Johnny's particular forte.

Mrs. Callini began to find that she could not concentrate entirely on her son. There was a division of labor between her mother-in-law and herself; dishes and cleaning had to be done. There were daily trips to her mother's home, where she not only enjoyed the fellowship of her family but undertook the household chores which she had performed before her marriage. She began to feel restless at the "temporary" residence with her in-laws, although it did not seem to bother her husband.

Johnny had a mild respiratory infection in his seventh month, and once more Mrs. Callini showed less than her usual perceptiveness. As soon as his fever abated, she inappropriately wanted to take him out on a cold wet day. During his cold he refused food, but otherwise his eating was reported to go "fairly well." He would feed himself a cookie or piece or bread but did not participate in table feeding. He slept well through the night and had long afternoon naps out-of-doors. Inside the busy house he found it hard to nap at all.

Johnny had always loved the roughhousing in which his parents happily engaged with him. But now, as he became more active, he demanded more and more of it. He started to be a "wiggler," and it became increasingly difficult to dress him. Also, he acquired the habit of scratching and biting, which was probably a game to him, but his elders became concerned about how to overcome these aggressions. Mrs. Callini was still at the "catching" level with Johnny's bowel movements. When his facial expression indicated that one was about to occur, his mother started chattering to him until they reached the bathroom. Her talking was effective enough to inhibit defecation until he was placed on the toilet.

At the well-baby observation in the eighth month Johnny's main contact with the adult was using her as a prop to help him stand up. Only when he was finally standing did he look at the adult's face. When he achieved the standing position he began to vocalize and smile. If he was unable to get himself to a standing position, his vocalizing took the form of whimpering and then crying. This did not subside when his mother spoke to him, but as soon as she was near enough for him to grab her dress he pulled himself up and smiled.

Johnny did not suck his thumb throughout the observation, but he mouthed play objects more than before. His mouthing had a specific pattern, showing some tension in the neck muscles, a pushing forward of the chin and an opening-closing of the mouth in a quick biting way. But there was nothing resembling a sucking movement. No smile was observed in connection with the mouthing. Johnny's expression was one of intense eagerness at the beginning, gradually fading to an empty stare.

The variety of his sounds had not increased very much since the previous observation, nor had he developed a greater specificity. However, the observer did get the impression of a better-developed vocal adaptation to distance. When his mother was quite near Johnny he vocalized softly, but when she moved away he became louder. In development Johnny showed no progress in imitation since the last visit.

On the Gesell test at the chronological age of 36 weeks his general maturity level was at 42 weeks, with a developmental quotient of 117. On the Viennese test he had a developmental age of 11 months, 3 days, with a developmental quotient of 133. His rate of development was quite consistently phenomenal.

Mrs. Callini became uneasy as soon as the pediatrician started the medical examination. She tried to distract Johnny with a toy and keep him from grasping the doctor's stethoscope. Her movements were quick and jerky. She talked so rapidly that her speech disturbance, a slight lisp, became quite marked. Johnny hardly reacted to the offered toy but showed a marked increase in his activity, wriggling almost continuously. Mrs. Callini asked the pediatrician if Johnny was to get an injection. When the answer was "no," she became slower in her movements and more relaxed.

Johnny could master situations extremely well, getting any object even halfway within reaching distance. He remained vigorous as long as the object was in sight, but if he lost sight of the object he became immobilized and lost interest. His stranger reaction remained unanxious and unperturbed. He responded according to the stimulation provided and the situation created. In contrast to the bland emotional attitude towards the stranger, his emotional response towards his mother was highly sensitive. Although he moved a great deal and touched different parts of his body with extreme ease, there was no touching of his genitals or attempt to do so. During the short time he was fully naked no erection of the penis was noted.

Johnny had been called "unattractive" as a newborn, and he still was not pretty. His features were coarse and had an un-baby-like quality. His body was rather too fat, and the color of his skin was dull. Nevertheless, he succeeded in enchanting every observer who met him. He seemed so well put together, so smoothly integrated, and so completely unaware of life's hardships that it gave pleasure to all around him. His lack of anxiety made him capable of approaching a stranger and leaving a contagious feeling of happiness.

Between eight and nine months Johnny began to crawl. The crowded home which had provided him with so much stimulation now began to limit him. He was constantly "getting into things," which made problems for his mother and pointed up her discontent with the living arrangements. The television set became a particular focus of struggle because the usually indulgent grandmother resented Johnny's fussing with the dials. Endless vigilance was required to assure the safety of the prized knick-knacks and religious statues. It began to harass Mary Callini.

In addition, Mrs. Callini's mother became ill and required her presence a good part of the day. The elder Mrs. Callini grew increasingly attentive to Johnny, and he enjoyed bouncing and playing on her ample lap. Mary Callini resented her role of having to force restrictions on Johnny to guard her mother-in-law's possessions while the grandmother became a refuge from those very prohibitions. Her repeated remarks about Johnny's preference for his paternal grandmother began to carry a more serious tone. Once, when his grandmother permitted Johnny to pull the venetian blind cords, which had always been forbidden, Mrs. Callini departed from her usual soft-spoken manner to say harshly, "You know Johnny isn't supposed to do that."

The crowded apartment began to oppress Mary Callini. "It would be nice to do what you wanted to for a change," she complained. The increased absence of her husband because of his job change further upset her. As time went on, her desire for an independent home became more compelling, and the search was begun for a separate home. Adding to her discontent was Mrs. Callini's lack of ease with the Italian language, and she began more openly to express irritation that her husband's family continued to speak a language she could not fully understand.

Her contentment in motherhood gave way to a sense of daily struggle. The easy-going but constant traffic of the household became more annoying, and the earlier attentions lavished on Johnny by relatives were now blamed by Mrs. Callini for his "slowness" in walking. "They hold him too much," she felt. Mrs. Callini said she was "tired of crowds" even though she recognized that "big families are nice anyway." Although she smiled, she complained how hard it was to keep up with Johnny's activity, how hard it was to dress him. There was little doubt that he was becoming increasingly difficult to manage as he became more mobile and less willing to conform.

In his ninth month Johnny had another respiratory infection with an asthmatic wheeze, but no special medication was required after a day or so. Near the end of his first year he had two bouts of "runny nose," not severe enough for Mrs. Callini to call the doctor. During his infection Johnny refused all food and fluids the first day but was soon back to normal. He permitted no one but his mother to feed him, and she was somewhat annoyed that he put his hands in the plate and grabbed the spoon. His sleep rhythm was regular except during illness and occasional awakenings when his father came home from work at 1 A.M. Mrs. Callini continued to "catch" Johnny's bowel movements and occasionally got him to urinate in the potty. At one well-baby clinic visit, when Johnny was put on the toilet, he was observed to finger his penis. After a moment Mrs.

Callini said, "That's not to play with," and held him so that he was unable to reach his genitals.

Mary Callini was ill for a few days when Johnny was between ten and eleven months old. Although her mother-in-law played with her grandson, she was unable to attend to his wants and had to call upon Mrs. Callini, who felt it an "unnecessary burden" to have to rise from her sickbed to feed and change her son. Even sickness failed to provide respite from the tensions of her situation.

In these months Johnny was active enough to exhaust both his mother and grandmother, but towards the end of his first year there was a striking slow-down in his gross motor development. He continued to enjoy social contact and delighted in making sounds. Mrs. Callini reported that he bit the crib bars, chewed the paint off, and had scratched her neck with his pinching.

The observation evaluation in the middle of his eleventh month (49 weeks) disclosed a surprisingly low gross motor performance for Johnny. He was not able to stand without support and not capable of walking unless both hands were held. On the Gesell scale, gross motor was at 48 weeks, fine motor 56, adaptive 52, language 56, and personal-social 57. General maturity level was 54 weeks, and the developmental quotient was 112.

Three different explanations suggested themselves for this gross motor slow-down. One was that he had not been born an active child but had been made so by his busy, attentive environment. Another was that his mother's prohibitions against moving around in the crowded apartment may have had an inhibiting effect. Third, the stimulation provided by bodily contact with his mother had diminished, since there was not as much physical interaction as before.

In contrast to the gross motor slow-down, Johnny's fine motor coordination had improved considerably. He was capable of imitating drumming with two sticks and was also able to spin a top by imitating. This was a motor performance requiring so much skill that it is not expected before the third year.

His own image in the mirror must have reminded Johnny of the sight of his own body because it stimulated genital masturbation. The hand went to the genital slowly and hesitantly, then he grasped it loosely. The contact between hand and genital was very short, however, and in every instance he suddenly withdrew the hand as if the genital were hot. He started genital masturbation again when his diaper was removed. At this point his mother actively interfered.

Johnny's incapacity to concentrate also appeared strongly at this observation. He was easily distracted from the object or material at hand by almost anything. It was hard to judge whether or not he remembered the rubber cat's missing protruding tongue because his attention had already turned to the door knob, the examiner, his mother, his own foot. His attention was caught more by human movement than by inanimate objects.

Johnny's parents reported that he said "mama," "dada," and "bye bye." He said "bad boy" fairly distinctly and also had an elaborate jargon, "telling long stories" with great intensity, with much modulation and varied inflection. Besides this "speaking" jargon he had a high-pitched triumphant squealing, which was sustained for a surprisingly long time and was accompanied by smiling and animation. There was a third kind of vocalization, somewhere between the other two, which was less high-pitched and was accompanied by a frown. It sounded like scolding or complaining and was always directed at his mother, as if he were quarreling with her.

There were further impressions that he was in opposition to his mother. He had developed quite a technique of resistance when she was dressing him. Despite her extreme skill she was forced to outsmart him for even the simplest ministration. Yet he was very sensitive to her reprimands. When she shushed him he started to cry as if his feelings were hurt.

Mary Callini was far less at ease with Johnny than before. He obviously did things with which she wanted to interfere, such as mouthing, masturbation, and making noise. During the observation she had a hard time keeping herself from interfering and she probably reacted more forcefully at home. She also reacted negatively to what he did not do, and seemed painfully aware of his lack of concentration. She strenuously tried to draw his attention back to the "task." But she had little success.

Johnny's second year was ushered in by two birthday parties, two being necessary because of the size of both parents' families.

Also, within three months, three major events took place in his life. He went on a two-week motor trip to the mountains with his parents, his father was transferred to a day job once more near home, and his mother went back to her old job in his fifteenth month. "I had to get out of the house," she explained. She worked from 3 o'clock in the afternoon until 11 P.M. During this time Johnny stayed at his maternal grandmother's home in the care of Mrs. Callini's sister.

The months brought increasing friction between mother and son. Johnny's insistence on feeding himself and the resultant messiness were exasperating. Mrs. Callini thought her son was old enough to obey commands, and she interpreted his independent behavior as "freshness." Both Mr. and Mrs. Callini became concerned with discipline. They found spanking, scolding, and banishment to his crib ineffective. While discipline was frequent, often it was inconsistent. The parents were sometimes firm and sometimes lax in enforcing their orders. With so many adults in the house it became a matter of many generals and conflicting orders. Johnny soon became adept at playing off one adult against another. Frustration developed as antagonistic struggle supplanted enjoyment.

The apartment seemed smaller than ever as Johnny grew. Escape from the confined living situation became even more imperative. Both the Callinis were unhappy about not having a home of their own, but now Mrs. Callini began to exert constant pressure on her husband to find them a place to live. He reasoned that they could only afford a cheap rental, and those were scarce. He felt that instead of showing so much concern for an apartment they should have another child quickly before he became too old. At that time he was twenty-six. His wife firmly refused to have a second child unless she had an apartment of her own. Thus, tensions began to arise in this hitherto serene relationship.

Although the contact between mother and child remained warm, Mrs. Callini was no longer able to anticipate Johnny's needs as readily as before. She once commented to a member of the staff, "The doctor gets such a kick out of Johnny, but it's not funny when you have to live with it all day long." Her skill with him continued to diminish in various areas of activity. Johnny objected violently to being bathed, and there was much struggle in this area. Mrs.

Callini reported that she tried to bathe him two or three times a day during the summer "to keep him cool."

She asked the home interviewer on one occasion what to do about Johnny's "freshness" and refusal to obey. When a decisive answer was not forthcoming she turned to Johnny and said, "She isn't going to give us a solution; we'll have to work it out ourselves." Although Mrs. Callini had not intended to go back to work when the baby came, she jumped at the chance when she heard there might be an opportunity to get her old job back. It became a means to financially expedite an apartment of her own and to resolve the social frustrations. However, her decision to return to work did not meet with her husband's approval. He strongly felt that a mother's place was in the home and that it was a surrender of parental responsibility to let someone else care for his son.

Mrs. Callini's feelings about working were ambivalent. She rejoiced in freedom from the tensions of her mother-in-law's home and in rediscovering old friends. While she was pleased that Johnny seemed to be less of a disciplinary problem with her mother and sister, she also ruefully observed that he obeyed them better than her. And she felt guilty because she shared her husband's feelings that parents should take care of their child. Also, in working full-time she had opened up a definite issue with her husband. Soon after her return to work Johnny had a brief illness, which made her guilt feelings even more acute. Furthermore, upon her return to work all efforts at toilet training were interrupted. "I don't have time any more for that," she said.

It was evident at a clinic visit that there was prohibition at home against Johnny's mouthing. At the clinic Mr. Callini firmly told Johnny to take his finger out of his mouth. When he made another try his father removed it himself. During clinic visits Johnny's play was remarkably independent. He moved from one activity to another and paid scarcely any attention to the adults. His interest was primarily in toys that he could actively manipulate, such as train, car, bell. His mother reported that he had a passion for pinwheels and now owned seven or eight of them. Johnny's development remained constant between the twelfth and fifteenth months. His jargon was elaborate and served for communication along with gestures. In the fifteenth month he started to walk, and his jargon became even more elaborate, but no new words were reported.

At the fifteenth-month evaluative observation Johnny showed himself to be a large sturdy boy who was definitely not pretty. His features were coarse, his large dark eyes too round and too thinly lashed for beauty, and his complexion sallow and pale. His hairdo had bangs in front and was cut too short in back. Nevertheless, he was engaging and had a rather comical appeal both in his appearance and attire. But mainly there was the impression that he laughed continuously except when he cried or screamed.

His laughter did not sound like a child's. It was loud and throaty, more like that of a man. The discrepancy between his appearance and his kind of laughter may have contributed to the comical effect. Also, the constant laughter seemed inappropriate and no longer moved observers to share his pleasures in the world. The laughter was interrupted when Johnny became upset. In one instance his arm proved too short to reach the ball in the Gesell box. He did not try another solution but increased his unsuccessful efforts to reach the ball and then started to yell.

He paid no attention to his mother, who demonstrated that the ball could be approached by moving the box. Even though the ball had now been placed within his reaching distance he tried to crawl into the box with his whole body, becoming even more angry when his shoulders were too broad for this. The observers were struck by his strong rage reaction, which made him incapable of adapting to reality. He was also quite upset during the medical examination. He cried heart-breakingly, hugged his mother, and tried to escape the threatening situation in her arms.

His approach to inanimate objects also tended to be unrealistic. When the massed cubes were offered, his sole activity was a brushing gesture, by which he moved them on the table top. Then he occasionally put one block on top of the other very sloppily. He laughed loudly, looked vaguely around, and hardly focused on the cubes at all. His manner suggested that this was his own unique approach to objects which held no emotional significance or interest for him. Or it could have been that Johnny became so absorbed with objects which did have emotional significance for him that he could not concentrate on others.

Throughout the examination Johnny kept pointing at the toy chest, saying "Mommy." The examiner finally realized that he was pointing to the toy milk bottle. He touched his chest and stomach with the milk bottle and then rubbed those spots with his left hand. The mother explained to the bewildered examiner that he was "powdering" himself as she powdered him after his bath. She also explained that when he became active and she couldn't handle him she would give him the powder box to quiet him down. Later, when he played with the teddy bear, it was obvious that he knew the real purpose of the milk bottle and that it was really no powder box.

His fantasy play was demonstrated vividly with the massed cubes, to which he had earlier paid so little attention. When a cup was offered, he immediately placed the massed cubes in it. In fantasy he suddenly transformed the cubes into "food," focused on them, grasped them eagerly, and put them to his mouth. It seemed that when he could make-believe and play out at the fantasy level the cubes assumed emotional significance for him and he was prepared to concentrate. The preoccupation with fantasy make-believe could well have been one of the factors which kept him from realistic use of the test material.

In throwing the ball Johnny showed vigor and glee, although he made a point of throwing it where he could not get it himself. Then he indicated by gesture and vocalization that the parents should get it for him. His demands were mostly directed at his mother. He threw the ball with amazing skill and showed far better motor coordination than he did in walking, which was still clumsy. The coordination in this one specific motor performance was above his age level, and he seemed to enjoy its mastery.

Johnny's vocabulary had not increased in the last two months. It still consisted of "mommy," "daddy," and "bad boy," with only "beer" added. In comparison with this poor number of words, he had a very rich jargon, which usually sounded like exclaiming or arguing but very rarely had the melodic quality of statements. It appeared to the staff that he used few words and much jargon because he was expressing emotional reaction and not objective communication.

During this observation Mrs. Callini was less intensely involved than before. She sat on a chair next to Johnny and talked occasionally to the examiner. She was mildly pleased when he succeeded in a task and mildly annoyed when he failed, but she did not try to manage things as she usually did. She volunteered her help only on two occasions, once to save Johnny's face with the Gesell box and once to help the examiner by reinterpreting her instructions to Johnny. Johnny did not pay any special attention to his mother except in the ball game. The impression prevailed that Mrs. Callini had removed herself from Johnny, that he knew it and used other objects to substitute for her.

In one situation, however, Mrs. Callini became her old self. During the medical examination she left her chair to be physically near Johnny in his anxiety. For the first time her face was soft and relaxed. Throughout the medical examination Johnny looked at her and tried to hug her whenever possible. The overall impression was that Johnny had psychologically separated from his mother and through fantasy play was trying to find his own gratifications. The mother became an interfering element in this gratification process and thus was an object for quarreling. On the basis of their past relationship this quarreling had emotional investment, so much so that it affected the development of his body image and body mastery. Only in extreme danger situations did Johnny revert to the original relationship with his mother.

For Mrs. Callini this development was extremely painful. Rather than relate to a child who was becoming independent of her, she gave in to her hostility and did not relate at all. Only if the old happy past could be restored would she be able again to assume fully her role as Johnny's mother.

Both parents remained disturbed by Johnny's "freshness" and disobedience. His mother said, "He knows when he's wrong but just goes ahead and does things anyway." She was particularly irritated one day in the clinic when he smashed his bottle to the floor. Her voice became tremulous and shrewish. When he was disciplined Johnny still had the habit of appealing to another member of the family, from whom he would gain comfort and thus offset any effective discipline.

In his seventeenth month Johnny began to awaken past midnight just after his mother returned from work. He insisted on having his bottle in her bed, where he would shortly fall asleep and then be returned to his crib to sleep without interruption until morning. Mrs. Callini "had not tried very much" to continue his toilet training, but his distinctive facial expression and vocalization permitted some success in catching his bowel movements.

Johnny did not like being wet or dirty but showed no inclination to use ordinary language to signal the adult. During a routine clinic examination he was observed to touch his penis several times, and on each occasion Mrs. Callini interceded, saying "Don't put your hand down there."

Johnny's activity in the communal apartment remained widespread. The birdcage and television set were still the chief sources of conflict and taboo with the grandmother. When he violated prohibitions he would run to the front door to escape his "crime." He now climbed expertly, enjoyed banging pots and pans, and maintained remarkable independence in his play. To communicate, he banged or pointed, scarcely using words at all.

At one play observation Johnny was left to himself with a number of toys at his disposal. The observer was struck with "how time had changed Johnny." All his animation and liveliness seemed to have disappeared, and he did nothing constructive with the material. Nor did he do anything destructive either. He just looked lost and bored. His reaction to a completely free and unstructured situation was quite different from that of the other study children, who became either immobilized on their own or went haywire with impulsive activity. Johnny reacted with neither of those extremes but remained lethargic, as if the life and flavor were drained from his actions because the adult did not instigate them. In his case it appeared that the adult was a necessary motivational source to make his actions personal, meaningful, and vivacious.

Despite his drive for independence he required active contact with his mother or a substitute adult to get him interested in what he was doing. Johnny's independence in relation to discipline appeared to have two polarities. At one end he protested and struggled against the prohibitions of banging, mouthing, and throwing. At the other were restrictions against which he did not struggle but had come to accept as an unchangeable part of the world in which he lived.

Similarly, Johnny's emotional expression showed two extremes. During much of the time he seemed neutral in his emotional expression. But when he did express emotion it was with his whole being, forcefully and definitely. If the emotion was pleasurable, Johnny chuckled, laughed loudly and throatily, his whole body shook, his head was thrown back, and his arms waved or rhythmically banged. If the emotion was the opposite, Johnny was mad all over. He screamed, frowned, tears rolled down his cheeks, he stamped his foot, and he threw whatever he could reach. The outbreaks of both pleasure and rage were short and terminated abruptly even at their peak if the cause was removed.

His motor actions also were of an extreme nature, with everything done at utmost speed. Even his walking was at the speed of running, although he did not bend his knees enough so one could call it running. He did not turn his head, he threw it around; he did not bend down toward an object but precipitated the upper part of his body toward it; he did not grasp objects but grabbed them; he did not dispose of them but lost or threw them away; his glance did not wander but brushed along things; he did not sit down but fell into a chair; he did not stand up but jumped up. Even his breathing seemed quicker than other people's.

All of these high-speed actions were not goal-directed to get somewhere or to get something but quick because he did not know how to be slow. He had not learned to wait or to master the coordination necessary to suspend an action. Also, he was quick because he enjoyed it that way. The very speed of his actions seemed to excite Johnny. It was also obvious that his quickness made it harder for his mother to catch up with him, and he made it an effective weapon in his struggle with her.

Johnny's perception was as quick as his actions. Despite his brief concentration on objects he had high accuracy in his perception of them. Even with the more difficult Viennese formboard he matched the right figure to the right hole immediately but left it at that without trying to finish the job by putting the figures into the holes. Obviously his speed did not interfere with discovery or solving of problems but only with sticking to them long enough to complete them properly.

It followed, therefore, that he was not receptive to non-motor activity, such as looking at picture books or building with blocks and cubes. When he tried building, the structure tumbled immediately not only as a result of his sloppy building but because the lower part of his arms leaned against it. He laughed heartily when the building fell to pieces. The construction itself was not an act of production but more an activity that excited. The process was rather closely related to the pleasurable sense of "throwing," which was still strong for Johnny.

At intervals during the test examination Johnny pointed to the chest of drawers which held the test material and said "Mommy." As in the last observation he referred to the milk bottle, which at that time he had pretended was a powder box. This time when he secured the milk bottle he put it to his mouth and pretended to drink from it. The examiner asked him to feed the teddy bear. He took the nipple off the bottle and approached the teddy bear with the reversed nipple. Mrs. Callini put the nipple back on the bottle, whereupon Johnny put it to his mouth again. When the request to feed the teddy was repeated, Johnny complied with the bottom of the bottle to the teddy's mouth. This incident was significant in that Johnny behaved as usual quickly and expertly in feeding himself, but when confronted by a task in which he had no emotional interest or involvement he moved slowly, absent-mindedly, and with boredom.

Around Johnny's nineteenth month Mrs. Callini heard about an apartment which was vacant near her mother's home. Hastily she called the owner and without even inspecting the place arranged to sign a lease. The new apartment was small, the walls were dingy, and there was no facility for hot water. The floors sloped and threatened the balance of the kitchen appliances. But there was space to provide Johnny with a bedroom of his own for the first time, and it would at least separate Mrs. Callini from her in-laws. Her husband was amazed that she had taken such an apartment, but he was reluctant to oppose her determination to move. One of Mrs. Callini's brothers papered the apartment, and the Callinis finally moved to a home of their own.

To solve the problem of no hot water they went to their respective family homes for bathing and shaving. This perpetuated family contact, and each continued to help out in their own parents' home as they had done before. However, the move did break up the constant interaction between Mrs. Callini and her mother-in-law, although in-law relationships remained friendly.

The deficiencies of the apartment became quite apparent. The sloping kitchen floor even bewildered Johnny. When he put a toy down, it rolled away toward the windows. But it was their own home, and the Callinis were markedly less harassed in trying to keep Johnny out of trouble. Mrs. Callini was dissatisfied that her husband now worked the day shift. On working days they saw each other only during the brief interval between Mrs. Callini's return from work and bedtime. It was necessary for them to leave notes for each other in order to keep the household functioning. Despite all this there was a warm, relaxed quality in their relationship to each other and to Johnny through this period which had been missing for several months. Mrs. Callini was fervent in her claim that life had greatly improved because of the move and that for the first time in their married life they could do as they pleased without considering the desires or schedules of others. Even Mr. Callini had to agree that it was good his family had moved into their own home.

Johnny adjusted well to the move. To his parents' satisfaction, his behavior began to improve, although he remained a very active child. The night-time demand to lie in his parents' bed with his bottle did not recur, and he slept through the night from 8 P.M. until 7:30 A.M. Mr. Callini's schedule permitted him more hours with Johnny while his wife worked. They had good times together, and more than once Mrs. Callini intimated that "the two of them got away with murder" in her absence. The staff felt that possibly Mrs. Callini was a bit concerned that her son might prefer his father to her. As for Mr. Callini, although he liked playing with Johnny, he continued to feel that baby-tending was "women's work," and he was never reconciled to his wife's working.

Johnny's second winter was less marred by wheezing coughs and colds than his first had been. He had only one infection which required the physician's care, an otitis media, and his recovery was typically easy and uncomplicated. Mrs. Callini stayed home from work for three days, although the illness would scarcely warrant such concern. And she questioned the pediatrician in detail about the causes of the infection, as if to ask, "Am I to blame?"

The ear infection did not disturb Johnny's feeding, and he was reported to eat very well. He liked everything except cooked cereal. On occasion he ate with a spoon, but the major share was still done rather messily by hand. He complained vigorously when wet or soiled but gave the adults no help in anticipating his need. Mrs. Callini was unable to catch his bowel movements with her former success.

The decreased tension between his parents resulted in an easing of Johnny's negativism. He no longer struggled against dressing, and the pediatrician remarked that "he was less involved in fighting with his mother." Johnny was vigorous and strong-looking. He took continuing pleasure in his own activity and was capable of amusing himself almost indefinitely. At twenty months he was reported to have some twenty to thirty words, walked up and down stairs by himself, threw a ball well, and did not show any shyness or stranger anxiety.

When Johnny entered the room for evaluation in the twentieth month he looked like quite an independent little boy who knew what he wanted and guessed what he was supposed to do. Nevertheless, after purposefully sitting down on the examining chair he turned around toward his mother saying "Mommy" and smiled. He was quite ready to look at the book alone, but his sitting posture was tense and he wriggled on his chair. When his mother looked at the book with him he relaxed immediately and quieted down. She showed him something in the book, and he followed her gesture, first with his eyes, then by rising from his chair as if he could better follow her gesture by doing so. When something about his fingernails was discussed, he spontaneously presented his hands to his mother.

Johnny did not respond to the examiner's request to point out the Gesell picture cards but did so at his mother's request. After solving the formboard a number of times he chanted "mamma-mamma" in a smiling happy way. His behavior showed that the mother was still the most important person in Johnny's life. Although he performed without her help, he needed to relate to her, and if the task was too difficult, he performed only with her assistance. If no assistance was given by her, any task might become too difficult.

There was some evidence, however, that the struggle between Johnny and his mother had not ceased completely. When Johnny was given the ball he first threw it to his father, then aimed it at his mother but changed his mind and threw it between the two parents. When he was asked specifically to give the ball to the mother, he did not bring it to her but threw it so that she had to bend down to get it. In contrast, when he was asked to put the ball on the table he placed it there slowly and carefully without throwing it.

He did not always enjoy contact with his mother when he was very busy with something. When she took his hand while he was busy at the formboard he pushed her hand away and said "no" energetically. When she asked him something while he was in a make-believe game with a key, he ignored her request. His position toward the interference was firm and energetic, with little hostility. But it was clear that in some situations he experienced his mother negatively.

Johnny was still a child who enjoyed moving. Even when he sat down he did so with a flourish, lifting one leg high and swinging it almost in full circle before sitting down. He kicked rhythmically with his feet against the bottom of the table, enjoying the movement as much as the noise. He repeated this same procedure while sitting on the crib. He most enjoyed rhythmically moving the Gesell box around the room, chanting as he went along. And he enjoyed throwing and kicking the ball with his leg. He was capable of doing this with both his feet, although he started with the right one.

While Johnny was a lively child, to whom moving about was important, he stayed on his chair or near the examining table most of the time. He completely left the table only when no material or attention was given him. In most instances he conformed when material was offered. He cooperated in building a tower and putting the cubes into a cup. But when the cubes were offered a second time despite his lack of interest, he asked firmly but politely that they be taken away. He did not put up any resistance to undressing and went willingly with his mother to the bathroom. Except for the mouth examination, against which he protested slightly and without real effect, he tolerated the medical examination well. He was even ready to lie down when necessary.

When the pellet was offered, he approached it to his mouth immediately. But he agreed promptly and good-naturedly to put it first into the bottle and then to eat it after he had taken it out of the bottle. Once he put a crayon into his mouth but took it out immediately at his mother's request. In contrast to Johnny's previous negativism he showed a new kind of freedom and efficiency by compliance.

There was little evidence that Johnny indulged in or enjoyed autoerotic activity. Except for the rhythmical kicking with his feet, nothing was seen that approximated rocking. He did not play with his genitals when he was undressed nor touch any other part of his body with his hands. However, he rubbed his navel with the stethoscope, then started to move it slowly and hesitantly to his genital but stopped before reaching his goal.

It seemed that as the struggle with his mother decreased, Johnny could function better on all levels. He was able to give his energies to solving problems of the outside world, and he became capable of applying himself to a variety of tasks. He "imitated" the "choo-choo" of the train even before the examiner demonstrated it. He closely watched her when she demonstrated the scribble, and then he imitated the horizontal and circular stroke successfully. He built a tower, filled a cup with cubes, solved the formboard. He took the ball out of the Gesell problem box without any difficulty and coped well with the examiner's attempt to interfere with his motion. His actions were just as clear-cut and efficient when he objected to a task as when he complied with it. Not liking the chimney on the train, he took it off each time it was shown him.

In solving problems Johnny still maintained his own personal touch towards the world. To him it was still a movable world, and he acted as if movability of his surroundings was a most important condition for solving problems. When the examiner reversed the position of the formboard Johnny did not attempt to fit the pieces but tried to adapt the position of the formboard so the pieces would be in front of the correct holes. When refused permission to do this, he tried to press the form into the hole with all his strength, then he tried to "hammer" it in. Failing in all this, he went back to his pushing attempt, again to no avail. He failed to solve the problem.

But Johnny didn't relinquish his interest in a task until it was solved. Much later in the session he got the formboard again and retackled it in his inimitable fashion. This time he adjusted it to his requirements, and holding all three figures under his left arm, he placed them on the board with his right hand. While trying to adjust the board and hold the pieces simultaneously he encountered many problems. He dropped some pieces, and he had to push the chair in order to sit and hold all the pieces at the same time. In spite of these obstacles he insisted on solving the formboard five times in a row until he finally lifted it triumphantly above his head.

Johnny's efficiency in solving tasks through action did not apply to language however. He spoke very little and for the most part his speech was unstructured and unvaried. He used language for naming the people of his immediate surrounding and to specifically request the ball. The word "no" and the demand "take it away" were also heard.

At the chronological age of 20 months and 7 days Johnny's performance on the Gesell examination showed gross motor at 24 months, with one item (walking on tip-toe) at 30; adaptive at 24, language 21, and personal-social between 21 and 24 months. General maturity level was close to 24 months, and developmental quotient was at 117.

As time passed, the sketchy furnishings of the Callinis' apartment were augmented by a television set, a goldfish bowl, an electric dryer, and a little table and chair for Johnny on one side of the kitchen. Because his parents worked different shifts, most of his day was spent with one or another of them. From Mr. Callini the interviewer heard extended and detailed discussion of his job, of the bad morale of his co-workers, and of the workings of the television set or the dryer. In the absence of her husband Mrs. Callini gave long accounts of their courtship, her family relations, the difficulty she had had while living for four years with her in-laws, and the concern she had about Johnny being raised by so many people. The interviewer had the strong impression that Mrs. Callini would continue to work even in the face of her husband's objections.

In handling Johnny Mrs. Callini was warm but firm. She had learned that "he listens better if you talk nice to him instead of yelling." The Callinis' primary discipline for Johnny was to make him sit in his little chair or stay in his crib for a few minutes. Apparently this bothered him more when his father did it. There was "no problem at all" when it came to eating. Johnny took almost any table food, supplemented once in a while by baby fruit, drank milk from a glass and also from the bottle. Mrs. Callini would feed Johnny at the start of the meal, but he always ended up wielding the spoon himself with no great efficiency. He slept well, although it was harder to get him to bed when the days were long and there was light outside. On the few occasions when he awoke at night he would no longer accept comforting by his mother but insisted on having his daddy.

Mrs. Callini had returned Johnny to diapers because he still failed to advise about his toileting needs. Near the end of his second year, however, his old pattern changed. He no longer complained when he was soiled, and he had begun to run away when Mrs. Callini went to change him. Johnny continued to be dominated by his own movement. He had a wild game in which he jumped and rolled around the floor laughing delightedly. He also was reported to enjoy watching other children at play. From home visit reports it was clear that Johnny was responsive to his mother's requests and showed great pleasure in physical contact with her.

The final evaluation took place when Johnny was 23 months, 11 days old. On the Viennese test his developmental age was 27 months, 18 days, with a developmental quotient of 116.7. He had still not developed into a handsome boy. All elegance and refinement were missing from his appearance. The dark straight hair was cut in a bowl shape and the saucer-like eyes lacked the softening feature of long lashes. His face was too round, and his husky figure, though not fat or flabby, did not appear graceful in any way. The mouth was neither delicate nor especially expressive. He gave the impression of "a husky little workman with a comic twist." Nevertheless he was not unattractive and presented childlike and endearing qualities. Although he looked as if he would stumble over his own feet, he did not do so. It was a demonstration of the "unrefined little man's" triumph over the traps and hazards which his environment presented.

Johnny entered the room purposefully and energetically, ahead of his mother, who "sneaked in" after him. With firm deliberation he sat down at the testing table and was ready to act only as he wanted to act. No amount of persuasion by either the tester or his mother could get him to look at the picture book or name the pictures. His reluctance was not due to incapacity to name the pictures but because the task was imposed on him and there was no room for choice. Also, Johnny tended to reject test items that required any prolonged receptive attitude because he would not interrupt his flow of action even for a short time to contemplate.

His transitions from one occupation to another were so quick that they gave the impression that he reacted immediately. Whether the reaction was a quick "no" or an acceptance of the task, literally no time elapsed between the request to do something and his response to it. This did not mean that he failed to stay with one activity for any prolonged time. He played with the hollow blocks for quite a time and tried many methods of nesting the blocks. But his transitions from one method of problem-solving to another were quick and decisive. The speed of solution did not necessarily interfere with its quality. After the merest hint by the pediatrician, he solved the formboard quickly and without any mistake.

Johnny's intellectual stature was about age-adequate when he had to deal with problems involving minimal motor efforts, as the formboard did. But it was above average when the intellectual solution involved a major motor effort. An object which attracted his interest (the top) was out of reach, and a stick was provided to get the top down from its high place above him. But the examiner did not notice that the stick was too short to get the top down. Johnny however noticed this immediately. He did not get upset or angry but pulled over a big chair, onto which he climbed, retrieved the top, climbed down, and started to play. His actions looked easy and natural. As a matter of fact, he solved a difficult intellectual problem extremely well for his age level.

During this evaluation Mrs. Callini spoke almost continuously, and so did Johnny. His talk was rich and varied, consisting partly of jargon and partly of English, all delivered with a delightful Italian intonation. Neither one seemed to listen to the other. This did not mean, however, that Johnny's language served a purely intellectual function. He used language mainly to express his wants, dislikes, needs, and objections. He did this with a refreshingly clear display of his emotions and a distinct enunciation of the words. He spoke very loudly, probably as an indication of awareness that he was not being listened to. The same pattern was seen in his mother, who talked without stop, encouraging him in tasks or prohibiting unruly behavior, but in a way that indicated she had no real hope of being listened to.

Johnny could not be induced to do what he didn't want to do. He refused to take the coat off the teddy bear and tried to distract the adults by bringing over the formboard or interesting them in the ball. When the adults forced the teddy bear on him he finally threw it energetically into a corner. Similarly, he ignored the request to feed the teddy bear with the little milk bottle. Instead he engaged in make-believe games of his own choice, such as pushing the little red car and making noises to reproduce movements and honks. He whistled as skillfully as boys of six or seven years. He also played a game with the top which impressed one as a make-believe game. After he had made it spin expertly he lifted it, still spinning, from the table "with a proud and serious face as if it were a flag."

His method of problem solution was just as determined as his selective process, and he became really angry when the examiner used the hollow blocks for building instead of for nesting, as he intended. So he destroyed the tower immediately. He went into a physical tussle with the examiner when she tried to prevent him from turning the formboard around instead of adjusting the figures to the reversed formboard. On the other hand, Johnny never objected if something was taken away from him. He came in with a measuring tape in his hand, but at the pediatrician's request he handed it to her, saying "Don't wanna." It was not clear whether he didn't want to give it up or didn't want to keep it anymore. He parted from other objects more clearly. There was no resistance to giving up the top, and he himself put the little red car back in the drawer. This was far different from the Johnny at four months, who was more interested in retaining than in getting.

At the beginning of his life Johnny was an outstandingly quiet and relaxed baby who was interested in and enjoyed the world around him. At two years of age he appeared to be an eager, hyperactive little busybody who rushed from task to task without being able to stop and look at the world or even to admire his own success. There was the firm impression that at two years the "active" Johnny was not the real Johnny at all. There was speculation by the staff that his activity seemed not inherent but a self-imposed borrowed role to link him more strongly with his mother, the most essential figure in his life. It was as if his actions and decisions were but an adaptation to the mother's desire for an active, vigorous baby who used his body easily and well, and with whom she had complete motor identification. Movement for the sake of movement therefore became vitally important in Johnny's development.

As with Johnny, one may speculate that it was equally difficult for both his parents to fully find their identification and assert independence from their own families. Theirs was a search for a way of life in which their new family could grow without crowding out filial roles and without sacrificing parental values for American ideals. Essentially the family process was in transition, and with the growth of Johnny, more demanding transitions were expected to be thrust upon the family. Only then would the quality of the adjustment be fully determined.

SUMMARY

A. EXPECTATIONS

1. Maternal Expectations. Mrs. Callini's anticipation of maternity appeared to be of a happy and pleasurable nature, untroubled by anxieties over assumption of the maternal role. She seemingly put a high value on motherhood but was very inarticulate about concepts of herself as a mother. She raised few anxious questions or fears about herself or the baby to come. She was eager to learn about the course of events and child care but had no feeling of inadequacy. There was no conflict about outside employment versus motherhood. In fact, she did not expect to return to work after the baby arrived. Pressures arising from life in the paternal grandparents' home and increased friction with her child because of his growing independence accounted for her return to work.

2. Specificity of Expectations. Mrs. Callini expressed few, if any, specific expectations. She seemed to feel that there was nothing special she could say which would be of any interest. Thus, she answered direct questions without elaborating on her feelings or introducing any new elements. Possibly, cultural factors in her background did not encourage self-introspection or verbalization. On the other hand, she felt that she had much to learn about pregnancy and child care, so she asked many specific questions of a factual nature and was eager to acquire all the precise information she could get.

She gave no elaborate thought to whether or not she would breast feed and expressed no special desire for the sex of the child. The only expectation which she emphasized was that she had expected to be uncomfortable during pregnancy and was pleasurably surprised to be free from any discomfort.

Although Mrs. Callini was one of the mothers who was most

gratified and satisfied with her approaching motherhood, she was also minimally expressive of her specific feelings.

3. Motivational Orientation. From the very beginning there was little question about Mrs. Callini's child-centeredness. Her child-oriented expectations fitted easily with her direct and unequivocal pleasure in the prospect of a child and her experiences with the infant. There was much pride in his appetite, growth, development, and response to her care. Almost instinctively a close rapport existed between mother and child, each seeming to adjust almost instantly to the clues of the other. This great attachment to the child was also shared by Mr. Callini.

But as the child grew older and more difficult to manage, some of the close rapport was lost. In addition, the restrictions of living in her mother-in-law's home complicated Mrs. Callini's management of Johnny. It made her submissive and dependent role in the elder Callinis' household far less palatable to her. With the increase of her own dissatisfaction there was a shift in her child-centeredness. She began to demand more from Johnny in the way of conformity, and she began to put more stress and value on social behavior, achievement, and performance. The combination of factors thus led to the decision to return to work.

When the Callinis at last moved to their own apartment some of the tensions diminished, and the conflict between Mrs. Callini and her child became less troublesome. Discipline was handled more effectively without the intervention of relatives, and Johnny became more compliant in his response. His mother came to see that "he listens better if you talk nice to him." The warm relationship between mother and son resumed its satisfactory course as the transitional adjustment was made between infancy and childhood. Despite the interim difficulties the motivational orientation of both Mr. and Mrs. Callini was decidedly child-centered throughout the study.

4. Role of Child in Fulfilling Mother's Expectations. In the early months of his life Johnny provided his mother with almost total pleasure, and he did nothing which diminished her joyous expectations of him. She felt competent in her role, and her son seemed to thrive by her ministrations. She had such strong expectations of a vigorous, healthy, and unproblematic baby that she could hardly adjust to periods of illness. Thus, when Johnny was ill at various times she seemed less able to handle him and could scarcely wait for convalescence to be over.

As Johnny emerged from early infancy, however, he began to present his mother with some major problems of adjustment, those posed by a vigorous little boy whose behavior was characterized by much physical activity. There was a discrepancy between the enthusiasm with which he explored the world and his mother's expectations of conforming behavior. For Mrs. Callini the task of giving up her early gratifications was very difficult. As Johnny's behavior began to create conflict there was some lessening of gratification and close interaction. But at the same time her child-centered values and the strong feeling of warmth remained, and she sought some compromise with the inevitable developmental changes. She tried to provide him with more opportunities for freedom of activity by moving into a separate home. But as he left infancy behind and became ever more independent from her, she sought additional satisfactions by going to work.

5. Paternal Expectations. Nothing is known about Mr. Callini's expectations before the birth except that he was highly gratified at the prospect of a child. The delight in his son was evident from birth throughout the study. He was eager to have more children and suggested to his wife that they have a second child rather than move to another apartment. During the two years he was fairly permissive in his attitude and showed consideration for the limitations of the child's ability to conform. He was tolerant of the child's activities and enjoyed roughhousing with him. However, he thought that Johnny could realize the difference between right and wrong and that he should do what was right. Like Mrs. Callini, he expected Johnny to be less mischievous and more docile than the lively one-year-old was inclined to be. On the whole, Tony Callini enjoyed his child and his paternal role.

B. BEHAVIOR

1. Communication. Mrs. Callini talked with her baby from the earliest days to express her feelings rather than to achieve specific goals. Her talking was accompanied by a good deal of physical contact, holding, and comforting. She was quick to respond to the child's clues relating to mood or effect. She felt that talking to Johnny even in infancy would have a salutary intellectual effect because with so many people talking to him "he would grow up to be smart." Johnny responded to the verbal communication by making his own sounds, vocalizations, and jargon.

As he grew older and situations developed that required more restraint, Mrs. Callini's use of language increased, particularly in the ninth-to-fifteenth month period. With a temporary deterioration of the close mother-child relationship there was much verbal prohibition, frequent angry shouting, and a change in physical communication to physical restraint and spanking. When Mrs. Callini returned to work there was less physical control and interaction. But by the second half of the second year the close active physical contact was again reported, including physical interaction, stimulation, and punishment.

To the very end of the study Mrs. Callini continued her verbal communication with Johnny. Even when he was busy with a task she spoke encouragingly to him or discussed the activity. Verbalization was an essential part of Johnny's environment.

2. Regularity and Flexibility of Scheduling. Regularity of the child's eating and sleeping schedules did not appear to be a matter of major concern, although it was not always achieved. For the most part there was regularity in sleep, but occasionally there were episodes of awakening, which were handled with a bottle or being taken into the parents' bed. Sleeping difficulties appeared for a short time when Johnny was around fifteen months old, associated with the general disturbance in the mother-child relationship at that time.

Feeding never presented a problem. Mrs. Callini was comfortable about feeding and took pride in Johnny's vigorous appetite and enjoyment of food. There did not seem to be any hurry to abandon the bottle or to force eating development. During the period of increased conflict Mrs. Callini objected to his messiness and efforts to feed himself. But for the most part regularity in sleep and feeding was established early.

3. Techniques of Management. Mrs. Callini used substitution to divert the child from forbidden activity. Thus, when Johnny tried to operate the forbidden television set, Mrs. Callini let him turn on the radio instead. But in her management she was not always consistent, partially because various adults in the house undermined her prohibitions. Johnny began to use the technique of playing off one adult against another, and Mrs. Callini felt frustrated in her attempts at discipline. During the second year scolding and threatening came into use when she found it increasingly difficult to control him.

For the most part generally permissive behavior was shown during the entire first year. In the second year non-permissive behavior reports increased, particularly relating to obedience and conformity. Nevertheless, the warmth and affection remained unimpaired. A high degree of variability was noted in the area of physical activity because of the high value put on infantile dependence. Mrs. Callini's management in almost all areas was on a reasonable level except for a variation during illness. In this regard she appeared unable to accept the fact of even a slight illness. She tended to deny the existence of illness and tried to hurry Johnny into complete recovery.

4. Relation of Expectations to Behavior. Although few specific expectations were expressed during pregnancy because of her comfortable, non-inquiring approach to the baby, Mrs. Callini looked forward to a rapport between herself and the baby which did indeed materialize from the beginning. Her manner and timing of activities was spontaneous, untroubled, and perceptive of the child's needs. Specific adaptations were made in feeding, naps, night sleep, bottles, play, and other areas without their becoming an issue. This was also true of toilet training, which did not become a source of conflict even though it was never entirely successful.

The expectation was implicit that the relationship with and care of the child would be a mutually satisfactory experience. Mrs. Callini's behavior clearly brought about its fulfillment.

As Johnny grew older, there was evidence of specific expectations tied to gratification from infantile dependence. The difficulties between mother and son began when Johnny became more active and less dependent on her. Mrs. Callini's contentment and placidity began to give way to expectations of obedience, conformity, and passivity from her child. In that unsatisfying period she implemented her behavior with more controlling methods, such as scolding, prohibition, and restrictions.

Although the initial warmth continued, the spontaneous intuitive ease of caring for an infant did not carry over to an older and more active child. The decision to return to work was further evidence of her ambivalence toward the emergence and growth of a helpless infant into an independent child.

5. Paternal Behavior. Mr. Callini appeared to be very devoted to the infant. In the early months he rushed home during coffee breaks to play with the baby, and at one point the baby's sleeping hours were rearranged to enable him to have more time with his son. Although he delighted in roughhousing with Johnny, Mr. Callini shared his wife's concern about the need to "tone him down" and exert some discipline. Like his wife, however, he was sometimes firm and sometimes lax. His participation in child care increased considerably when his wife went back to work and he was at home alone with the baby. Mr. Callini felt strongly that it was the parents' responsibility to care for their child, and to the end of the study he was not reconciled to his wife's going to work.

C. SOCIO-CULTURAL INFLUENCES

1. Socio-economic Status and Values. In terms of upward striving, the Callinis would be considered in the non-mobile group. They were a low-income family living with parents who were first generation immigrants to America. Both came from large Italian families where there was an underlying atmosphere of friendliness, warmth, and sharing. Despite the language difficulty in Mr. Callini's familial home, Mrs. Callini felt accepted and comfortable. Joys and sorrows were shared by all members of the family, hardships and deprivation were cushioned in the security of the family circle.

There was little drive for economic or prestige status, and Mr. Callini seemed more interested in having a job which allowed him to see a lot of his family than one which offered higher pay or a chance of promotion. Both the Callinis worked in factories, and Mr. Callini remained content in this role. To a small degree his wife had ambitions more in keeping with the urban norm than he did. She was more anxious to live independently, and she was more concerned about Johnny's performance in the well-baby clinic. Generally she seemed to value achievement in the occupational and educational world more than her husband, but this was not dominant and brought no overt conflict.

The social-psychological climate into which Johnny was born was not characterized by intellectual interests. Television was a prized possession in the in-laws' home and was one of the first acquisitions in the Callinis' new apartment. Books and reading played a small role in the cultural life of the family. Despite the problems inherent in being associated with large extended families of low income, there was the impression that they were inclined to take things as they come and to live each day without looking into the future.

Their Roman Catholic faith did not seem to make undue demands on the Callinis, and there was no indication of great religious zeal. Johnny was baptized in due course, but there was no expression of concern for his religious upbringing. As with other cultural processes, it was taken in stride. Surrounded as they were by large families, there did not seem to be need for a large circle of outside friends. Little reference was made to friends beyond the fact that Mrs. Callini enjoyed meeting them when she returned to work. There was no evidence of much social life outside the family circle.

2. *Extended Family.* There was minimal separateness of identity between the Callinis and their families of origin. This was emphasized by Mr. Callini's continued residence with his parents after marriage and his wife's continued performance of chores at home for her mother. Living with the extended family increased the emphasis on filial roles and the importance of obligations to parents. These arrangements of helping with housekeeping in both grandparents' homes continued even when Mrs. Callini was working and finally had her own apartment.

Prior to Johnny's birth a sense of dyadic togetherness on the part of husband and wife was not thoroughly established, nor was there an opportunity to resolve interpersonal tensions and conflicts which were created while living in the paternal grandparents' home. Hence, the achievement of separate living quarters became highly desirable for Mrs. Callini.

The comings and goings, anticipations and activities of all persons in the family were mostly shared by all. Generally the in-law relationships were not conflictful. However, during the period of greatest difficulty with Johnny, Mrs. Callini was resentful of her mother-in-law's inconsistent behavior with him, which was at times over-indulgent and at times prohibitive. Also, she blamed Johnny's slowness in walking on the fact that so many relatives held him, and she thought that he would "be spoiled" with so much attention. She also felt somewhat uneasy in her in-laws' home because of ineptness with the Italian language.

None of these problems, however, became significant sources of conflict, although they entered into Mrs. Callini's determination to have an apartment of her own. Yet the move to separate quarters was only a partial break with the families, since activities and responsibilities in the parental homes continued.

3. Spatial Arrangements and Values. Despite the severe spatial limitations and management problems in shared living, the Callini family exhibited fewer disagreements than did many of the other families. Management difficulties and over-crowded conditions posed a serious problem when Johnny reached the point where he needed room for his crawling and walking explorations. Prohibitions to protect furniture and certain objects, such as the television, were zealously enforced but Mrs. Callini attempted to substitute by permitting freedom with other objects, like the radio.

As Mrs. Callini's own relationship with Johnny ran into difficulty, she intensified restrictions upon his use of space and at the same time sought to change their living conditions to permit him more freedom. Despite many disadvantages, their own apartment provided a real improvement in Johnny's opportunities for movement and space in which to play and explore. There was little evidence of any special prohibitions or restrictions in the new apartment.

The Callini Family

D. FAMILY RELATIONSHIPS

1. Marital. Marital compatibility was predominant, and there was no unusual amount of unresolved emotional tension or anxiety appearing between husband and wife. They greatly enjoyed sharing their activities, feelings, and possessions with one another. When Mr. Callini changed his job they missed the former frequency of contact, and Mrs. Callini became less content with her status in the in-laws' home. Despite this, observers continued to note that the solicitude between husband and wife remained, usually the sign of happy marriage.

When Mrs. Callini went back to work an area of disagreement was opened with her husband that was never quite resolved. Throughout the study he remained opposed to it, although he was cooperative. The overall impression of the marital relationship was that of relative contentment and personal support.

2. Mother-Child. The infant was one, but not the only, source of satisfaction for Mrs. Callini. She also had a satisfying and supportive relationship with her husband and with members of both their families. As so frequently happens in tradition-oriented family structures, the child was treated as a favored person by the whole household, which provided Mrs. Callini with further gratification and self-esteem.

She placed a high value on the child from the beginning and considered him her primary vocation. She thought he was a "wonderful baby." His eating, sleeping, and growth were all gratifying to her, and she was not unduly apprehensive or anxious. When his activity began to pose management problems, however, he was somewhat less emotionally satisfying than before. As the intensive early absorption gave way to struggle over his independence, and disagreements with the paternal grandmother arose regarding management of his activities, Mrs. Callini turned to work and contact with others. At this time the household relationship ceased to provide a full measure of the satisfactions she had hoped for. But the basically positive mother-child relationship remained unimpaired and was warmly demonstrated.

3. Father-Child. From the beginning Mr. Callini had a high investment in fatherhood, and there was positive interaction with the baby. He was a proud and joyful parent and participated to some extent in child-care routines. Although he was concerned with "getting Johnny to do the right thing," he was not unduly prohibitive and recognized the child's limitations. When his wife went to work Mr. Callini took over a considerable part of the child's care. The child was a source of considerable satisfaction to Mr. Callini and an integral part of his family.

E. PERSONALITY CHARACTERISTICS

1. Handling of Anxiety and Hostility. Although Mrs. Callini was fairly non-communicative about expressing or revealing her feelings, she showed few overt signs of anxiety. There was little apprehension during pregnancy or after the baby's birth, a seeming expectation that "all would go well." Only in the area of illness was there evidence of possible suppressed anxiety in her haste to have it done with. There were no unusual inhibitions about expressing her feelings toward the child or significant adults in her life. Mrs. Callini was easily able to express her feelings of love and also annoyance in interaction with the child.

Similarly, in interaction with her husband and other family members she could express both love and occasional anger. Although she recalled the rigidity and strictness of her own childhood, she never felt alone in her large family of origin and felt favored as the "baby" of the family. Much of the emotional warmth and closeness of her own childhood family was perpetuated in the present, and she was able to demonstrate openly her satisfactions and dissatisfactions as they occurred.

2. Dependency and the Sense of Security. Dependency posed few problems for Mrs. Callini. She had a keen sense of filial obligation to her parents and tended to perpetuate the closeness and warmth of this many-membered family of origin. She performed chores for her mother because of a sense of responsibility and obligation rather than because she was clinging to old securities. The same filial ties existed with her parents-in-law, but she strove to be in some measure independent of them. However, even when physical separateness was achieved, the extended family ties were maintained. Mrs. Callini had no unusual reliance upon authority figures and was able to limit the intensity and expression of her dependency needs. She accepted child-care advice and medical care as reasonable aids but did not rely upon them as a demonstration of dependency. She mainly wanted factual understanding from authoritative sources, which she incorporated into her activity.

The extent and character of Mr. Callini's dependency was not known. It was not clear whether his willingness to continue joint living was a dependency need or arose from practical considerations and filial loyalty. He had a strong sense of family obligation to his parents in the traditional sense, but when the move was made to separate quarters there was no dysfunction in his own nuclear family.

3. *Feelings of Adequacy or Inadequacy.* Feelings of inadequacy did not present major problems in the Callini family. Mrs. Callini rarely expressed feelings that reflected on inadequacy, self-devaluation, or self-criticism. She wanted specific information about pregnancy and child care as a matter of scientific information, with no evidence that her own adequacy was in question. Her relationships with those close to her were natural and easygoing, without indication of stress. She showed a matter-of-fact approach to her family and to the social world, consistent with taking life as it came from one day to the next.

4. *Self-Assertion.* This question did not, by itself, appear to be a source of difficulty. Mrs. Callini felt free to express dissatisfaction with certain aspects of her situation and was critical when events warranted. She took a positive stand to assert her demands when necessary, such as the determination to move to more satisfactory living quarters, and she was critical of her mother-in-law when she interfered with her efforts to manage Johnny.

5. *Planning and Impulsiveness.* Mrs. Callini appeared to be confidently flexible in meeting life situations. She was not impulsive in her marriage because, as the youngest daughter, she felt obliged to help her mother. When she reached twenty-one she felt it was time

to act and she did so. In terms of infant care she did not need to maintain a rigid schedule in her activities or to insist on specific routines. As a matter of fact, she changed quite readily to accommodate needs as they arose. Although she finally rented an apartment "sight unseen" in her eagerness for separate quarters, this was the result of months of consideration and a long-standing determination to move.

6. Recapitulation of Past Experiences. There was no evidence of the extent to which recapitulation of past experiences assumed major prominence in child-care routines.

F. EMERGENCE OF FAMILY INTEGRATION PATTERNS

1. Family Structure. Because Johnny was warmly welcomed into a vast network of relatives, his relationships were effective and satisfying to all concerned. The dyadic relationships of husband-wife, mother-child, father-child were also emotionally satisfying to all concerned. Thus, the integration of this child into the family was achieved in the triadic nuclear family group and also in the larger extended family group. The Callini family was one in which the parents were able to fulfill their parental roles with the child and maintain their own filial roles as well.

Their daily activities were shared with Johnny. He went with them on shopping trips, vacations, rides, and family gatherings. He shared coffee breaks with his parents, and even his sleep was adjusted to his father's work schedule so he could spend time with him. In this non-intellectual, unsophisticated, and non-striving family Johnny fitted into a web of satisfaction shared by all. With satisfying parent-child relationships, ethnic-oriented, and more or less comfortable extended family relationships, Johnny became well integrated in a unitary nuclear family and also in the extended family pattern.

2. Division of Labor and Balance of Power. The family seemed to maintain a balance of power that could best be described as sharing. The division of labor included the fulfillment of respective filial roles by both Mr. and Mrs. Callini. In his own family Mr. Callini assumed household tasks and child care as called for in addition to his job. Mrs. Callini managed her household and child-care tasks in addition to her job. Most of the family activities and decisions seemed to be joint undertakings, with Mrs. Callini taking more initiative than her husband in deciding family affairs.

3. Development, Achievement, and Social Behavior of Child. According to the developmental tests Johnny was more than age-adequate on an overall basis. Mrs. Callini found it difficult to conceptualize the specifics of inevitable developmental change in her son. She had a general concept of developmental stages, but this was more a rationale of current behavior than an anticipation of behavior to come. She thought that Johnny would be more easy to manage when he could walk, yet she limited his opportunities for walking. She found it hard to accept his developmental changes from an infantile dependence to more aggressive self-sustained activity. Her non-recognition of these factors was partially responsible for the conflicts that developed between herself and Johnny. Mrs. Callini was eager for Johnny to achieve and perform well, and she was also quite conscious of his social behavior. But her efforts in pushing him in these directions were not extreme.

4. Prospect of Siblings. During pregnancy and soon after birth Mrs. Callini spoke of having more children. However, she refused to consider another baby until they had their own apartment. On the other hand, her husband was eager to have another child before he became too old (he was 26) and suggested this as an alternative to getting an apartment. However, Mrs. Callini was adamant about the apartment. Even after the move she did not become pregnant, and nothing was made explicit about the prospect of siblings

5. Status of Family in Community. The Callinis were well integrated in the maternal and paternal grandparental settings in a neighborhood where they had lived most of their years. They were familiar with the community, which housed their friends and whatever activities in which they engaged. There was no evidence of the extent of involvement in broad community life, and their chief community participation was through the extended families.

6. Types of Parent-Child Adaptation. The Callinis showed the child-centeredness and permissiveness generally associated with the unitary families. While Mrs. Callini was somewhat inconsistent in her permissiveness, she remained basically permissive throughout the study. Mr. Callini was also characterized as largely permissive and child-centered in orientation. The Callini family emerged as a unitary, child-centered, permissive family.

POSTSCRIPT

Passage of time accented the impression that members of the Callini family had not yet found their full identification in the family process, themselves, or each other. Although her husband looked with disfavor on it, Mrs. Callini continued to work the major part of the time, spurred on by determination to buy a house. She remained eager to have another baby but was deterred by the inadequacy of the apartment and the immediate stress that Johnny presented.

Much of the time Mrs. Callini found Johnny "hard to live with" and "out of control," to which her own management, involving impulsive anger, scolding, and inconsistent discipline, seemed to contribute. It was observed that both parents were wont to engage the child in a teasing and exciting kind of physical interaction, which heightened his undesirable behavior. The impression of the staff grew stronger that the "active and driven" aspect of Johnny was more an external facade of behavior triggered by the environment than an internal mechanism. In moments of self-evaluation Mrs. Callini was aware that Johnny responded better when she didn't "nag and holler so much," but life styles are not easy to change.

Mrs. Callini continued to feel considerable guilt about working. Opposing work schedules allowed the Callinis little opportunity for togetherness, and a degree of estrangement took place. Differences became magnified, and dissatisfactions developed. During the hours when Mr. Callini had the major care of Johnny, the study staff came to know him better. He impressed them as a quiet, self-effacing, and passive man who chose a course of compromise with his more dominant wife rather than an assertive one.

In his handling of Johnny two distinct characteristics appeared.

For one, Johnny was more tractable and responsive to his father's management because Mr. Callini quietly but firmly set consistent lines of behavior. However, Mr. Callini asserted himself all too rarely. Before taking action he tolerated much aggression by the child, including hitting, biting, and provocation. The role reversal in the household was pointed up by Mr. Callini's threats to tell Johnny's mother about his transgressions upon her return from work. Clearly, Johnny was more vulnerable to his mother's anger, although he actually conformed better with his father. Mr. Callini attributed this to the fact that he didn't "holler so much" and that "Johnny knows I mean what I say."

Both parents were highly disturbed that Johnny developed overt masturbation and nail-biting. The conspicuous masturbation, which continued over a period, caused them embarrassment and concern about his normality. In nursery school Johnny was seen as a sober, rather cautious and anxious child who preferred to play independently. In close interaction with his peers he expressed himself in clowning, teasing behavior as a cover for his apprehensions. The aggression and belligerency which he released on his parents was held in check with children, and he seemed to need adult help in various situations. Mrs. Callini feared that he would become "a mama's boy."

By three years of age Johnny was fully toilet-trained, ate and slept well, and was generally competent. It took a long time for his speech to emerge clearly and understandably despite his copious verbalization. In play therapy, as at home, Johnny tended to be destructive with objects to provide himself with aggressive release. The hitting and physical assaults on his father were seen as an identification with the controlling role of the mother.

As Mr. Callini capitulated to his wife's dominance, his own tension and anger erupted in ulcer symptoms and digestive disturbances. Aware of the psychological implications, he pointed out that his own passive role had not helped Johnny. The child began to show evidence of ambivalence in identification with mother and father, taking the form of anxiety, over-caution, object destruction, aggressive negative behavior at home, and overdependence on adults.

Mrs. Callini's ambitions for a home were finally realized when Johnny was about five years old. They purchased a nice residence in a suburban development, replete with appliances and modern comforts. With improved living conditions the family relaxed into more gratifying and consistent patterns. When Johnny was next seen he was no longer an anxious, depressed boy. Although still unspontaneous and unassertive, he began to appear more capable of handling himself and his experiences. Nor did he show the disturbance in self-concept which was seen before. In his new environment he adjusted well to playmates and to school.

The intervening years served to blunt the sharp corners of family interaction. When Johnny was close to eight years old, his sister was born, followed in approximately three years by another sister. Mrs. Callini ceased work and returned only briefly when her husband had another bout of ill health.

At fourteen Johnny appeared to be a handsome, clean-cut boy who did average work in school, socialized with his peers, was actively motivated, and had specific plans for college. He was comfortable with himself, confident about his ability to accomplish his goals and to get along well with other people. The two girls seemed to be attractive, vigorous children who were closely attached to their mother. At this age Johnny seemed to feel closer and to identify more with his father in the sharing of male interests and pursuits.

Although Mr. Callini remained rather quiet, relaxed, and less intense than his wife, he did not hesitate to express himself or his points of view. Mrs. Callini appeared confident, friendly, seemingly happy, and proud of her family and home. Both parents were clearly interested in and closely involved with their children and family life.

It seemed that the process of family integration and self-identification had been fulfilled in the course of the years and that the Callini family was restored to the happiness and contentment which had been evident at the study's beginning.

Comparative Summary of Families

A. EXPECTATIONS

1. MATERNAL EXPECTATIONS

Expectations concerning their children and the experience of motherhood showed a wide range among the mothers. The areas, qualities, and characteristics of expectations varied from family to family, from one area of child care to another, and from one time to another. In some families various attitudes and anticipations expressed during pregnancy remained consistent throughout the following two years. In other families there was a gradual change of expectations in response to life with the child.

In some families it was possible to recognize the specific points at which changes occurred. These were at points of crisis or of important environmental occurrences. Sometimes they were contingent on the mother's first awareness of changes in the child relative to her own specific expectations. Such changes may not have been recorded at the time the mother first communicated an awareness of change in her feelings or attitude toward the child or the maternal role. It is also possible that such points of change became known as the result of changes in communication between the mother and the observer.

Findings. For two mothers (Cyrenski, Callini) the advent of pregnancy and the anticipation of maternity appeared to be a happy and calm experience, untroubled by anxiety over the assumption of the maternal role. A third mother (Grasso) also evidenced great satisfaction at the prospect of a child but was fairly inarticulate at revealing expectations of herself in the role of mother.

Four women expressed concern about their adequacy as mothers. Two of them (Silver, Bjornson) anticipated their children with considerable pleasure but suffered generalized anxiety and concern about their own adequacy. Two other mothers (Fallon, Harris) did not verbalize satisfaction but did express considerable anxiety concerning their adequacy. However, Mrs. Harris seemed eagerly happy for motherhood, but Mrs. Fallon appeared to regard it with foreboding.

One mother (Neville) was clearly reluctant to assume the maternal role. She emphasized the disruption to her life which the child would cause and the negative quality of her anticipations.

1A. INTEREST IN OUTSIDE EMPLOYMENT

It is important to assess whether interest in outside employment has a bearing on maternal expectations. In this connection one must differentiate between consideration of employment because of economic or psychological environmental stresses and consideration because of negative or ambivalent attitudes towards motherhood. It is also of interest to know whether mothers with negative maternal expectations tend to be motivated toward outside employment or whether their dissatisfactions take other forms. A further question is whether prior employment experiences provided the mother with satisfactions of needs which were unmet in family relationships.

Findings. Employment became an issue for the three women who approached motherhood with the most satisfaction and the least ambivalence (Grasso, Callini, Cyrenski). It became an issue during the second year of the child's life, when economic necessity or escape from pressing family situations turned their minds away from home. Economic necessity accounted for one (Grasso), and frustration from living in the paternal grandparents' home accounted for a second (Callini). The third (Cyrenski) needed relief from a dominating mother-in-law and became discontented as the child left the infancy stage, which was most pleasurable to her.

There was no question of seriously engaging in work after the baby was born for three mothers (Silver, Harris, Bjornson). A fourth mother (Fallon) had derived much satisfaction from employment prior to marriage and felt that she could always return to work in case of emergency. But she was never actually motivated to do so despite family dissatisfactions.

Mrs. Neville, who did not view motherhood with any satisfaction, did consider the conflict between a mother's employment or intellectual pursuits and her responsibility to the child. Although she had ambitions for outside employment, the value of motherhood became more acceptable through compensation afforded as the child grew older.

2. SPECIFICITY OF EXPECTATIONS

The basis for specific expectations stems from several factors, including cultural standards and values, established ways of facing new situations, and personal characteristics. Expectations may be expressed as detailed specific questions about particular items of concern or in broadly vague ideas about motherhood, children, and child-rearing or about being adequate as a mother. Diffuse anxiety may express itself not only in general doubts about oneself as a mother but also in preoccupation with particular aspects of management and care of the child.

It was not surprising that the most urgent expectations during pregnancy were expressions of thoughts and feelings about the forthcoming maternal role. Those who had few anticipations in the beginning about such details as infant feeding, discipline, health, or sleep became more specific as these areas became activated. In fact, all the parents became relatively more specific in their expectations about child-care areas during the infants' first two years of life. The overall difference between parents was one of degree rather than of kind.

A variety of factors doubtlessly influenced the presence or absence of verbalized specific expectations. One such factor was the character of communication between mother and interviewer. An expectation may have existed which was not voiced by the mother and was undetected by the interviewer. On the other hand, the mother's way of dealing with new experiences may have been to let them unfold rather than to anticipate them in detail. Furthermore, the characteristics of introspection, imagination, self-evaluation, curiosity, communicativeness, the pressure of specific anxieties or the need to deny them, may influence a mother's readiness to anticipate specific problems and situations.

Findings. There was little relationship between the expression of specific concerns and the character of maternal anticipations. In the non-specific group were two most contentedly expectant mothers (Cyrenski, Callini), one who was inarticulate on the subject but evinced great satisfaction (Grasso), and one who was outspokenly negative about the prospect (Fallon).

The expectations of four mothers were quite specific and were related to the child's health and development or the details of child care. The specific expectations of two (Silver, Bjornson) were influenced by their diffuse anxiety; one (Neville) by established ways of focusing on new situations, and one (Harris) by her methods of dealing practically with problems.

During the study period two characteristic shifts appeared in expectations. First was the shift from general to specific expectations as the realities of living with and caring for the child became part of the mother's experience. Secondly, as the child developed and moved from one phase of growth to the next, the mother's expectations moved with him, bringing into focus new and specific expectations.

3. MOTIVATIONAL ORIENTATION

An examination of parental expectations and their goals of behavior showed that orientation of the parents may be toward the self or toward the child, i.e., their satisfactions may come from fulfillment of either their own needs or those of the child. Needless to say, these two orientations are by no means necessarily opposed. Indeed, a mother's gratification may be derived in large measure from satisfying the needs of the child, both because nurturing is a kind of expressive behavior and because she derives her satisfaction from those of the child.

However, when a mother's goals of satisfaction do not coincide with those of the child, a choice is made. As was shown in some instances, the mother failed to consider one or another of the child's satisfactions because of her own pressing needs, her anxieties about the child, or her unawareness of the latter's needs. Therefore, the term "motivational orientation" refers to whether the satisfaction of interests or the gratification of needs is "parent-centered" or "child-centered." The source of such gratification is another matter. It may stem from the mother's own behavior or the child's, and either may lead to her own or the child's gratification.

Closely related to motivational orientation is the appropriateness of the mother's expectations. Mother-centeredness is often expressed in age-inappropriate expectations. A mother may expect behavior from the child which is more suitable to a later age because parental gratification depends on more adult behavior than the child is capable of at the time. In some instances the mother may expect continuation of the infantile period after the child has outgrown it because her conceptions of a child are attached to a specific age or because the period of infancy itself holds the greatest measure of pleasure for her.

The study mothers fell into three apparent categories: those who were consistently mother-oriented, those who were predominantly child-oriented, and one who fluctuated between mother- and child-centeredness. To a considerable extent, as we have already seen, the expectations of the mothers kept pace with the development of the children, and for most of them there was some degree of change in their expectations which grew out of experience itself.

The child's ability to understand and to do more provided the mother-oriented women with increased satisfactions in their own role and that of the child. Upon gratification of their mother-centered goals there was an increase in child-orientation. Growing satisfaction with her child and with her own fulfillment of the maternal role also accounted for expectation shifts in the mother who showed both mother- and child-centeredness.

The most child-oriented mothers also demonstrated shifts in expectations, but these generally were not shifts away from child-centeredness. Rather they were redirections of some interests from the children to themselves and were related to other circumstances in the family life, such as health or family difficulties.

The most striking effect on the mothers' expectations was the experience of daily living with the child. The mothers differed greatly in their sensitivity to this force. Some responded with relative ease to changes in the child and to living with him, while others responded more as the child adapted to the demands made on him. Still others attempted to keep the early status quo of mother and infant during most of the two years. But many preconceptions had to be abandoned if they were found to be irrelevant to the facts of the child's existence.

The major differences found in respect to expectations were those between mothers whose expectations were modified to fit their experience and mothers who induced the children to make experience fit the expectations.

Findings. Two mothers (Neville, Fallon) were clearly and consistently mother-centered in terms of their expectations. They were intolerant of the child's demands on their time, activities, and attention. They wanted their infants to respond to the routines of child care in a way more reasonably to be expected from older children. Mrs. Fallon became somewhat less mother-centered in the eighteen to twenty-four month period and showed more tolerance for her child's behavior. Mrs. Neville became more satisfied with pleasing qualities which developed in her child, but she was consistent in setting values in terms of her own satisfactions.

Five mothers (Harris, Grasso, Cyrenski, Callini, Silver) were predominantly child-centered in their expectations throughout the period. However, some shift appeared with each of them because of particular circumstances. For Mrs. Harris it was because of a second pregnancy and family difficulty; for Mrs. Grasso, because of management problems with the child and economic difficulties; for Mrs. Cyrenski, because of family conflict and the child's development out of infancy, and for Mrs. Callini, because of difficulties in shared living arrangements. Mrs. Silver also showed some change by focusing inward concern about her own health. Despite these shifts and refocusing from time to time there was no substantial change in the child-centered orientation of any of these mothers.

Mrs. Bjornson fluctuated between mother-centeredness and child-centeredness. As her role become more familiar, the shift was towards child-centeredness, with growing recognition and acceptance of child-oriented needs. However, there were also areas where mother-satisfactions were stressed. The shift was not unequivocal, and there was evidence of both approaches during the study period.

4. ROLE OF CHILD IN FULFILLING MOTHER'S EXPECTATIONS

While the mother's expectations and values were primary factors in establishing her behavior, the child's course of development during the first two years obviously affected her success in carrying out such expectations and also influenced the shifts in expectation that occurred. The child's individuality, the way in which he made his demands felt, and his specific abilities for adapting and compromising were contributing factors. The determinants of mother-child interaction were clearly found in both individuals.

There is no simple relation between the kinds of expectations that mothers hold and the personalities of their children. Nor is there a simple relation between the problems encountered by the mothers and their ways of dealing with them. The variables of maternal expectations, child's personality, and behavioral patterns must be seen in configuration rather than in any linear relation.

Findings. The development of their babies into vigorous little boys posed problems for two mothers (Grasso, Callini). Mrs. Callini tried to preserve her gratifications by restricting Johnny's behavior, but she maintained her child-centered values and warmth of feeling. Mrs. Grasso developed a highly variable and inconsistent relationship, with rigid control in certain areas and permissive behavior in others.

For two of the mothers (Cyrenski, Fallon) the passivity of their sons was in accordance with their expectations of infants, but as both boys developed out of infancy the expectations of their mothers were shaken. Mrs. Fallon became more friendly and accepting as the child veered away from her former expectations, while Mrs. Cyrenski found it difficult to adjust to a child who was leaving infancy.

The girls of two mothers (Neville, Bjornson) demonstrated a capacity to respond to their mothers' expectations for social behavior, even though the demands were rather high. The other two girls (Harris, Silver) also responded well to their mothers' expectations, although the demands in these instances were more child-centered.

While it appeared that the girls had more success in fulfilling maternal expectations than did the boys, one cannot on the basis of this evidence generalize about sex differences in the process of family integration

5. PATERNAL EXPECTATIONS

Paternal data are limited because the fathers typically regard child-rearing as the woman's domain, and they viewed the study as basically involving the mother and child. This, combined with practical difficulties due to work schedules, precluded a penetrating examination of fathers. Within these limitations, however, a determination was possible of the range in which the fathers operated.

Some fathers reflected keen and pleasurable anticipation of a child, and others expressed apparent indifference or even displeasure at the prospect. Often these expectations were expressed in defining the relation between the father's and the mother's role or were implied in expectations of the family as a group.

During the first two years the fathers' expectations were largely related to the children's behavior and development. Some fathers were primarily concerned about the child's conformance to social and intellectual standards; others with the desirability of permitting a child to grow without imposing specific requirements. Still others showed a combination of these two kinds of expectations.

Findings. Three fathers (Grasso, Cyrenski, Callini) shared in their wives' high degree of investment in having a child and expressed their pleasure at the forthcoming birth. A fourth father (Silver) had many anxieties about the child and about his own ability to fulfill the paternal role adequately. One father (Harris) was pleased at the prospect of having a child and anticipated his future role in terms of both the child's needs and his own responsibility for satisfying them. Another father (Fallon) reported expectations concerning religious training for the child and a hope that the child would be different from himself. One father (Bjornson) shared some of his wife's pervasive concerns about the forthcoming child, and one father (Neville) thought in terms of a family of three or four children, like the one in which he grew up.

B. BEHAVIOR

1. COMMUNICATION

The mothers showed certain clear differences in their modes of communication with their children, particularly during infancy. Some mothers "talked" to their babies from the beginning. Without waiting until words were understood, they conversed with their babies for the purpose of expressing their feelings rather than for achieving specific goals.

With these mothers speech was accompanied by a great deal of physical contact, especially during the first year, and was evident in active play and enjoyment of the routines of feeding and bathing. As the children became able to respond to the meaning of words, language was increasingly used as an instrument of control, teaching, training, or encouragement by the mother.

A second group of mothers used verbal communication from the beginning to direct and control the behavior of their children rather than as a mode of expressing maternal feelings of pleasure in the child. They used language variously to teach, scold, prohibit, and threaten. Language assumed more the function of providing a means of control, ineffective though it actually was, than of providing contact between mother and child. Physical contact in this group was also more limited, sporadic and not well defined.

Finally there were three mothers who could not be categorized with either group. One verbalized as a substitute for physical communication because of concern about ability to handle the child. A second mother showed intense and concentrated physical communication, with a marked paucity of verbal expression, and a third was variable in her use of verbalization.

Findings. Three mothers (Harris, Callini, Silver) were in the group who "talked" to express loving maternal feelings; they also had important physical contact with their children throughout the two years. Some shift was observed in Mrs. Callini, who encountered activity struggles with the child during a particular period of development. At this time there was an increase in verbal prohibition and frequent angry shouting; she later returned to the close mother-child interaction. Physical contact diminished somewhat for Mrs. Silver as the child grew out of infancy and she was more able to substitute verbal for physical contact. There was some decrease in both verbal and physical interaction by Mrs. Harris as family difficulties and a second pregnancy intervened, but no appreciable weakening of the relationship.

A second group, of two (Neville, Fallon), did not use verbal communication to express maternal feelings of pleasure. Mrs. Neville talked as a substitute for physical contact with her child. She also yelled and scolded when she was intolerant of the baby's screaming. But as the child began to provide some satisfaction for her, verbal communication was increasingly used for teaching and directing her activities. Mrs. Fallon also used language as a substitute for physical contact, and later used it in an attempt to control her son's activity. From the time Ross was eighteen months old and developed in a way more satisfying to his mother, there was a softening of behavior, and words were used for comfort and entertainment.

The last three mothers (Bjornson, Grasso, Cyrenski) could not be defined with either group. Mrs. Bjornson had difficult and uncertain communication in the beginning, mainly because of her tension in handling the baby. Although evidences of verbal communication were limited, she appeared to use it as a substitute for her fearfulness in physical contact. As Lorna developed, however, language became an important bond between them. Mrs. Cyrenski, on the other hand, had an extraordinarily close physical contact with her baby during the early period but produced almost no report of verbal communication. Joey's language remained meager throughout the study, and verbal communication even in the later period did not play a substantial role between mother and son. Mrs. Grasso had warm and loving physical communication with her son but verbalization was quite varied. At first she used words more to scold and prohibit, but then she also used words to praise and persuade. As the baby picked up words, his mother enjoyed facilitating the language exchange.

1A. USE OF CLUES

An important aspect of communication between mother and child is the giving, perception of, and response to clues from one to the other in order to indicate a need, a wish, or the expectation of particular kinds of behavior. The mother's perception of clues from the child depends on her ability or readiness to anticipate the needs of the child and upon her awareness of the child's way of acting and reacting.

Clue responsiveness indicates sensitivity to the child's way of experiencing his environment and to his physical and emotional status at any given time. The mother's ability to perceive and to interpret such clues indicates her recognition of the qualities and characteristics of the child's individuality and her readiness to respond to the child. In turn, clues given by the mother to the child provide a way of helping the child to understand the parent and are a guide to appropriate responses that he may learn to make.

Clues are effective if they are definite enough to be understood by the receiver and to evoke a response. They may be vague and general in nature, or precise and definite. They may be directed toward the accomplishment of a particular activity or toward expression of mood not associated with any specific activity.

The perception of clues appeared to be immediate and intuitive for some mothers from the earliest days of the child's life. For other mothers it appeared to develop with experience from daily contact with the child. Similarly, the interpretation of clues came with apparent ease to some mothers, while others were aware that the child was communicating something but could not tell what it was.

The range was wide among the mothers from frequent and sensitive perception of clues to almost complete absence of perception, unawareness, or inability to make use of them. A relation was seen between clue-perception and mother-centeredness. Those mothers who were the most child-centered were also the most perceptive of and responsive to clues given by the child, whereas the mother-centered parents were either unperceptive of, or non-responsive to, the child's clues.

Findings. Four mothers (Silver, Callini, Grasso, Cyrenski) were quick to respond to the child's clues. These mothers were characterized as being the most child-centered. Mrs. Grasso was aware of and used clues mostly in relation to specific areas of activity. Mrs. Silver alerted herself to any indications of the child's need for care or wish for attention. Mrs. Callini interpreted restlessness and fussiness as clues of the baby's need for comfort. Mrs. Cyrenski responded immediately and intuitively to mood and effect clues.

Reports on clue perception from two mothers (Bjornson and Harris) were too sparse and indefinite to permit analysis. However, it was evident that Mrs. Bjornson's insecurity about her adequacy as a mother blinded her to many of the baby's clues. Mrs. Harris' rapport with Heather, however, suggested a keen perception of, and response to, clues.

For two mothers (Neville, Fallon) a low range of response to clues was evident. Both these mothers were characterized as predominantly mother-centered. Mrs. Neville reacted negatively to the clues, with annoyance and frustration, and showed little or no appreciation of the child's moods and needs. Mrs. Fallon was impervious to the child's expressed clues, choosing largely to ignore them

2. REGULARITY AND FLEXIBILITY OF SCHEDULING

Regularity was considered in reference to the systematic organizing, scheduling, and carrying out of activities related to child care, including the timing and amount of food, day and night sleeping, bathing, play with the child, and management of the child's own activities. Flexibility is the mother's capacity to modify or adapt her requirements of the child or the situation to suit the circumstances.

A mother may be very regular in the scheduling of her daily program but at any given time will make allowances for the child's readiness or unreadiness to respond, for his shifting preferences, or for the occurrence of events that may interrupt the schedule. Illness of the child, for example, is often an event that modifies a mother's ordinarily systematic and repetitive practices. These practices may be accompanied either by rigidity that allows for few exceptions or by a flexibility that permits variation in the details.

Although the mothers varied widely in their degree of regularity or irregularity, flexibility or rigidity, this did not appear to be a determining factor for most of them. In most cases it was clear whether the mother adapted to the child's preferences or was inflexible in her motivation for regularity. There was also variation in respect to different areas of child care. A mother who could be flexible about sleep might be less so in regard to feeding. The extent to which actual regularity and scheduling were achieved also varied in each case.

Findings. For seven mothers (Silver, Cyrenski, Harris, Bjornson, Grasso, Callini, Neville) regularity per se was not observed to be a dominant force or to present undue problems. Mrs. Silver achieved regularity because her baby was remarkably regular, although she was prepared to adapt herself completely to the baby's preferences. Mrs. Harris did not achieve regularity because of Heather's sleeping difficulties, nor did Mrs. Bjornson because Lorna was irregular in both feeding and sleeping, at least in the early period. All of these mothers were prepared to accede to the demand schedules of their babies. Rita Neville also had considerable irregularity in feeding and sleeping, which was a source of annoyance to her mother but not a great problem. In time these irregularities diminished for all mothers and more regular patterns ensued.

Mrs. Callini and Mrs. Cyrenski seemed to have no regularity problems, and Mrs. Grasso was flexible with Vince's schedule and routine.

In contrast, Mrs. Fallon was seen as outstandingly inflexible; the achievement of regularity became a determining factor in her management. She showed both compulsiveness and inflexibility, ranging from marked lack of acknowledgment of the baby's needs to rigid "regularizing" of scheduling. Her child managed to adapt in a number of ways to her inflexibility, mainly by non-intrusion.

The Firstborn

3. TECHNIQUES OF MANAGEMENT

The elements which facilitate relationships between parent and child are to be found in the daily care of the child and in the specific interaction. A number of categories describe the differing techniques developed by the mothers in managing their children. These categories attempt to distinguish the degree to which parents allow autonomy to their children or impose restrictions on them in order to establish desired modes of behavior.

Permissiveness includes a number of techniques primarily directed to meeting the child's wishes and establishing opportunities for him to satisfy them. These include tolerance, compromise, and giving in, but they may be limited by protective watching to see that he does not get hurt or by a compromise between what the child wants to do and what the mother wants him to do. But even in the latter the mother takes into account and acts in terms of the child's wishes.

Among these permissive techniques are diversion, substitution, and accommodation. Through diversion one may distract a child to something permitted in order to turn him away from disapproved behavior, i.e., story telling at mealtime to distract him from messing in the food or refusing to eat. Or one might substitute a permitted object for something forbidden, i.e., substitute a coloring book for pulling out books from the shelf.

Accommodation is a technique of adapting the environment to the child, or creating a situation that will enable the child to function in the desired way or with a minimum of conflict. It is directed toward manipulation of the environment to induce the child to behave in the desired way or to lessen the possibility of anticipated undesirable behavior. An example is the advance placement of toys in a playpen to induce the child to spend time there alone.

Non-permissiveness includes techniques for direct control of the child, which will probably frustrate some of his desires. Among these techniques are restriction and avoidance. Restriction covers physical restraint of his activities, specific verbal prohibitions, establishment of highly regulated schedules to which the child is required to conform, or disciplining by scolding, threatening, or physical punishment.

Avoidance is a technique demonstrating either unwillingness or inability of the mother to adapt her own activities to the situation. The situation is avoided by ignoring or denying it, or by delaying doing anything about it. Such behavior may be evidenced by delay in preparing a bottle, leaving a room so as not to get involved in the child's behavior, failure to remember the child's needs, or unawareness of realities such as illness.

In evaluating the parents' behavior a number of limitations must be recognized. The amount of detailed reporting by either the mother or the staff observer varies widely from family to family and from time to time. Hence, the available observations may not correctly represent the frequency with which specific kinds of behavior actually occurred or the emphasis placed by the family on particular aspects of daily experience. We may assume, however, that the evidence available from the mothers' reporting and the two-year observation period generally does represent the relative importance of different areas of activity for the family.

Findings. The permissive type of behavior was clearly predominant for the two-year period in six families (Silver, Grasso, Bjornson, Harris, Cyrenski, Callini). In these families it was reported from almost two to almost four times as frequently as non-permissive behavior. This predominance of permissive versus non-permissive behavior follows the general cultural norm of our society.

In two families (Fallon, Neville), where the mothers were predominantly adult-centered, the pattern was quite different. With Mrs. Neville the non-permissive acts were reported about one and a half times as frequently as the permissive, and with Mrs. Fallon they were of equal frequency.

A significant aspect of child-care behavior by the mothers was the shift between the first and second years. There was an increase from 40 percent to 60 percent in reports of both permissive and non-permissive behavior during the second year. This reflected the mothers' increased rapport with the study staff and also an increase in situations which required permissive or non-permissive reactions because of the developing mobility of the children.

Significantly, there was little difference between the first and second years in the proportion of permissive reports from the eight mothers as a group, but there were pronounced changes for some individual mothers. In the first year there was a relatively greater amount of reported non-permissive behavior by both Mrs. Neville and Mrs. Fallon. This was consistent with their expectations of conformity by the children to their own adult-oriented values.

However, in the second year the increase in the proportion of permissive behavior for Mrs. Fallon is most marked and is noticeable also for Mrs. Neville. This corresponded with the fact that in these families the child began to provide greater satisfactions in the later period.

For the other six families there was a decline in permissive behavior reports during the second year, consistent with the increased mobility and development of the children. The largest decreases in the proportion of permissive behavior in the second year occurred in the families of Harris, Cyrenski, and Bjornson. This accorded with the qualitative changes in those families, with growing emphasis on social control for Mrs. Harris and Mrs. Bjornson and a breakdown of the intense mother-child relationship in the case of Mrs. Cyrenski.

4. RELATION OF EXPECTATIONS TO BEHAVIOR

Of major interest is the extent to which behavior can be seen to relate directly to expressed expectations of the mother. As patterns of behavior have been established that satisfy certain expectations, attention is directed to other ones. On the other hand, new expectations may arise, and with them new kinds of behavior, because of dissatisfaction or frustration in carrying out earlier expectations.

In the ordinary process of the child's growth and development we note that shifts in expectations occur which move the parents' concerns and interests from infantile to childhood expectations. But we are also aware that there are shifts in expectations, behavior not clearly consistent with expectations, and inconsistencies in behavior which may arise from a number of circumstances. In some instances we have also seen changes from mother-centeredness to child-centeredness or the reverse, and these changes in turn may affect both expectations and behavior.

We shall therefore look at the data as far as possible to discover the degree of fulfillment of expectations in behavior, and the changes in expectations which are related to changes in behavior. We shall be guided by the understanding that the most giving, permissive, responsive, and child-oriented mother is not wholly so; nor is the opposite pattern consistently and unequivocally present.

Findings. Of the four mothers who had specific maternal expectations, two (Silver, Bjornson) reported most frequently on those behavioral areas of interaction in which they had expressed most of their specific concerns and expectations. These related to the normality and well-being of their babies, with intense and diffuse anxieties about their abilities. Mrs. Harris's activity with the child followed her permissive and lenient expectations, and Mrs. Neville acted in terms of what she regarded as her responsibilities to the baby and her baby's responsibility to her.

In all of these mothers certain shifts and redirection of behavior were noted as the babies went from infantile to childhood activities. Mrs. Silver, Mrs. Harris, and Mrs. Bjornson became slightly more directive and controlling, while Mrs. Neville became somewhat less so as she gained more satisfaction from her child.

The behavior of four mothers who had few specific expectations was consistent with their pleasurable or unpleasurable attitude towards motherhood. The three who had in common a pleasurable anticipation (Callini, Grasso, Cyrenski) were adaptable in all areas of child care. Mrs. Callini demonstrated an easy interaction with her baby; Mrs. Cyrenski's intense relationship with her baby was evidence of her instinctual mothering; and Mrs. Grasso, after the first surprises of motherhood, responded positively to her maternal role.

However, the fourth mother, Mrs. Fallon, was as non-adaptive to her baby as she was non-specific in her expectations, but her behavior was consistent with her negative approach to maternity and her severe doubts about motherhood. Interestingly, as the babies went from infantile to childhood activities the shift was towards less permissive and less adaptive behavior by Callini, Cyrenski, and Grasso but a somewhat more adaptive reconciliation of behavior for Mrs. Fallon.

5. PATERNAL BEHAVIOR

The evidence of paternal participation in child-care activities is generally sparse. However, it was clear that none of the fathers assumed major care of the child, although all fathers participated to some degree in child care, some minimally and others more extensively, especially upon illness or employment of the mother.

Even the most demanding and adult-oriented fathers did take some active part in the rearing of the child. Despite strictures placed on the child for behavior to satisfy adult convenience, there was real paternal giving and responsiveness. The "rejecting" aspects of some of the fathers' attitudes are only part of the story. They may fit in very well with the idea that fathers can love and take care of their children but at the same time expect their own adult interests and conveniences to be respected.

Findings. In the two families in which the mothers were most clearly mother-centered (Neville, Fallon) the attitudes of the fathers provided a balance to the demands which the mothers made. The fathers were more demonstrative toward the children, shared some enjoyment of activities with them, were more able to recognize their limitations, and were slower to push them toward achievement. They served to put a check on the mothers' demands and to give something which the mothers apparently could not give. This made for a more secure parent-child structure than the child would otherwise have experienced. There were no comparable data concerning the moderating influence of mothers against excessive paternal demands or conflicting relationships on the part of the fathers.

Five families in which the mothers were basically child-centered (Silver, Callini, Grasso, Harris, Cyrenski) showed varying degrees of paternal behavior and involvement. Mr. Silver was anxious and panicky in care of the child but thoroughly enjoyed playing with his adored Ruth. Mr. Callini romped with his son and handled him well. There was little call on Mr. Cyrenski's paternal qualities in a home where he himself was still the recipient of maternal attention. Consequently the relationship with his son was more like a sibling.

Mr. Harris enjoyed his daughter and was able to care for her rather well when called upon, and Mr. Grasso shared substantial care of the child, especially when his wife worked. In these families the fathers were a further supportive factor for the child.

In the Bjornson family, which fluctuated between mother- and child-centeredness, the father also tended to moderate the mother's high demands for achievement and perfection and also provided loving companionship.

C. SOCIO-CULTURAL INFLUENCES

1. SOCIO-ECONOMIC STATUS AND VALUES

The life goals and social orientations of the parents are assumed to be crucial factors that bear directly and indirectly upon child-care patterns. The arrival of an infant may be consistent with the life goals and orientations of the parents. Often enough, however, the infant's arrival may not fit in with parental goals, and indeed the hierarchy of family social values may not include a child among the most important things in life.

Of social value also are the parents' families of origin, which may or may not serve as models for the many cultural alternatives that influence the parents' experiences with their children. Contact with extended family is partly contingent upon whether the parents are moving away from an immigrant, tradition-oriented extended-family culture or whether they continue to identify their own goals with the culture of their family of origin.

Family income may be viewed as a basis for evaluating social importance or primarily as the determinant of a more or less healthful level of living. Parents who stress upward mobility may view continual increases in income as the vehicle for raising their social status. If income is only a means of maintaining a level of living, climbing the ladder of success may not be important.

There is good reason to believe that where upward striving is thought to be important, child-spacing and indeed the economics of child care result in family integration problems that are different from those in families where such values are not held. In the latter case, childbirth and child-raising may be seen as desirable accompaniments of married life, with or without recourse to child-spacing.

Findings. Two families (Bjornson, Neville) were considered to have upward mobility aspirations. In these families both parents were characterized by an identification with the social amenities and customs of the upper middle social and occupational classes. The importance of proper behavior, decorum, and achievement were stressed, as were expectations of more than age-adequate developmental levels from the child. In these two families neither of the first children were planned.

In three families (Harris, Fallon, Silver) the social aspirations were sometimes ambiguous or contradictory, and these families were characterized as having equivocal mobility aspirations, without the intense feelings for such achievement that dominated the first group. The Harrises' aspirations for social and economic advancement were crippled by the husband's work history, with its financial ups and downs. In the Fallon family there were many inconsistent statements about the mother's social strivings, but these were mainly associated with income and the things that money could buy. The Silvers were indecisive about seeking prestige advancement but tended intellectually to accept "middle-class" standards of child-rearing rather than those by which they had been raised.

The three remaining families (Callini, Grasso, Cyrenski) did not indicate a desire to change their level of living or social status and were considered the non-mobile families. The Callinis were inclined to "take things as they come" and to live each day without looking to the future. The Cyrenskis showed little interest in social advancement or attainments and continued their isolation in Old World ways. The Grassos were a non-striving lower-income family experiencing a great deal of economic insecurity, with no intense drive towards higher aspirations.

2. EXTENDED FAMILY

Where families share living arrangements with grandparents it is important to examine whether this is a source of strength and comfort or a basis for conflict. Shared living arrangements are intimately tied in with the socio-economic status of the extended family as well as of the parents, and it would be expected that each set of parents and their child would have their individual ways of adapting to such home situations. If the parental scheme of values includes a moving away from one's family of orientation, it seems unlikely that parents would share living arrangements after the child is born. Yet this may be modified if financial necessity intervenes or if the grandparental hold on them exceeds the need to move.

With two adult generations in the same household there is frequently occasion for personality differences to be expressed more often and with perhaps more sharpness. It is also true, however, that family cohesiveness may be enhanced if the ways of handling such differences and tensions are effective. The helping function of grandparents in the family, by providing a wider source of affection and interest for the child, may contribute to such cohesiveness.

For those families living separately there is a more simple pattern of relationships without involvement of two generations in the conduct of a single family unit. Parents can be free from conflicting situations with their parents and more successful in achieving adult independence. On the other hand, the absence of grandparents in the home may mean a loss of emotional support. One cannot generalize concerning the psychological or emotional effects of grandparents in the home; one can only say that this is a highly variable matter.

The important aspect is how the parents themselves perceive their relationships with their own families. If the perception is one of a conflicting relationship, then a source of ego support is lost and may intensify the mother's own doubts about her abilities. If the relationship is emotionally comfortable, then it continues to provide support even though physical presence is minimized. The relationships are never simple. For the parents they are at times comforting and at times conflicting, and frequently both at once.

Findings. In the two families who lived with members of their extended family (Callini, Cyrenski) the goal of separate living arrangements was paramount with the mothers. In these families the shared living was with the husband's family of origin. Mrs. Cyrenski had intense conflict with her mother-in-law about care of the infant, and Mrs. Callini had difficulties managing a lively child in the crowded home of her in-laws. There were also problems for both families in regard to cooking, mealtimes, and sleeping arrangements. Furthermore, in the shared living there was a tendency toward increased emphasis on filial roles, and prior to the coming of the child a sense of dyadic togetherness between husband and wife was not established.

In two families who lived apart from their extended families (Fallon, Neville) there was considerable conflict with at least one of their families of orientation. In the Fallon family stress occurred mainly in relation to both grandmothers. In the Neville family conflict was mainly with the paternal grandmother. Because of the separateness of living arrangements this did not intrude directly upon the care of the child but that is not to say that extended family conflict was unimportant. It may well have been a contributing factor to the tensions and dissatisfactions which were prominent with these mothers. A third family (Harris) lived separately but later lived in the maternal grandparents' home. Here sibling and extended family conflict added to the marital stress.

Two families with separate living arrangements (Bjornson, Grasso) showed no appreciable extended family conflict. For them the separateness provided the advantages and disadvantages. The Bjornsons were successful in maintaining warm and active contacts with their parents while at the same time widely departing from their social and cultural patterns. The Grasso family secured some close and supporting relationships from their families of origin as well as practical assistance.

The final family (Silver) was in a unique category, with practically no sustained extended family relationships, complicated by the problem of mixed religions, and sharp political cleavage. The absence of family relationships added to Mrs. Silver's loneliness and isolation.

From the experience of these families it appeared that separate living did not guarantee the absence of extended family conflict, and that inter-generation conflict could not be ascribed simply to sub-cultural differences between the generations. It also indicated that accommodative techniques and deliberate insulation from potential areas of disagreement were required to avoid conflict. Finally it may have significance that the three families who were unable to avoid marked extended family conflict also experienced difficulty in achieving a "unitary" organization in their own nuclear family.

3. SPATIAL ARRANGEMENTS AND VALUES

The way in which a home is organized and the utilization of different parts of the home strongly reflect the individual personalities and the psychological needs of the arranger and of those living within the home. Although the space available is contingent on socio-economic status, it nevertheless is indicative of the family's sense of social values and motivational orientation.

The advent of a baby into these various household environments poses special problems of integration for each of the parents. In shared living arrangements with grandparents there is a good likelihood that spatial problems become more complex. But there is no assurance that there will be an absence of spatial problems even where families do not share living space with extended families.

What is most important about spatial arrangements is how the parents or other significant adults perceive its use and social purpose. In an adult-centered home a dwelling unit is a place where grown-ups live and where the child may be considered an intruder. In child-oriented families there is emphasis on the infant's needs for use of at least some areas in the home.

The division of household labor also reflects parental personality, social values, and life experience. The families showed wide variability in the extent to which fathers felt it part of their household responsibility to help provide infant care. Virtually all the fathers enjoyed some play with their children, but traditionally some fathers looked upon household repairs and lawn maintenance as their major home responsibility, while other fathers entered more actively into the feeding, bathing, and dressing processes.

Findings. The two families who shared living arrangements with grandparents (Callini, Cyrenski) did indeed have spatial difficulties and disagreements. The Callini family had fewer overt disagreements than the Cyrenskis, but limitations of space and restrictions for the baby motivated a move to separate quarters. The Cyrenskis put up with unreasonable living restrictions imposed by the paternal elders and severe spatial limitations which affected the baby's opportunity for development. This characterized some of the interpersonal relations of all family members, including the grandparents.

In their use of space the families with separate living arrangements reflected to a large degree their personalities and value-orientations. The Fallons did not reorganize their apartment to provide a nursery as planned because "the baby would be too hard on the furniture." They "accommodated" him elsewhere. When the Harrises had their own home there was no evidence of restriction for the baby, but when they had to share living arrangements temporarily there were sharp restrictions and limitations.

The Bjornsons managed a skillful compromise between maintaining their attractive home and allocating freedoms for the child. Mrs. Neville made little effort in spatial arrangements for the pleasure or safety of her child. Mrs. Silver geared every household arrangement and rearrangement for the comfort of the child, even at great inconvenience to herself and her husband. Mrs. Grasso tried to organize her apartment to consider the child's needs, and she was acutely aware of the space limitations which made for difficulties with her active son.

D. FAMILY RELATIONSHIPS

1. MARITAL

The marital emotional atmosphere may have significant influences upon the growth and development of the child. We do not know very much about these general perceptual effects, but we do know that they operate. Emotional tension and anxiety from marital discord may be more influential than feelings of well-being in the home and may reflect on the infant's development and growth in two ways. The ministering adult may be incapable of handling routine processes with the child because the tension and anxiety is so great. Or emotional tension in the home may create an atmosphere which is perceived by the infant in a general and diffuse way, in reaction to raised angry voices, drawn, unsmiling cold expressions, and stiff bodily postures.

On the other hand, as we have seen in some families, a compatible marital relationship does not guarantee a smooth mother-child or father-child adaptation, or problem-free integration of the child into the family.

Findings. Three families (Bjornson, Neville, Callini) could be characterized as having predominantly compatible marital relationships in which there were not unusual amounts of unresolved tension or anxiety. The Callinis enjoyed sharing activities, feelings, and possessions, content in their traditional orientation. The Bjornsons had common cultural backgrounds and shared similar values and ambitions. Their different personalities merged, for different psychodynamic reasons, into a compatible marital relationship. The Nevilles had common intellectual and artistic leanings and were mutually ambitious in social striving. Despite marital compatibility the mother-child relationships of Mrs. Neville and Mrs. Bjornson were hardly free of tension and anxiety, although for different reasons. Mrs. Neville was characterized as definitely mother-centered, but Mrs. Bjornson fluctuated between mother- and child-centeredness.

In two families (Cyrenski, Silver) the marital relationship was not in jeopardy, but there was a considerable amount of unresolved tension. Mrs. Cyrenski had many emotional difficulties stemming from the domineering paternal grandmother and the immaturities of her husband. However, there was no overt marital conflict, as Mr. Cyrenski lent himself to her need and enjoyment of mothering. Both Mr. and Mrs. Silver had many emotional difficulties, but their marriage functioned as smoothly as possible within the limits set by their respective personalities. There was also a fair amount of agreement on life goals.

Three families (Fallon, Harris, Grasso) showed evidence of marital conflict and degrees of incompatibility. Mrs. Fallon's severe emotional problems were hardly diminished by her husband's intolerance and lack of understanding. Their marriage had much volatility and was deficient in providing Mrs. Fallon with a secure emotional base. The vacillations and uncertainties of Mrs. Grasso were compounded by her husband's illness and lack of economic responsibility. The Harrises had a basic lack of sharing or agreement on life values and goals as well as extremely sharp conflicts between personalities. Of all families in the study they came closest to disintegration.

A number of factors operated in these three couples characterized by marital conflict: lack of wholehearted sharing in life goals; discord between basic personality patterns in the dyadic relationship; and difficulties in the socialization process. For each of these individuals one might visualize marriage partners with whom they might have been more compatible and with whom the marital relationship might have been more emotionally satisfying.

Nevertheless, it is significant that the Grasso family, despite marital problems, did achieve a unitary form of family organization, while the Nevilles, on the other hand, did not achieve a unitary family organization despite a predominantly compatible marital relationship. It seemed to indicate that the marital relationship is one, but not the only, significant factor which determines the emerging family organizational structure.

2. MOTHER-CHILD

Again this is not the only significant factor in the integration of the child into the family, but it is certainly one of the most important. The extent to which the mother accepts the child and the way in which she reacts emotionally to the demands of child care have an important effect on the interpersonal development of the family. These processes are completely interwoven with the mother's personality and the degree to which she finds satisfactions in other areas of her life.

The mother-child relationship may be one area of emotional satisfaction, along with gratifications from husband, friends, or relatives. On the other hand, the relationship between mother and child may be the only area of satisfaction in a life of stressful and conflicting interpersonal relations. This may result in a situation where emotional investment is concentrated on the child as a substitute for conflict and stress in other relationships.

Finally, the mother-child relationship may be only a limited one, where the infant is lost in the burden of other emotional or situational problems. The child's birth may not have been timed fortuitously in relation to the life goals, values, or deeply rooted personality needs of the mother, or with the parents' household or social activities. Under such conditions the mother may focus on other life situations and give the infant a low priority. However caused, situations of rejection may be associated with either satisfaction or dissatisfaction in various aspects of a mother's life.

Findings. In four families (Silver, Grasso, Cyrenski, Harris) the child seemed to be the most important person for the mother. Mrs. Silver invested much of her emotion in the child because of a great need to have someone all her own and a difficulty in sharing loved ones. Vince Grasso was a major source of emotional satisfaction for a mother whose marital relationship was rather ambivalent and conflict-ridden. More than any other mother Mrs. Cyrenski was the most intensely absorbed in her child. The immaturity and dependency of her husband, the conflict with the paternal grandmother, the physical and emotional isolations from her own family and friends, tended to make Joey the major source of emotional satisfaction for Mrs. Cyrenski. In her baby Mrs. Harris found a self-confidence, warmth, and satisfaction which other relationships and past experiences had failed to provide.

For Mrs. Callini and Mrs. Bjornson the infant was one, but not the only, source of satisfaction. Mrs. Callini had general happiness and contentment in marital and other relationships. Johnny became a new and additional source of satisfaction. Mrs. Bjornson was able to find gratification in her baby, but the child was never completely or exclusively absorbing. She continued to turn to her husband for companionship and had other strong interests.

On the other hand, Mrs. Fallon and Mrs. Neville did not find emotional or psychological satisfactions in relationships with their children. It was difficult for Mrs. Fallon to provide any positive and protective mothering in view of her emotional volatility. In turn Ross's passivity actually reinforced his mother's detachment and non-involvement. Mrs. Neville's negative responses to Rita, and her rigid expectations that the child conform to her wishes, created a sharply unsatisfactory relationship.

In these two families, where the mother-child relationships were the least satisfactory, there was indeed staff concern that the basic physical and emotional needs of the children would not be met. However, the mothers managed to perform their functions with respect to physical care of the child and by the end of the two-year period Ross Fallon and Rita Neville were apparently restored to at least minimally adequate functioning. We cannot say to what extent this minimal mother-child relationship will be followed by later symptoms of early deprivation.

3. FATHER-CHILD

Again the paucity of data permits only limited evaluation. However, as already noted, there were a number of ways in which the father-child relationship was established. These were demonstrated by the father's role of physical care and protection of the child, interaction with the child, and strength of the father-child attachment. For some fathers positive interaction with the child in play or child-care activity began at birth, for others it came only after the child had achieved a certain degree of independence and had grown out of the infant stage. The extent of physical care and responsibility for the child was minimal with certain fathers and greater for others. Significantly, even the most forbidding fathers sometimes behaved in a way that indicated positive feeling and acceptance of the new third member of the family, and all fathers were involved to some degree in interaction with their children.

Findings. By the end of the second year seven of the eight fathers were involved to a considerable degree with their children. The ways in which this interaction was experienced, however, were highly varied. For two fathers (Silver, Cyrenski) the involvement was mainly in a high investment of feeling for the child; emotional rather than physical involvement. Mr. Silver played with Ruth and enjoyed her enormously, but he was overly anxious and unsure of his adequacy in the paternal role to the point where he was practically immobilized. Mr. Cyrenski seemed to relate to and identify with Joey in a sibling rather than a paternal fashion. Although the interaction was basically warm and responsive, it did not reflect a strong father-son identification.

From the beginning three fathers (Grasso, Bjornson, Callini) participated to a considerable extent in child care and play with their children. Mr. Grasso, in particular, assumed many aspects of the mothering role because of his continued presence in the home during the day. Within the limits of his leisure time Mr. Bjornson gave special attention to his daughter, and Mr. Callini even came home from work on his lunch hour to play with Johnny.

Two other fathers (Harris, Neville) had smaller parts in child-care routines but shared experiences with the child in play, outdoor activity, teaching and learning exchanges. Mr. Harris's relationship with Heather was on a high level of pleasure and interaction, and he was able to establish an empathy with his daughter that was lacking in his adult relationships. Mr. Neville was also quite responsive to Rita from the beginning, although absorption in his work allowed minimal time with her.

In contrast, Mr. Fallon was rather unresponsive to his child. He was often derogatory about Ross's appearance and accomplishments and quite rigid in his expectations. His values and orientation were primarily adult-centered. Nevertheless, Mr. Fallon was better able to meet some of his child's needs than his wife. Occasionally he also assumed some active responsibility for the child and provided some indulgence, such as buying a puppy.

When the pattern of father-child relationships was combined with difficulties in mother-child interaction, there resulted a close alignment of father and child, with marked evidence of the child's preference for the father. This was especially noticeable in the Neville and Grasso families despite the very different mother-child relationships. In the case of the Nevilles, where the early mother-child interaction was unpleasurable and unsatisfactory, Rita seemed more at ease and happier with her father. With Mrs. Grasso the generally pleasurable and satisfactory relationship with Vince became conflicting in the period of his vigorous mobility, and the child seemed to show preference for his father.

E. PERSONALITY CHARACTERISTICS

1. HANDLING OF ANXIETY AND HOSTILITY

It has already been indicated that certain personality characteristics are intimately associated with the parents' attitude toward their baby and with the mechanics of their behavior in child care. The way in which a mother copes with anxiety, anger, or hostility does not only color her attitude to, and behavior with, the baby but is a strong factor in the emerging family structure, whether along unitary or segmental lines, child-centered or adult-centered orientation.

In general, all the mothers had a degree of anxiety, but some could handle the tension that did exist in such a way as to build toward a reasonably functioning family organization and gratifying relationships. For these mothers it was apparent that the child was one, but not the only, source of personal gratification and that there were other sources of ego support and sharing of tension. Hence the child was not called upon to carry the prime burden of the parent's emotional need. Here the mother-child relationship was less demanding and permitted a more pleasurable interaction.

The handling of anxiety presented a vastly different picture for other families, where it was pervasive to the point of infringing on reasonable family functioning. The techniques for handling anxiety were either inadequate or insufficient to bring satisfaction or prevent dissatisfaction. Sometimes the child was the chief source of satisfaction, with no other gratifying relationships, or the child was a chief source of dissatisfaction, along with unsatisfactory marital relations. For some mothers, who otherwise had gratifying interpersonal relationships, the child became the chief source of dissatisfaction and a divisive family force. Sometimes the amount of tension was beyond the capacity of the mother to deal with it, and so intense that it could not be alleviated by other relationships.

Findings. The handling of anxiety by four mothers (Callini, Bjornson, Silver, and Grasso) permitted reasonable family functioning. The considerable anxiety of Mrs. Silver and Mrs. Bjornson did not become disruptive of their family life; Mrs. Grasso's volatility provided her with adequate tension release, and Mrs. Callini had few overt signs of anxiety. For all of these mothers there was a pleasurable and satisfying mother-child relationship, and the families tended to operate on a unitary basis.

The other four mothers were less successful in coping with anxiety. Mrs. Cyrenski's suppressed hostility and conflict with her mother-in-law heightened her anxieties and prevented her from resolving personal relationships. Mrs. Harris's dysfunctional way of handling tension led to prominent fears, repression, and inhibitions which affected all relationships except with her child. Mrs. Neville's anxiety and hostility led to mother-child detachment and depression. Mrs. Fallon's anxiety produced emotional extremes and unstable personal relationships.

Two of these mothers (Cyrenski, Harris) had pleasurable mother-child relationships but other relationships were unsatisfactory. But for Mrs. Neville and Mrs. Fallon the lack of pleasure in their children added to other areas of dissatisfaction. Whatever the source, the handling of anxiety by these four mothers was not adequate for a harmoniously functioning set of unitary interpersonal relationships involving mother, father, and child. These families all tended to develop along segmental lines of organization.

2. DEPENDENCY AND THE SENSE OF SECURITY

In this connection we want to consider how parents handled their needs to look to others as sources of security and help, and to whom they looked for such support. Since all parents have dependency needs in some aspect of their life experience, we are interested mainly in the intensity and pervasiveness of those needs, their influence on parental functioning, and the manner of handling them.

Dependency need not imply personal inadequacy or pathology but may be part of mutually interdependent relationships and a highly integrative force in the family. Therefore, such feelings must be considered along with other aspects of each parent's personality, life situation, and sense of security.

An analysis of dependency patterns must also include their influence on the integration of the family unit. It appeared that when dependency needs were associated with inadequate techniques for handling anxiety and with excessive reliance upon the child as the chief source of emotional satisfaction or dissatisfaction, the resulting climate lessened the likelihood that a strong triadic family integration would occur. Generally there were fewer dependency problems among the families able to move in a unitary direction and greater dependency problems in those developing a segmental structure. However, it was also clear that the absence of dependency problems did not of itself give assurance that a family would move in a unitary direction, or conversely that the presence of such problems would prevent unitary organization. The ways in which dependency feelings were handled varied considerably among the individual parents.

Findings. Strong dependency needs appeared for five families (Bjornson, Silver, Cyrenski, Fallon, Neville), but the satisfaction of these needs were diverse. Mrs. Bjornson relied on authority figures and had great need for reassurance, but she secured certain dependency satisfactions from her husband and others. Mrs. Silver's strong dependency needs were only partially resolved by her husband, and in her isolation there were few other resources upon which to call. Mrs. Cyrenski's needs would have been less acute were it not for the extended family conflict and the passivity of her husband. Mrs. Fallon was ambivalent in her dependency. She did not want to be dependent on her husband but yet was unable to find dependency satisfactions in other relationships. And finally, Mrs. Neville's early sense of loneliness and parental deprivation required greater dependency satisfaction than her busy husband could provide.

Such dependency needs did not interfere with family functioning or prevent unitary structure for Mrs. Silver and Mrs. Bjornson. But for Mrs. Cyrenski, Mrs. Fallon, and Mrs. Neville, it was an additional factor which led towards a segmental family organization.

Three families (Callini, Grasso, Harris) showed no unusual amount of dependency. Mrs. Callini was able to limit the intensity and expression of her dependency needs. There was no unusual reliance upon authority figures, and she derived support from a many-membered family of origin. Mrs. Grasso found support in her mother, who also served as a model for her own maternal role. The marital stress was not around dependency needs but rather around the unreliability of her husband as a breadwinner. On the surface Mrs. Harris's mother seemed to provide support, and severe dependency problems did not seem to be part of the marital difficulties which characterized the Harris family. Of these families, only the Harris family evolved along segmental lines.

3. FEELINGS OF ADEQUACY OR INADEQUACY

While it is difficult to make a judgment of no feeling of inadequacy, the amount of difficulty from such feelings can be fairly accurately assessed. It was clear that the feeling of inadequacy created operational problems for some mothers in their maternal role but did not necessarily influence the unitary or harmonious functioning of the families. Inadequacy feelings were not major for three unitary families but were marked in a fourth. Feelings of inadequacy were major in two segmental families but were not significant for two other segmental families.

Findings. Three mothers (Bjornson, Harris, Fallon) were characterized by marked feelings of inadequacy. Mrs. Bjornson in a number of ways expressed guilt over her possible failure to meet family and social demands made upon her. Each new situation was looked upon as a possible threat to her concept of self. She said that she expected too much of herself as well as of others and that she never seemed to be satisfied with her own achievements. Hilda Fallon depreciated herself in all areas of life, including the maternal role. She chronically hungered for approval and was sensitive to any reflection on her adequacy as a person and a mother. Each new social demand produced uncertainty and indecision. Irene Harris was quite revealing of her inferiority feelings and sense of inadequacy. She had difficulty in new relationships and believed that she had little to offer which would be attractive to others. She also perceived herself as "rejected" in many areas of life.

Feelings of inadequacy were not a major problem for five mothers (Callini, Silver, Grasso, Neville, Cyrenski), although such feelings were indeed present to some degree in each. Mrs. Silver characterized herself as a rather mediocre person with no outstanding talents, and she was disparaging of her abilities. Although her inadequacy feelings were at times severe, her handling of them did not operate toward family disunity.

Eleanor Grasso felt quite threatened by the necessity to assume family financial responsibilities and the wage-earning role as well as management of her son. Her vacillation, however, did not operate against family integration. Although Maria Neville felt much dissatisfaction in her role as a mother, it was not accompanied by depreciation of self or her own adequacy. There was, in fact, evidence of assurance and adequacy in other aspects of life. Rose Cyrenski felt fairly adequate with her son but was ambivalent regarding her adequacy in other areas of life because she was constantly undermined by her mother-in-law. Mary Callini was the only one for whom expression of inadequacy, self-devaluation, or self-criticism was rare.

4. PLANNING AND IMPULSIVENESS

These personality characteristics were expressed quite differently and to varying degree in each family, but there was no clear distinction between developing unitary or segmental families in this regard. Its importance was clearly related, however, to the process of child care, to the type of interaction among family members, and to the developing environmental climate of a family. Where the mother's planning need is impervious to the needs or desires of other family members, it may create a tense and conflict-ridden family environment. The impulsive, volatile, and unpredictable behavior of a mother may establish an uncertain environment which affects family interaction and integration.

Findings. The question of planning or impulsiveness emerged more prominently for two families (Grasso, Bjornson) than for the remaining six. Mrs. Bjornson carried her need to plan almost to the point of compulsiveness. She had a tremendous need for scheduling, orderliness, and predictability, but it did not prove to be disruptive of the family organization. Eleanor Grasso was more impulsive and less of a planner than the other mothers. Furthermore, Vince's irregularity of behavior also contributed to this inconsistent and impulsive behavior by his mother, even though she adapted in many ways to his needs. For Mrs. Grasso these characteristics served to reduce tension and did not become disruptive of family life. Both these families tended to develop a unitary form of organization.

Planning was not significant for the remaining six mothers. Mrs. Callini appeared confidently flexible in meeting life situations; Mrs. Silver devoted her energy to matters of the day and was future-oriented only as it was associated with her general feelings of dependency and insecurity; Mrs. Cyrenski's pattern of life held little planning incentive due to the controlling grandparental influence, and she gave no evidence of impulsiveness. Mrs. Harris was not given to intensive planning or impulsive decisions in her life situations. Mrs. Neville also had no problems in this connection. It was not inability that prevented effective scheduling of special care routines or play periods with Rita but Mrs. Neville's lack of emotional gratification in doing so. Mrs. Fallon was able to plan effectively and was not given to impulsiveness despite her view to the contrary. In many ways she proved herself a careful, well-ordered housekeeper and manager.

5. SELF-ASSERTION

This was another area of personality which was individual and varied for mothers in both unitary and segmental family organizations. Its significance was in terms of effect on interpersonal relationships, and it contributed to the creation of problematic emotional interactions in certain families. Where this characteristic was combined with other problems, such as feelings of inadequacy or inability to handle anxiety, it became a factor in segmental family organization. However, a lack of self-assertion was not always associated with strong inadequacy feelings.

Findings. Five families were characterized by problems of self-assertiveness (Bjornson, Silver, Harris, Cyrenski, Fallon). Edna Bjornson found it extremely difficult to take the initiative in interpersonal relationships with others, and this detrimentally affected initial contacts with her child. It was hard to assert herself in routines of child care, but these became less important as Lorna became more responsive. Mrs. Silver asserted herself by conveying the impression that she was culturally superior to her environment, but this did not significantly impinge on family relationships. Mrs. Fallon wanted and expected help from others, but could not bring herself to ask it. When it was not forthcoming she felt rejected and hurt. Mrs. Cyrenski had difficulties in self-assertion from her early years and tended to repress her feelings in adult relationships. This was also the case with Mrs. Harris, who could not assert herself openly on matters of great importance to her, such as the baby's baptism. In neither case, however, did it influence or impair the mother-child relationship.

Although other personality problems affected the remaining three families (Callini, Grasso, Neville) the question of self-assertion did not by itself appear to be a source of difficulty.

6. RECAPITULATION OF PAST EXPERIENCES

Since past socialization experiences are an important ingredient of human personality and behavior, their influence was apparent in the study. Some mothers verbalized about past experience and made demonstrable effort to emulate or depart from it. Other mothers verbalized about past experience but gave no evidence that it assumed prominence in their own child-rearing patterns. Finally, some mothers in their behavior automatically demonstrated the influence of their own past experiences. Whether demonstrable or covert, verbalized or unarticulated, it served all mothers as an antecedent of attitude and behavior towards their children.

Findings. Three families (Bjornson, Harris, Silver) were consciously aware of past experiences and gave evidence relevant to it. Mrs. Bjornson vividly recalled her own deprived and restricted childhood. She was actively determined that it should be different for Lorna. Mrs. Silver was keenly sensitive to the sense of maternal loss upon her mother's remarriage. She vowed that Ruth would have the love and maternal security which she had been denied. Mrs. Harris bitterly recounted tangible hardships and emotional insecurities from a mother who failed to provide warmth or intimacy. In her close and perceptive relationship with Heather she established a markedly different base of experience.

Three mothers (Callini, Grasso, Neville) did not verbalize but followed patterns consistent with their past experiences. Mrs. Callini expressed the warmly close congeniality of a many-membered family orientation, and Mrs. Grasso followed patterns of mothering and behavior set by her own mother. Mrs. Neville provided minimal maternal attachment, reflecting the absence of a mother figure from her own life.

Two mothers (Fallon, Cyrenski) verbalized about unhappy past experiences but gave no evidence of altering their own patterns on the basis of these. Mrs. Fallon spoke of her moody, disturbed father and her harshly dominating mother. Her own attitude and behavior with Ross were critical, withdrawn, and conflicting. Mrs. Cyrenski referred to her unhappy school experiences and the feeling of being culturally apart. There was no evidence, however, that she consciously attempted to provide a different cultural or emotional climate for Joey.

It should be noted that of the six personality characteristics outlined above, four did not appear to distinguish unitary from segmental family organization. These were the presence or absence of feelings of inadequacy; planning and impulsiveness; problems of self-assertion; and the influence of past experieces. The two characteristics that did seem to distinguish between unitary and segmental family organization were the handling of anxiety, and dependency and the sense of security.

F. EMERGENCE OF FAMILY INTEGRATION PATTERNS

1. FAMILY STRUCTURE

The quality of the dyadic relationships (husband-wife, mother-child, father-child) is a base for evaluating the combined relationships and the manner in which the child can be integrated into the pre-existing family structure. The type of total relationship which emerges may be defined as either a unitary or segmental structure of family organization. The presence or absence of emotional difficulty is not a realistic criterion for judging family unity. The crux is rather in the configuration of the predominant emotional atmosphere into which the child is born and the personal and familial patterns for handling each member's psychological problems in the presence of emotional difficulties.

Many factors may be observed in the fabric of the triadic relationships that vitally influence the family towards either unitary or segmental organization. This study did not attempt to delineate any single factor or combination of factors as the decisive element in family structuring. It sought only to observe those features which produced inter-relationships or the reverse, on the assumption that this undoubtedly influenced the pattern of organization. In some families a unity could and did persist despite obvious relationship stresses. In others the stresses led to divisive, disconnected, and segmental operation. Since patterns of life and interaction are not always explicit, the overall evaluation of family climate and relationships are at best the objective judgment of its interpreters.

Findings. The study staff judged that four families tended toward unitary organization (Callini, Silver, Bjornson, Grasso). The Callinis' baby was warmly welcomed, and the dyadic relationships of husband-wife, mother-child, and father-child were emotionally satisfying to all concerned. In the Bjornson family the husband-wife relationship was an emotionally supportive one, and there was considerable sharing with the baby. Also, they had close and genial relationships with extended family members. Despite emotional uncertainties, the Silver family early established themselves as a tightly knit threesome, with much common satisfaction in their baby. The Grasso family was included in this group although it had pronounced elements of marital stress. However, it appeared that a certain unity persisted on the part of the three nuclear family members, in that the parents shared similar life goals, cultural background, and pleasure in their baby. In these four families it could be said that the dyadic relationships were generally supportive but that the Grasso family was at the low end of the continuum in qualifying as a unitary family. (Subsequent follow-up of this family revealed deeper elements of marital conflict and consideration of divorce by Mrs. Grasso.)

The remaining four families (Harris, Cyrenski, Neville, Fallon) had in common the emergence of a segmental family system, characterized by the relative isolation of at least one family member in dyadic relationships. The Harrises' baby became the focus of her parents' world, but marital dissatisfactions were such that there was no genuine pattern of three-person sharing. The Cyrenski marital relationship was not supportive enough to overcome extended family problems or the personality immaturities of each. The negative character of Mrs. Neville's relationship with her child made a satisfying triadic nuclear family impossible, although the marital relationship seemed secure. And finally, the Fallons had marital conflict as well as unsatisfactory parent-child relationships.

2. DIVISION OF LABOR AND BALANCE OF POWER

These factors may facilitate unitary family functioning or may become a further focus of conflict in a segmental family operation. Some families seemed to contain a family balance of power that could be best described as a joint enterprise and a sharing of responsibilities and management. In other families, however, the lack of sharing and the dominance of one or the other partners were apparent.

Findings. The unitary families (Silver, Callini, Bjornson, Grasso) were inclined to share, divide, or allocate respective household tasks. In decision-making there was either sharing or the acceptable dominance by one of the partners. In these families there was also a balance toward marital compatibility, despite the considerable strife between the Grassos. The Callinis handled family activities and decisions as a joint undertaking, with Mrs. Callini showing more initiative in deciding family affairs. The Bjornsons had mutual security in the home, with Mr. Bjornson in charge of the remodeling process and his wife of the household. The Silvers had a sharing but anxious partnership. Mrs. Silver managed the home and child almost exclusively, and her husband assumed a slightly more dominant role in decision-making. The division of labor was rather ill-defined in the Grasso family because of the husband's constant presence in the home, but there seemed to be a sharing of household duties and decision-making.

In the segmental families (Harris, Cyrenski, Fallon, Neville) there was far less sharing or agreement on household roles and decision-making. Mr. Harris played the dominant role in his family, often making decisions which were unsatisfactory to his wife. The Cyrenskis were dominated by the paternal grandmother, who held the balance of power. Mr. Cyrenski had little or no part in household duties or family management. Mrs. Neville was the dominant force in her family, and her husband played a slender role in household management. Mr. Fallon was the authoritative member of his household and served as caustic critic of his wife's management. In all these families there were apparent marital discomforts, with the exception of the Nevilles, where the mother was the dominant force.

3. DEVELOPMENT, ACHIEVEMENT, AND SOCIAL BEHAVIOR OF CHILD

High growth and achievement standards of the mothers did not determine the success or failure of their children to be above-age in development. In general, high development standards were more prominent in the segmental families, where they tended to become a problem. The unitary families were generally more lenient towards the individual limitations of their children and less demanding of them. There was no simple relationship between mothers' expectations in regard to their children and the children's personalities or development. Nor was there a simple relationship between the problems encountered by the mothers and their ways of dealing with them.

Findings. Children of all the unitary families (Bjornson, Silver, Callini, Grasso) were all slightly above-age in developmental achievement. After a slow start Lorna Bjornson met her mother's high standards of achievement, and her development proceeded at an accelerated rate. Ruth Silver was especially advanced in language development and was an appealing and attractive child. Vince Grasso's level of performance was somewhat advanced, and he was described as a lovable, active boy. Johnny Callini was more than age-adequate on an overall basis, even though his mother was quite conscious of his social behavior.

Of the segmental-family children only Heather Harris was above-age in almost all developmental areas, and her achievements were matched by her winning social behavior. In this case the mother did not pose unusually high goals for her child. Rita Neville was not outstanding on an overall basis in developmental tests despite the unusually high standards for growth and development held by her mother. The Fallons' high standards were confronted by a child whose development, achievement, and social behavior was slow or below average in several respects. Joey Cyrenski was passive but age-adequate, even though his parents held no high standards. Children from all of the unitary families were somewhat above-age developmentally, but only one from the segmental families was outstandingly so.

4. PROSPECT OF SIBLINGS

Although all the mothers spoke of future children, there was a rather clear difference between the two groups of families on this score. With one exception the unitary families all looked favorably and with positive feelings upon a larger family, but for one reason or another there were no second pregnancies among them during the two year study. Among the segmental families, however, the desire for a second baby seemed more pressing and was based on a number of negative feelings or dissatisfactions. For some mothers a second child was seen as a panacea for existing personal or family difficulties. Two of the segmental families had a second pregnancy during the study, whereas none of the unitary mothers became pregnant.

Findings. Among the unitary families, both Mr. and Mrs. Grasso were eager for a second child despite marital and economic difficulties. Mrs. Bjornson stated her desire for a second child when

Lorna would be three years old. The Callinis favored more children, but Mrs. Callini wanted to solve economic and housing problems first. Mrs. Silver gave no evidence of desire for a second child. In fact, she was eager to learn about contraceptives. Mr. Silver also did not express any desire for a larger family.

Among the segmental families, Mrs. Fallon and Mrs. Harris both had second pregnancies. Although Mr. Fallon ridiculed his wife's wish for another child, she hoped to obtain satisfactions which Ross had failed to provide. Mrs. Harris strongly felt that Heather needed a sibling and hoped the marital situation would benefit from a second pregnancy, although Mr. Harris was opposed to it. Mrs. Cyrenski had, but did not dare indulge, a desire for another infant because of the mother-in-law's adamant opposition. Mrs. Neville spoke of a second child as a source of possible satisfaction which she had not secured from Rita.

5. STATUS OF FAMILY IN COMMUNITY

The community status of a family may be derived from relationships within their families of origin and/or from the community or neighborhood in which they have spent most of their life. In the unitary families there was no pronounced family conflict, and consequently there was more pleasurable family social status and contact. In the segmental families there was pronounced conflict with one or more extended family members, with consequent dampening of social relations.

The extent of community status and participation in social clubs, church, friendship, and service organizations may stem from socialization and status accorded their families of origin or may reflect the independent goals and value of the nuclear family. This did not appear to distinguish between segmental or unitary families but pertained rather to the personalities and social strivings of the individual families.

Findings. In the unitary families the Callinis lived in the same neighborhood as their parents and were socially integrated within its framework and a familiar community. The Grassos found some satisfaction in their family associations and in their lifelong neighborhood, but with minimal community involvement. The Bjornsons maintained close extended family relations despite differing values, and they established broad independent community participation. The Silvers were quite removed from close family ties and were also culturally remote from community associations. Two of the unitary families (Callini, Grasso) were nonstriving, lower-income families, one (Silver) had equivocal social aspirations, and the Bjornson family was upward-striving.

Since all the segmental families had an area of extended family conflict, this impaired sustained and gratifying intrafamily social relations. The Harrises were also quite isolated from church and community affairs. Young Mrs. Cyrenski was isolated both from the American community-at-large and from the Bulgarian orientation of the paternal home, which regarded her as an intruder. The Fallons had strong discontents with both their families, and despite Mrs. Fallon's social activity with friends there was little evidence of wide community participation. Mrs. Neville, however, was active in community life outside the family and aspired to a prestigious social and professional life. One of these families was characterized as upward-striving (Neville), two equivocally so (Harris, Fallon), and one (Cyrenski) not at all.

6. TYPES OF PARENT-CHILD ADAPTATION

The relationship of parental orientation to family structure disclosed four rather clear family types: child-centered, unitary; intermediate-centered, unitary; child-centered, segmental; and parent-centered, segmental. Child-centered orientations were generally found in unitary families. Three of the four unitary families were mostly child-centered (Callini, Silver, Grasso), and the fourth unitary family (Bjornson) was intermediately so. In none of the four unitary families was there a decidedly parent-centered motivational orientation.

In the segmental families two were decidedly parent-centered (Fallon, Neville), and two were child-centered (Harris, Cyrenski).

The relationship between family organization and the extent of parental permissiveness shows three rather clear family types emerging: permissive-unitary; permissive-segmental; and non-permissive-segmental. The four families characterized as unitary were all permissive, including the fathers as well as the mothers (Callini, Silver, Bjornson, Grasso).

Two segmental families were permissive (Harris, Cyrenski) but tended to become somewhat less permissive as the children matured. These two fathers were also highly involved in their children's lives and were relatively permissive.

The two non-permissive segmental families (Fallon, Neville) were sharply so in the early period, but the mothers made some significant shifts toward greater permissiveness as the children matured. These fathers also were the least involved in their children's lives. Although Mr. Neville seemed to be more permissive than his wife, Mr. Fallon was clearly non-permissive.

RÉSUMÉ OF FAMILY INTEGRATION AND ADAPTATION

Fallon: segmental, parent-centered, non-permissive
Bjornson: unitary, intermediately child-centered, permissive
Silver: unitary, child-centered, permissive
Grasso: unitary, child-centered, permissive
Cyrenski: segmental, child-centered, permissive
Harris: segmental, child-centered, permissive
Neville: segmental, parent-centered, non-permissive
Callini: unitary, child-centered, permissive

Observations

Of the numerous observations which were recorded in this study, we have selected for listing in a summarized fashion those which appeared most significant to us in terms of the elements with which we were concerned. On the basis of this small sampling of families we do not suggest these as hypotheses but only as items which may warrant further investigation.

EXPECTATIONS

1. The fact that some mothers seem wholly happy and satisfied with approaching maternity does not guarantee that life with the child or development of the child will actually be completely satisfactory or untroubled.

2. Mothers who are the most reluctant and negative about the approach of maternity continue to find the most disruption and dissatisfaction in life with the child.

3. Whether or not a mother has previously been interested in outside employment or career is not the determining factor whether she turns to jobs outside the home after the baby is born.

4. Mothers who are the least pleased with approaching maternity consistently remain the least child-centered, suiting their behavior more to satisfy themselves than the child.

5. The experience of life in general and with the child in particular causes changes in all mothers, allowing even the least child-centered mother to become more child oriented over time.

6. Regardless of the mother's expectations and behavior, the unique personality and individuality of the child serves either to enhance the mother's gratification or to conflict with it.

7. A major difference between mothers is that some can modify

their expectations to fit their experience while others try to induce their children to make experience fit the expectations.

BEHAVIOR

1. The more maternally gratified mothers are generally more perceptive of and responsive to their child's clues and actions. The range of response from the least child-centered mothers is lowest.

2. From the beginning some mothers "talk" to their babies to express warm maternal inner feelings, while others "talk" to direct, control, and substitute for warm physical contact.

3. The achievement of regularity and flexibility of scheduling in care of the child stems more from the mother's personal flexibility and capacity to adapt than on either satisfaction or dissatisfaction with the child or the maternal role.

4. Child-centered mothers are generally more permissive in their management techniques than parent-centered mothers. Nevertheless, with all mothers there are shifts in one direction or another as the child develops and as maternal adjustments take place.

5. Mothers tend to behave along the lines with which their expectations are most involved, particularly in their anxiety, feeling of adequacy, and attitudes towards specific care routines. The past life of parents clearly determines their style of parenthood.

6. Child-centered mothers derive greater gratification from infantile dependency. As the child grows older, mother-child conflicts heighten for these mothers.

7. Where the mother's behavior with the child is the least "giving," the fathers in those families present a behavior which may serve as a balance and check for excessive maternal demands.

SOCIO-CULTURAL INFLUENCES

1. Having a child is not included in the plans of families with strong upward social strivings.

2. Families having the greatest conflicts and problems with

their extended family also have the most difficulty in achieving a unitary family of their own.

3. How parents arrange their households and use of space reflects not only their own personalities but also their child-oriented or adult-centered values.

4. Separate family living does not insure that a family can achieve a unitary organization of its own, nor does shared family living preclude the development of a firm unitary family integration.

FAMILY RELATIONSHIPS

1. Neither marital accord nor marital incompatibility are the determining factors in adequate development of the child during the first two years.

2. An unsatisfactory mother-child relationship gives rise to evidences of early deprivation. However, even those children with the least satisfactory maternal relationship can achieve at least minimally adequate development within the first two years.

3. The quality and degree of a mother-child relationship basically depends on other aspects of the mother's life, becoming a focus for either satisfactions or dissatisfactions with the total life situation.

4. Where the mother-child relationship is the most unsatisfactory, the father-child relationship assumes a quality which may serve as an antidote or balance in support of the child.

PERSONALITY CHARACTERISTICS

1. The characteristic which plays the most decisive role in whether a family can develop along unitary lines is the manner in which it is able to handle anxieties and dependency so as to prevent disruption and disunity.

2. The dependency need affects family development patterns only when it is associated with inadequate ways of handling anxiety.

3. The areas of adequacy, planning, self-assertion, or past experience affect family integration only to the extent that their interaction with each other and with the two above characteristics may prove incapacitating to family wholeness and unity.

FAMILY PATTERN CHARACTERISTICS

1. Unitary family integration is possible where each of the twosome relationships are satisfying to some degree (husband-wife, mother-child, father-child). It is not achieved in families suffering from a totally unsatisfying relationship in one or another of the twosome relationships.

2. Unitary families have more pleasurable anticipations toward the coming child than do segmental families.

3. Unitary families face fewer serious problems of child care relating to regularity, handling of illness, sleeping, and feeding than do segmental families.

4. Unitary families achieve a balance of sharing and division of power which is lacking in the segmental families.

5. Unitary families have less pronounced extended family conflict.

6. Unitary families are more permissive towards their children, while the segmental families tend to be either intermediately permissive or non-permissive.

7. A family may be segmental and yet be child-centered or intermediately so. A family may be unitary and yet not wholly child-centered.

8. Segmental families attempt to improve family and/or child relationships and satisfactions by producing an additional child. Segmental families produce a second child sooner than unitary families.

9. There is less satisfaction with the development, achievement, and social behavior of the child among segmental, parent-centered families and more effort to make the child conform to standards and expectations.

Commentary

This study concerned itself with the lives of married couples and their first children. It was an attempt to describe the way these families came to terms with a variety of stressful circumstances.

The study was long term. There was contact with some of the families for over fourteen years. The method was clinical. It proved impressively that interviews, conversations, and observation techniques over an extended period do reveal more pertinent information than questionnaires, no matter how foolproof their structure. We learned, for instance, that mothers are prone to "forget" distasteful episodes. Mrs. Neville at times stated that she didn't believe in spanking and never spanked, which was at variance with facts related on many other occasions. We learned of vital facts which inadvertently came to light quite late in the study only apropos of some conversational gambit in the many discussions. Thus, towards the end of the study we happened to learn of Mrs. Silver's prior marriage and aborted pregnancy.

Much depended, of course, on the staff members' ability to pursue productive avenues of investigation, to observe astutely, and to extrapolate with insight. This was accomplished to a surprising degree. Often they penetrated deeply despite meager specific information. A good case in point was the Grasso family, where staff reports hinted strongly that the marital situation and relations with the maternal grandparents held more stress than met the eye or was evident on the surface. In following years, as the postscript indicates, this was verified.

The aim of the study was not to make a psychiatric survey but rather to examine the experience of ordinary men and women as they approached one of the normal crises of life. This is not to say that the people described did not develop a variety of symptoms in mind and body which on occasion indicated the need for psychiatric intervention. But the authors were not interested in disease or psychopathologic processes as much as in the study of the lives of normal people and the assessment of the ways in which they met problems and maintained relative stability.

Such a study posed two exacting moral and philosophical questions, which have relevance to all such studies. First, does the goal of "seeing and hearing" people *in situ* take priority over corrective or therapeutic action? Secondly, what is the obligation of the study to present their findings forthrightly to those involved? How far does one go in telling a mother that her nurture of the baby is detrimental to his development? How direct can or should such intervention be? In the final analysis, what is paramount to staff members, the intactness of the study, or the people themselves?

The study staff was motivated to intervene when it became clear that immediate action was required to safeguard the child or mother herself. Then specific and precise recommendations were made. In several instances psychiatric therapy was suggested and even urged. When supportive aid was required, more frequent contacts by the psychiatric social workers took place and help was provided. Whether such intervention detracted from the study's objectivity was of less moment than the welfare of the people involved. In this sense, the study took the calculated risk of possibly sacrificing some scientific accuracy and objectivity.

The persons from different professional disciplines who carried out this research combined the interests and skills of clinicians as well as those of social scientists. The clinician is interested in what goes on inside people and too frequently is not aware of what takes place in their environment, particularly social and economic influences. The presence of social scientists in this research made it possible for the group to pay special attention to the factors in the environment, including the direct and personal influence of the clinicians on the study.

Because of the variety of disciplines represented, the study group was well qualified to go back and forth from the intrinsic to the extrinsic, from the inside world of the individual to the outside world. The fact that practical problems of living make for emotional problems is well borne out in this study. The move to a better home can ameliorate emotional distress, as in the case of the

Callini family, or financial problems can create family dissension, as with the Harris and Grasso families.

The detailed written records of the lives of eight randomly selected families of white, middle- and working-class women coming to a university prenatal clinic serve as valuable teaching material for students of human behavior. Possibly it is also of some worth to future historians interested in knowing how a few Americans lived through a critical period in their lives. Certainly it has relevance to those lay persons who daily face the responsibilities of parenthood and may see in this material the assurance that they are not alone in having problems. The study reported here is only a beginning in demonstrating some of the influences that determine why or how parents rear their children as they do. The biographies represent the core of basic material for future study, as there is a minimum of theory provided.

The arrangement of the material, and particularly its assessment, mainly follows a psycho-sociological pattern despite the fact that psychoanalysts were members of the study group. The study later became more psychoanalytically oriented, with play and psychiatric therapy for some children and parents. The postscript material owes its existence to that. In terms of this study, it was proved that psychoanalytical insights could and did reveal considerably more fundamental and complex pathology than was earlier disclosed, but that this did not alter the premises or implications of the family integration study. Rather, the psychoanalytic material validated those problem areas which had been pinpointed or suggested by the first two years of study.

For example, the psychoanalytic material substantiated the problems of Vince Grasso's hyper-motor and uncontrolled activity, the vicissitudes of the mother-child interaction, and the variability of the marital relationship. Thus, in juxtaposition to each other it may be said that the socio-psychological insights were actually solidified and complemented by the psychoanalytic interpretations. At least one of the cases, that of Cyrenski, is a classic description of the development of separation anxiety and the Oedipus complex as seen not in retrospection of psychoanalytic theory but as it was observed directly by non-psychoanalytic observers.

The most noteworthy findings from the study are that any parental act in rearing a child is the result of multiple interwoven factors which follow an exchange of influences between parent and child. The dominance of any of these influences is determined by elements in the total situation. We may know that all pregnant women have forebodings about the coming child, based on superstition and folk lore, but the influence of these dire apprehensions is determined by the sum total of the mother's personality and situation. Because of neurotic mechanisms in some mothers, their forebodings are borne out as behavior which is directed to make these dire anticipations become realities. In other mothers extrinsic influences and healthy psychological defense mechanisms intervene constructively.

A striking aspect of the data was that the developmental observations made immediately after the baby's birth pinpointed the unique "personality" characteristics and responses of each newborn. On the basis of this, certain extrapolations were made concerning the environment and nurture which would be most desirable for each infant. For example, the newborn evaluation of Ross Fallon characterized him as a passive infant who faced the world's discomforts by withdrawal. It was noted that such a baby required a mother who would be particularly alert, perceptive, and responsive to his needs or they would go unrecognized. In his case the maternal climate hardly met those requirements, and the record of Ross' first two years bore out the prediction.

On the basis of these important newborn developmental observations it would seem warranted to suggest that every newborn be given such an examination, and one periodically thereafter, to help parent and professional advisors better understand the behavior of each child and ways of coping with his particular needs.

The readers, like the research team, may be concerned about the degree of neurotic and emotional problems seen in this random selection of normal Americans. In a way, it is a sad commentary on the emotional health of people generally and on the state of our society and its culture. On the other hand, equally impressive is the degree of resilience and the effectiveness of psychological defense mechanisms which permit people not only to survive but even to rise above stressful circumstances.

Index

Index

Index

Index

Index

Bei Fragen zur Produktsicherheit wenden Sie sich bitte an:
If you have any questions regarding product safety,
please contact:

Walter de Gruyter GmbH
Genthiner Straße 13
10785 Berlin
productsafety@degruyterbrill.com